CONTROVERSIES IN EXERCISE SCIENCE

Controversies in Exercise Science introduces a series of selected unresolved issues in the field of human exercise science. The common thread to all of these topics is that, in their ultimate resolution, they offer promise of insights into the essential principles of physiological systems and how these respond to the stresses of exercise. Each case study includes an examination of research surrounding each issue; the innovative aspect, however, is that each of these controversies is presented in the context of an historical and/or philosophical perspective.

These chapters include topics related to basic exercise physiology, sports, physical activity, and exercise health. Underlying each of these debates lie clues which may offer insights into the basic nature of living beings.

Aimed at both academics and practitioners in the fields of exercise science, biology, and related sports science disciplines, *Controversies in Exercise Science* provides arguments for both sides of several selected contemporary controversies in the field of exercise science and, while no ultimate resolution is provided, the goal is, rather, to offer the reader sufficient "raw material" on which he or she might make their own judgment on the matters presented.

Thomas Rowland, M.D., is the retired Chief of Pediatric Cardiology at the Baystate Medical Center in Springfield, Massachusetts, USA, where his research focused on exercise cardiovascular physiology in children. He is the author of over 200 peer-reviewed articles and ten books, including *Children's Exercise Physiology* and *Biologic Regulation of Physical Activity*. He was the founding editor of the journal *Pediatric Exercise Science*, a post he served for 23 years. He was a member of the Board of Trustees of the American College of Sports Medicine and has served as president of both the North American Society for Pediatric Exercise Medicine and the New England Chapter of ACSM. He received the Honor Award from the latter organization in 1986.

CONTROVERSIES IN EXERCISE SCIENCE

Thomas Rowland

Routledge
Taylor & Francis Group
NEW YORK AND LONDON

First published 2019
by Routledge
711 Third Avenue, New York, NY 10017

and by Routledge
2 Park Square, Milton Park, Abingdon, Oxon OX14 4RN

Routledge is an imprint of the Taylor & Francis Group, an informa business

British Library Cataloguing-in-Publication Data
A catalogue record for this book is available from the British Library

Library of Congress Cataloging-in-Publication Data
Names: Rowland, Thomas W., author.
Title: Controversies in exercise science / Thomas Rowland.
Description: Abingdon, Oxon ; New York, NY : Routledge, 2019. |
Includes bibliographical references and index.
Identifiers: LCCN 2018024840 | ISBN 9781138311725 (hardback) |
ISBN 9781138311732 (paperback) | ISBN 9780429458668 (ebook)
Subjects: LCSH: Exercise—Physiological aspects. | Sports sciences.
Classification: LCC QP301 .R6935 2019 | DDC 612.7/6—dc23
LC record available at https://lccn.loc.gov/2018024840

ISBN: 978-1-138-31172-5 (hbk)
ISBN: 978-1-138-31173-2 (pbk)
ISBN: 978-0-429-45866-8 (ebk)

Typeset in Bembo
by Apex CoVantage, LLC

CONTENTS

FIGURES

TABLES

PREFACE

As far back as recorded history can take us, human beings have sought to make "sense" of the world surrounding them. As the ancients observed the flow of natural phenomena—the tides, the motions of the heavenly bodies—distinct patterns of change were obvious, but just how to go about explaining such events was not at all clear. Surely, they reasoned, the gods were responsible, but by what rules, what principles did such natural phenomena occur? As they are today, such questions were prompted not simply out of intellectual curiosity, but, equally important and in a deeper sense, by a need to search out the meaning of their own existence in the Grand Design of the universe.

Concepts of "truths" that would explain the real world have proceeded historically in a step-by-step progression, each "advance" deemed to invalidate its predecessor. One might start with the ideas of the Greek philosopher Pythagoras, who considered that truth in the universe was founded in numbers, particularly the ratios between numbers, as indicated by the harmony of sounds produced when a string is plucked at certain ratios of its length. Such harmony was reflected in the functional reality of the universe, he said, and the motions of the planets were explained by numerical ratios.

Then in 300 BC, Euclid's geometrical precepts—the same ones learned by high school math students today—became accepted as the benchmark of ultimate truth, the foundations by which the actions of nature could be explained. As expressed in a quote attributed to Johannes Kepler, "Geometry is unique and eternal, a reflection of the mind of God." All were so convinced until the universality of these principles was invalidated by the advent of non-Euclidean geometry (such as that which occurs on curved surfaces, where the shortest distance between two points is no longer a straight line).

In the 17th century, Newton's laws of motion—the principle of inertia, the contributions of mass and acceleration to force, and the equal and opposite reaction to every action—indicated a predictable, pre-determined universe. Here were certain, fixed principles defining physical reality that held true locally from shooting baskets in one's driveway to universally in the mutual attraction of celestial bodies. But then Einstein demonstrated that Newton's laws did not hold in conditions of extreme velocity, like the speed of light. The governing principles of physics, he revealed, were not absolute but relative.

All of this falls apart in the world of quantum mechanics, where nothing is predictable or certain. Here subatomic particles can alter their form, occur at two places or states simultaneously, and resist having their location and momentum measured at the same time. Here is a bizarre world—hidden beneath our visual experience—which is completely foreign to our sense of reality in our everyday lives.

Even today as physicists seek to identify a simple, unified truth which will encompass all these disparate realities—a Theory of Everything—it is apparent, then, that physical "truth" depends on conditions. The concepts of Newton, Einstein, and quantum mechanics are all valid and predictive in describing the principles of the behavior of matter, but only within the realm of a specific context (i.e., macroscopic, high velocity, and subatomic, respectively.) Within their own domain, each accurately expresses reality. Beyond this, no. The lesson learned is that a truth, or physical law, must be considered in respect to a particular reality.

It is intriguing to note that while physical laws may provide a certain immutable determinism, in the end these laws are largely *descriptive* in their predictability, and what remains obscure is the *meaning* that underlies them. Take gravitation, for example. We learned from Newton that the force attracting two bodies, say the planet Mars and the sun, is proportional to the product of the masses of the two celestial bodies, and inversely as the square of the distance between them. Mathematically, that's

$$F = G\left(mm'/r^2\right)$$

But *why* should this be so? How does this work? The eminent physicist Richard Feynman spoke of this conundrum during a lecture at Cornell University back in 1964.

> What does the planet do? Does it look at the sun, see how far away it is, and decide to calculate on its internal adding machine the inverse of the square of the distance, which tells it how much to move? This is certainly no explanation of the machinery of gravitation! . . . So there is no model of the theory of gravitation today, other than its mathematical form.
>
> *(4)*

Physics Envy

In this search for unraveling essential principles within the mysteries of natural phenomena, biologists have not fared well. Indeed, in seeking similar governing principles which define the nature and behavior of living matter, they can only regard their physicist colleagues with a certain sense of envy. A physicist will assure us that a ball dropped in a vacuum will fall with an acceleration of precisely 9.80 m per second squared. For mathematicians, the length of the hypotenuse of a right-angled triangle will end up, with no discussion, to be the square root of the sum of the squares of the two sides. On the other hand, biologic phenomena—including clues to the central mystery of the essence of life itself—are shrouded in variability, unpredictability, and heterogeneity. To wit: When Lortie and colleagues in Quebec measured changes in maximal oxygen uptake following a 20-week endurance training program in a group of previously sedentary adults, improvements ranged from 5% in some individuals to 83% in others, a 16-fold variability in response (7). While baffled by the complex of genetic and environmental factors which might account for such inter-individual differences, biological researchers are accustomed to such ambiguous outcomes.

Certainly, biological systems must comply with physical and electrochemical laws. But in the confounded intricacies of such systems, what biological principles hold forth to establish the uniqueness of living matter? In fact, after centuries of search, and despite giant leaps in our understanding of the biochemical processes surrounding the life process, such laws, or primary truths, continue to be elusive. As the chemist Addy Pross has succinctly concluded, "The difference between living and non-living entities has remained provocatively out of reach" (11).

Not that there haven't been many efforts to pin down such defining features. Every high school biology student has learned the same list of characteristics of living matter—living matter reproduces, grows, utilizes energy for cellular functions, moves, can sense and respond to their surroundings, and acts to adapt to its environment. Plants and animals are all composed of enveloping membranes. Living matter seems to exhibit a certain sense of purpose. "All living things behave as if they have an agenda" wrote Pross (9), though just for what is not at all clear. But all these descriptors are in truth simply characteristics, and hardly provide any insight into the essential nature of living matter.

This idea of the apparent uniqueness of biological matter was expressed by Claude Bernard almost 300 years ago in evolutionary terms:

> Every living being indeed appears to us provided with a kind of inner force, which presides over manifestations of life more and more independent of general cosmic influence in proportion as the being rises higher in the scale of organization. In higher animals and in man, for instance, this vital

> force seems to result in withdrawing the living being from general physico-chemical influences[. . .]
>
> *(2)*

In this statement Bernard was tip-toeing closely to the idea of *vitalism*, a concept—now discredited—that holds that living beings are possessed with a particular fundamental principle that sets them apart from those which govern physical actions. In fact, no process or activity in living beings has ever been described that does not conform to recognized physical-chemical laws. What sets biologic functions apart is the manner in which such activities are *organized* (6). And that organization exhibits bewildering intricacy, the outcome of an extraordinary length of evolutionary time. George Gaylord Simpson wrote that "Life . . . is not necessarily considered as nonphysical or nonmaterial. It is just that living things have been affected for . . . billions of years by historical processes. . . . The results of these processes are systems different in kind from any nonliving systems and almost incomparably more complicated" (12).

Perhaps the closest thing to a biological principle is the process of Darwinian natural selection, holding that genetic variability is acted on by environmental stressors to permit survival of the fittest. Despite naysayers and its "tweaking" even by main-line biologists, the modern-day version of Darwin's grand idea remains the bedrock for explaining the contemporary existence of anatomic and functional features of living matter. It is a "truth" that provides a descriptive mechanism for the evolutionary development of such features, and it is a process in which all living matter—and only living matter—participates. But, again, it is descriptive rather than predictive, and it reveals nothing of the intrinsic "rules" by which the living is differentiated from the non-living.

As the role of deoxyribonucleic acid (DNA) in directing function in living matter was revealed, expectations rose that here, in this biochemical model, would finally be a means of truly defining "life" itself. Such hope was fueled by the Human Genome Project, in which mapping of the human gene complement was expected to open new horizons not only on the essential nature of life but also on the application of such information for its therapeutic value. Unfortunately, however, it is increasingly apparent that the idea of a primary action of genes in the life process is a far over-simplistic one. Human behavior—physiologic or otherwise—reflects instead a combination of multiple genetic, epigenetic, environmental, psychological, and social factors. "The more we learn about human biology, the more we find that DNA is just one partner in a very complicated dance" (10).

As this scenario has unfolded, gene action is now seen to be dictated by genetic, non-genetic, and environmental influences, supporting a suspicion that the process of life is far more complicated than was ever previously imagined. As Oxford emeritus professor Denis Noble has pointed out, physiological systems may dictate gene function instead of the other way around (9). "Clearly the simplistic view that genes 'dictate' the organism and its function is just plain silly" he writes in his book *The Music of Life*. "The greatest challenge of [21st] century biologists is how to account for the phenotype in terms of systems level interactions of proteins. About this, molecular genetics tells us very little" (9).

Beauty and Scientific Truth

An idea which has been long-entrenched in scientific lore is that an essential truth or principle can be recognized by its eloquence, or "beauty." That is to say, an idea which strikes to the essential nature of natural phenomena is one which is simple (following Occam's razor) and unified, characterized by harmony and symmetry. Strange bedfellows, indeed!—science (the objective) and beauty (the subjective). But in the final analysis, goes this traditional premise, ultimate truth surrounding natural phenomena forges a juncture of the two. The reading of such insights should evoke an "Ah, yes!" response.

This focus on beauty as a link to scientific truth has suffered in recent decades by a growing awareness that biological processes largely function as *complex systems*. As will be described in several chapters in this book, this means that they operate at multiple hierarchical levels and display emergent properties—new outcomes that cannot be predicted by the features of any of its component parts. Key aspects of system function involve interactions not only between the hierarchical levels but also between systems, feedback loops, dependency on initial conditions (chaos), and non-linear relationships. In reality, biological systems, far from exhibiting the beauty of simplicity, are a messy business. And to quote the mathematician David Orrell, we need a "shift in aesthetics from order and symmetry to something more complex, organic, and messy. . . . Whether a theory or experiment is in some sense ugly or attractive should not enter the calculation. All that matters is whether it works. Beauty is the province of art museums" (10).

Complex systems have displaced beauty as a criterion for scientific proof with a truer vision of a universe characterized by imbalances, asymmetries, and imperfections, one which "is fluid and curved rather than square and static" (10). Orrell expressed this neatly in his book *Truth or Beauty. Science and the Quest for Order*:

> Complex organic systems are dominated by emergent features as well as interlocking feedback loops, which are difficult to capture using predictive models. One could say that the systems have evolved in such a way that they elude prediction. Clarity and certainty are in short supply. . . . In biology, the only things that are stable are dead.
>
> *(10)*

No biological laws or principles have yet been defined for complex adaptive biological systems. It is not difficult to assume that 1) these will involve the dynamics of *interactions* between and within systems, and 2) they will be extraordinarily challenging to decipher. Some would say, in fact, that no laws can universally define the interaction of multiple complex systems in the human body, and that no ultimate biological truths exist, or at least, are discoverable. As far back as the mid-17th century Bernard wrote that "there is no truth apart from mathematical principles; in all natural phenomena the principles from which we start, like the conclusions which we reach, embody only relative truths" (2).

But, as one witnesses in the relative nature of physical laws, that doesn't mean the quest is fruitless. To quote Joan Fontcuberta, "Science is based on the idea that there is truth, whether or not we have access to it. What we know depends on systems of knowledge, and we may never be able to get to specific truths, but the idea is that there is a reality; there is a way humans evolved, or cancers grow, for instance. And science is a way to get to that" (5). So here, at least, biological systems might imitate those of the physical world—truths may be relative, depending on conditions.

Nigel Goldenfeld and Leo Kadanoff are physicists, but what they contend could certainly be applied to biological systems as well: "Up to now, physicists looked for fundamental laws true for all times and all places. But each complex system is different; apparently there are not general laws for complexity. Instead, one must reach for 'lessons' that might, with insight and understanding, be learned in one system and applied to another" (6).

The Measure of Biological "Truth"

In this quest for ultimate biological truths, one inconvenient fact must be faced: our means of interpreting the realities within living systems is limited by the capacity of our cerebral thinking machinery. The question was raised succinctly by the title of an editorial in the journal *Nature*, "Can biological phenomena be understood by humans?" (1). To which Dean Buonomano has replied, in respect to understanding the nature of time, "Our ability to answer questions pertaining to time is constrained by the nature of the organ asking them. Although the gelatinous mass of 100 billion brain cells stashed within your skill is the most sophisticated device in the known universe, it was not 'designed' to understand the nature of time [. . .]" (2).

Within the chapters of this book, the reader will be not infrequently confronted with this disturbing perplexity. The nature of biological functions as complex systems implies an incomprehensible tangle of inter- and intra-system relationships. So does the intrinsic variability which characterizes all biological systems, one whose nature can only be divulged by computer analysis. Are human beings—limited by insights of an extraordinarily complicated but still limited central nervous system—capable of understanding all this?

Mysteries, Controversies, and Insights

Such "lessons" are what this book you are holding is all about. The chapters that follow provide a series of randomly selected dilemmas that have challenged exercise scientists. This book surrounds the idea that essential biological truths might well be revealed in resolving such mysteries of exercise science. But why exercise? What opportunities does it offer? Here's the idea: Physiological stability is a hallmark of living systems. A myriad of finely tuned mechanisms serve to control the *milieu intérieur*—body temperature, cellular pH, fluid balance, blood pressure, blood glucose levels, and so forth. There is probably no single "insult" which so globally threatens this stability as much as physical activity. Indeed, it is difficult to think of a body system that is not perturbed—pushed outside the "status quo"—in some fashion by an acute bout of strenuous exercise. Studying the body's responses to this "disturbance" might well provide a unique means of recognizing essential biological principles—or, at least, lessons that form part of an overall truth.

There exists no cohesive "story line" in the chapters that follow, no narrative arc, no conflict resolutions. Indeed, the topics are widely diverse, ranging from controversies over the subconscious control of racing pace to sex differences in physical activity levels to baseball hitters trying to strike a 100-mph fastball. The common thread to all of these topics, however, is that in their ultimate resolution they offer the promise of insights into the essential principles regulating physiological function and how these respond to the stresses of exercise. Behind each of these mysteries, then, rests a unique opportunity to define the fundamental realities of biological systems.

References

1. Anonymous. Can biological phenomena be understood by humans? *Nature*. 2000;403:345.
2. Bernard C. *An Introduction to the Study of Experimental Medicine*. New York: Dover Publications; 1957.
3. Buonomano D. *Your Brain is a Time Machine*. New York: W.W. Norton & Company; 2017.
4. Feynman R. *The Character of Physical Law*. Cambridge, MA: MIT Press; 1965.
5. Fontcuberta J, Ruiz I, Altaba A. Objectivity and the image. In:, Bly A, editor. *Science is Culture*. New York: Harper Collins; 2010.
6. Goldenfeld N, Kadanoff LP. Simple lessons from complexity. *Science*. 1999;284:87–89.
7. Lortie G, Simoneau JA, Hamel P, Boulay MR, Landry F, Bouchard C. Responses of maximal aerobic power and capacity to aerobic training. *Int J Sports Med*. 1984;5:232–236.
8. Mayr E. How biology differs from the physical sciences. In: Depew DJ, Weber BH, editors. *Evolution at a Crossroads. The New Biology and the New Philosophy of Science*. Cambridge, MA: MIT Press; 1985. pp. 43–63.
9. Noble D. *The Music of Life. Biology Beyond the Genome*. Oxford: Oxford University Press; 2006.
10. Orrell D. *Truth or Beauty. Science and the Quest for Order*. Yale: Yale University Press; 2012.
11. Pross A. *What is Life. How Chemistry Becomes Biology*. Oxford: Oxford University Press; 2012.

ACKNOWLEDGMENTS

Chapter 6 is based on the contents of my book *Biologic Regulation of Physical Activity* (Human Kinetics, 2017). The section on the grunting of tennis players in Chapter 14 draws heavily from *A Philosophy of Tennis, or You Kant Be Serious* (Kemper Conseil Publishing, 2018). Chapter 4 was written in conjunction with George R. Biltz, M.D., Senior Lecturer in the School of Kinesiology at the University of Minnesota, to whom I am grateful for his invaluable guidance over some difficult scientific terrain. Todd Rowland, Ph.D., provided assistance in the mathematical interpretations of Zeno's Paradox in Chapter 3. I am especially indebted to those who have provided me with inspiration, not only for writing this book but throughout my professional career. The list of such names (certainly not inclusive) would include Oded Bar-Or, Bo Fernhall, Denise Smith, Vish Unnithan, Robert Malina, Steve Siconolfi, and Rainer Martens. The author also expresses his thanks to Sandy Savenko and the staff of the Medical Library at the Baystate Medical Center without whose assistance in obtaining resource materials this book could not have been written.

1

WHAT LIMITS TRAINING-INDUCED IMPROVEMENTS IN ATHLETIC PERFORMANCE?

At the 2012 annual meeting of the American College of Sports Medicine in San Francisco, Claude Bouchard and Anders Ericsson squared off in a debate surrounding the issue of what limits improvements in performance with exercise training. The former took the traditional position that one's genetic endowment set such limits, while the latter proposed a theory of deliberate practice in which one's ultimate progress was dictated only by one's commitment to a proper path of training.

At least that's what they thought they were doing. In fact, these two experts were engaging in a discussion which has been at the heart of human inquiry for as long as there has been recorded history. It might have begun in a corner of the Acropolis, then moved on to places like the ivy halls of Oxford, and eventually at the smoke-filled back tables at the Café de Flore. The central question: Do humans have the capacity for free will, to make conscious decisions which govern their actions? That is, do they possess the ability—some would say the *responsibility*—to define themselves through such conscious decision-making? Or, on the other hand, is it true that all events, all actions, all decisions are fixed, or pre-determined, by biological and cultural forces, and that humans are deceived in being convinced that they control their decisions when, in reality, all are in fact dictated by a pre-ordained destiny? Human freedom of conscious choice, if such is the case, is nothing but an illusion.

It's a very popular philosophical question, one ranking right up there with "Is there a God?" and "Why are we here?" and "Why is there the universe instead of nothing?" And all card-carrying philosophers have weighed in on the issue. Some of their important points:

- The question is particularly poignant because it speaks to the issue of individual freedom. And "to be undetermined is to be free, and everyone wants to be free" (5). What affronts most people who believe in free will "is the suggestion that he is only a machine, a big foolish clock that seems to itself to be acting freely, but whose movements are controlled completely by the wheels and weights inside, a Punch-and-Judy show whose appearance of doing things because they are right or reasonable is a sham because everything is mechanically regulated by wires from below" (5).

- Sigmund Freud contended that in this matter our minds are easily deceived, since the subconscious brain in fact directs our apparent conscious decision-making. In contemporary times this claim has been backed by some good scientific evidence—based on brain imaging studies—that our day-to-day decisions are likely to be influenced by such subconscious motives (38). Yet, it has been claimed that "the introduction of the unconscious as an explanation does not help the determinist at all. Far from it: for the unconscious, when it is truly creative, is far more unpredictable than the conscious mind" (3).
- Many of the greatest thinkers—Plato, Descartes, Kant—considered human reasoning and cognitive ability to weigh options to be the emblem of the human spirit. "One of the main motives in the rebellion against determinism, not only on the part of ordinary people but also of those modern philosophers who have been most vigorously opposed to the determinist position, [is] the desire for freshness, novelty, genuine creation—in short, an open rather than a closed universe" (3). But, on the other hand, it has been argued that is it not the subconscious, independent of conscious effort, that provides the spark of human creativity? As Blanshard recognized, "Many an artist and musician have left it on record that their best work was done when the whole they were creating took the brush or pen away from them and completed the work itself" (5).
- Determinism is frightening, since it necessitates an abrogation of all social responsibility. The morality of human behavior—crime, anti-social activity—become meaningless if an individual cannot be held personally responsible. If such were the case, "how can anyone be responsible for his actions, since they grow out of his character, which is shaped and molded and made what it is by influences—some hereditary, but most of them stemming from early parental environment—that were not of his own making or choosing?" (33).

And so forth and so forth. Indeed, as NYU's William Barrett has noted, " a subject like this . . . has been so long discussed that nothing new is likely to be said" (3).

So here in room 210 of the San Francisco Convention Center one heard the arguments on each side of an ages-old debate. Here was a proponent of genetic determinism, arguing that, yes, one could certainly expect to improve performance with training, but there was a fixed limit, one pre-determined and dictated by a factor out of one's control, the genetic information inherited from one's parents. On the other side, an argument for free will. Not only could one improve with training, but the individual possesses the capacity for adopting certain training regimens, the outcomes of improved performance which are not associated with any particular ceiling or limit. The choice, and the degree of training-induced improvements, are under one's personal control, a matter of free will.

What makes this debate particularly novel is that here is a classic philosophical problem which just might possibly be solved through the process of scientific research. By its very nature, "philosophy" is considered to address questions which are surrounded by uncertainty. "Philosophy is to be studied," contended Bertrand Russell, "not for the sake of any definitive answers to its questions, since no definitive answers can, as a rule, be known to be true, but rather for the sake of the questions themselves" (53). Maybe here is an exception.

Assuredly neither Professors Bouchard and Ericsson nor their audience had the above thoughts in mind as the debate unfolded. The arguments presented were not new, as both had long personified opinions on both sides of the question, which had become highly popularized among athletes and scientists alike. Predictably, at the end of the debate there was no "winner," and it could have been suspected that the members of the audience departed with the same opinion as they had when they first sat down. But it was clear that both had defined intriguing ideas surrounding directly opposing viewpoints, ones which went to the roots of both exercise physiology and questions of the relative importance of free will and determinism.

The Training Effect

The controversy surrounding the limits of athletic training adaptations rests on the foundation of a more basic concept, upon which both sides of the argument would find common ground: Repetitive muscular activity, within certain limits of frequency and intensity, will trigger specific positive adaptations in human physiologic function and/or anatomy. So this is where the story must begin.

That trained athletes are characterized by greater muscle strength and endurance compared to untrained individuals has been recognized since antiquity. However, the mechanisms underlying the physiologic/anatomic effects of such training and the means by which these adaptations to training are translated into improved athletic performance remain incompletely understood to this day. Such adaptive mechanisms must reflect the accumulated responses to repetitive exercise bouts; hence, clues to their nature might at least initially best be sought in an examination of biochemical/metabolic changes that occur following a single bout of acute exercise.

The nature of such responses to individual bouts of exercise have traditionally been considered in the context of a lineage of seminal publications which have described the body's adaptations to acute stress. It starts in the mid-1800s, when Claude Bernard placed human physiological function on a scientific footing by introducing the concept of the necessity of body systems to maintain the stability of the *milieu intérieur*. By this he meant that perturbations of the physiological steady state induced by the external environment (such as that occurring during physical exercise) must be met by compensatory adjustments (i.e., thermoregulation, acid-base status, blood glucose levels) to sustain the internal equilibrium essential for living tissues (24).

(In addition, it must be recognized here that in *An Introduction to the Study of Experimental Medicine* Bernard decried what has been called the "tyranny of the mean," contending that researchers should avoid interpreting an average finding as indicative of biologic truth. As an example, he cited the folly of the physiologist who "took urine from a railroad station urinal where people of all nations passed, and who believed he could thus present an analysis of *average* European urine!" (4). Bernard emphasized, too, that good scientific research is laborious and not always easy. He described such work in words (as would certainly be appreciated by any modern-day grad student) as being like "a superb and dazzling lighted hall which may be reached only by passing through a long and ghastly kitchen.")

Walter Cannon served as chairman of the Department of Physiology at Harvard Medical School until 1942. In his book *The Wisdom of the Body* he expanded on Bernard's concept of the *milieu intérieur*, outlining the specific physiological processes that served in the objective of maintaining physiological stability, which he termed *homeostasis* (11). In these chapters he described now-traditional processes by which cardiopulmonary, thermoregulatory, fluid balance, and acid-base status were maintained during exercise. He placed emphasis on sympatho-adrenal responses to stress and was the first to coin the term "fight-or-flight response."

It remained for Hans Selye, the Austrian-Canadian endocrinologist, to regard changes triggered by the stress of exercise as positive functional adaptations rather than homeostatic responses (54). In his *general adaptation syndrome* model, he proposed that adaptations to progressively increasing physical stressors occurs in three stages, an initial fatigue, or decrease in function, followed by a second phase of positive adaptation, and, then, if stress reached sufficient levels, a third stage of exhaustion and performance decline.

Modern-day precepts of training regimens follow this model, particularly in athletic events that involve strength and muscular endurance. That is, the physiological, anatomic, and biochemical events culminating in the positive "fitness effect" reflect reactions to the stresses of training overload. And such adaptations consequently form the basis of enhanced physical performance. Excessive stress to body systems beyond a certain threshold, however, are counter-productive, culminating in tissue damage and performance declines (i.e., the genesis of "overtraining" or sports overuse injury).

This scenario of positive adaptations to exercise training (within limits) effecting parallel improvements in physical functional capacity is characteristic of the process of *hormesis*, defined as the biological phenomenon in which beneficial effects of a stressor are gained in a linear dose-response fashion up to a certain threshold level, beyond which the stressor becomes harmful. The term has most commonly been employed in describing the actions of chemicals on living beings—like caffeine and alcohol—which are stimulatory or beneficial at low doses but toxic at higher doses. In exercise physiology, hormesis has been described in respect to the effect of physical training on immune function (protective at low-moderate training levels but diminished resistance to infection with intense training) and the similar effects of exercise on protection from the oxidative damage of free radicals (23,49).

The particular anatomic and physiological adaptive responses to a period of physical training, of course, depend on the physical activity involved. What is remarkable—and not often appreciated—is the "intelligence" displayed by the body in making anatomic and physiologic adaptive changes to athletic training which are specific to those underpinning the performance of the particular form of exercise. If one regularly engages in exercise involving large muscle groups over a sustained time duration (running, cycling), mitochondrial aerobic metabolic capacity is enhanced along with expansion of the cardiovascular system (cardiac enlargement, increased plasma volume), both features essential for endurance exercise performance. In resistance training, on the other hand, repeated bouts stimulate adaptive cellular protein synthesis and intensify neuromuscular stimulation which promote muscle strength. Repeated 10-mile training runs do little or nothing to promote muscle size and strength, while free weights lifted on a regular basis cannot be expected to improve one's 10K race times.

This specificity of training response is evident even within the confines of a particular form of exercise. During resistance training, for instance, adaptations resulting in augmented strength are limited to the muscle group employed in the training protocol as well as its angular position and movement velocity (36).

In emphasizing the hormetic nature of Selye's stress theory, Radak et al. made two critical observations (49). First, exercise training must achieve a certain level of stress in order to trigger adaptive changes. And second, chronic stress (i.e., highly intense training periods of long duration) can be deleterious unless sufficient rest periods are included. It is during rest that compensatory positive adaptations occur in response to the stresses and microdamage experienced in the training bouts themselves. Sustained training without periods of rest can be expected to push the training athlete onto the maladaptive regions of the hormetic curve.

The mechanisms underlying visual-motor performance improvements with training in skill sports such as tennis and baseball are different and are just beginning to be understood (51). Imaging studies suggest brain regions specific for certain visual-motor skills shift from purposeful cognitive attention centers to those governing automatic, subconscious play with training. Animal studies are consistent with a model of neural training adaptations such as changes in neuron firing patterns, increased amplitude of cellular electrical potentials, and augmented synaptic connections.

Considerable progress has been achieved in understanding the biochemical/metabolic processes that underpin these phenotypic expressions of response to physical training. Most of these concepts have been developed through animal studies, but new information has recently become available in human beings as well (43). Yet, "most of the mechanisms underlying the adaptation of human skeletal muscle to exercise still remain to be discovered" (20). (This despite the fact that the process by which human beings improve with physical training has long served as a fundamental question in exercise science. In their year 2000 review, Hamilton and Booth noted that over 15,000 articles had been published in the preceding 30 years that included the words "exercise" and "muscle" in their abstracts [30].)

Some have placed emphasis on the potential role of heat shock proteins, whose intracellular action is upregulated by the stresses of exercise (43). While these appear to serve to maintain cellular homeostasis and protect against the disturbances of subsequent exercise stress, their role in triggering functional and anatomic adaptations to the training regimen remain uncertain.

Mechanisms underlying muscle adaptations to repeated bouts of exercise may relate to the presence or absence of cellular injury incurred during training. It has been suggested that during endurance exercise, in which no overt cellular injury is typically observed, adaptive responses may surround reaction to factors such as redox signaling (oxidation of muscle proteins), while in the presence of structural damage to muscle cells, as occurs with resistance training, the response to cell inflammation may be key.

Other potential physiological signals that could be instrumental in triggering the adaptive response to exercise stress have been suggested. Increase in muscle temperature with exercise has been established as a reliable stimulant of heat stress proteins and reactive oxygen species, but such findings have not been consistently substantiated in humans (43). The role of the metabolic byproducts of exercise stress (such as acidosis and substrate depletion) have long been suspected of playing a role in training adaptations, but conclusive evidence remains elusive.

Finally, one mustn't ignore the question of *why* humans should demonstrate positive adaptations to repeated bouts of exercise. From a Darwinian perspective, it might be expected that the biological "meaning" of the human to improve physical performance with training reflects evolutionary pressures to escape predators and enemies, track down fast-fleeing food, and avoid environmental extremes. Some authors, however, have been skeptical of such facile explanations (9,32). For example, although certainly there exist animals with physical abilities exceeding that of humans, out on the primate branch of the evolutionary tree only human beings are capable of endurance running. The fossil evidence indicates that this was first evident between 1.5 and 3.0 million years ago, so just why humans became endurance athletes dates that far back. Hunter-gatherers began to utilize weapons—bows and arrows, spears—about 40,000 years ago. So, if the traditional explanations are true, little survival pressures to avoid predators by distance running occurred this recently. The bottom line is that the evolutionary origins of mankind's ability to improve performance with training—at least in distance running—are not entirely clear (9,32).

The Controversy

So much for the mysteries surrounding the well-documented realities of improvements in athletic performance gained from periods of event-specific exercise. On now to the essential question: What limits the magnitude of this training response? We now examine the two opposing viewpoints at hand.

Genetic Determinism

The oft-cited argument for a genetic determination of athletic prowess is bipartite, involving two processes which are presumably independent of each other: 1) the actions of genes in defining sports performance in the untrained individual, and 2) the genetic influence on one's capacity to improve physical fitness in response to a period of exercise training. Before delving into a discussion of each, it is important to place these purported genetic influences in the context of the evolving history of our understanding of how genetic material governs phenotypic characteristics (anatomic, physiologic, metabolic, and so on). So, a brief digression . . .

An Historical Perspective

A recounting of mankind's various explanations for the obvious transmission of familial characteristics from one generation to the next could (and has) filled many volumes (see reference 57 for a concise overview). Since early recorded history, Divine Direction has taken a central role—from Plato, to the Stoics, to the Romans, and then the early Christian writers. To all, reproduction was considered a creation of a Supreme God. Presciently, the Greek followers of Hippocrates in the 4th century B.C. considered that this was achieved by the process of *pangenesis*, meaning that newborn infants were an expression of a physical mixing of substances contributed by both parents. It wasn't until nearly 2,000 years later, however, that William Harvey (he of circulation-of-blood fame) proposed, based on his examination of dissected fowl and deer, that reproduction and transmission of parental characteristics occurred by the union of the male's semen and female's egg.

It awaited the invention of the microscope—which permitted direct observation of chromosomes, as well as their duplication—and the astute observation of the outcomes of selective breeding of animal and plants, for the development of ideas concerning the means by which inherited material is expressed phenotypically. And in the early 1900s that the activity of a specific locus on the chromosome (gene) action could account for a particular phenotypic outcome was established through observations of the effects of change in gene change (i.e., mutation) on certain characteristics of fruit flies. Such observations indicated the fixed nature as well as plasticity, through mutations, of one's genetic complement. The latter neatly filled the conceptual gap in the Darwinian construct of natural selection, offering a means of variation upon which the forces of such selection might act.

The concept of "the inheritance of acquired characteristics" introduced in the late 18th century held that behaviors and functions of animals acquired during life could be passed on to one's offspring. The giraffe—and its progeny—possesses a long neck because it stretched out to reach nutrition in the tree's high branches. This theory has been traditionally attributed to the French biologist Jean-Baptiste Chevalier de Lamarck, who, after being rejected by the army, moved on to the Royal Herbarium in Paris in 1793 to study insects and worms. The concept prevailed for over 200 years, adopted by mainstream biologists, including Charles Darwin. It's a story historically important to mark, since "Lamarckism," later strongly discredited, has, as will be seen below, in recent times re-surfaced "despite the strong distaste of most biologists" (58).

It was generally agreed by 1940 that genes were discrete units of information situated on chromosomes. The major breakthrough that became the turning point in understanding of gene action came, of course, with the description of the structure and function of deoxyribonucleic acid (DNA) by Watson and Crick in the 1950s. DNA is comprised of two helical strands consisting of a sugar-phosphate lattice on the outside with interior-facing complementary nucleotides, thymine pairing with adenine and cytosine with guanine. In a scenario quickly recognized by all high school biology students, DNA serves as a template for ribonucleic acid (RNA), which enters into the cellular cytoplasm and by its sequences of nucleotides triggers the production of proteins which then perform activities of the cell. And the self-replication of DNA was assured as each strand could form a template for the other.

This elegant description provided a seductive sense of finality, explaining the essential mechanism by which genetic material dictated the operation of living matter—perhaps offering insight into the meaning of life itself. The gene was paramount. In controlling phenotype, genetic information is transmitted from generation to generation, can organize its own duplication, and includes in its nucleotide pairs the "experiences" of all human ancestors (40). Here was the ultimate "blueprint of life" by which all human function could be ascribed and many disease states explained. The primacy of the gene was emphasized by Richard Dawkins in his book *The Selfish Gene*, in which he pointed out that, contrary to the rest of human flesh, the gene, in reproducing itself, does not grow senile, and, in fact, is immortal (12). All these considerations generated eventually the Human Genome Project, which offered to provide a "library" of the location of specific gene loci by which such function and dysfunction could be described. In any event, Lamarckism was now defunct.

As the investigative tools of molecular biologists became more sophisticated, however, it became apparent that all was not that simple. This, it turned out, was not the way living beings actually worked. To wit:

- Of the approximate 3 billion base pairs in the human genome, only about 1% function in the coding of proteins. The Human Genome Project identified only such 20,000 active genes, far lower than the number needed to encode for protein production. This discrepancy has been accounted for by the process of "alternative splicing," whereby a single gene produces multiple RNAs via different combinations of exons (coding sequences) (50). Too, some genes can generate different proteins depending on the situation. What the remainder, which are inactive—so-called "junk genes"—are doing still remains uncertain.

- As Waller concluded, "in practice so many traits arise from the complex interaction of multiple [gene] loci that it has proven difficult to show clear links between [genes] and particular phenotypes" (57).
- As early as 1950 research had indicated that there exist factors which control which, and to what extent, a particular gene functions. (This was, in effect, obvious, since some such mechanism was required to explain how embryonic stem cells possessing a full genetic complement evolved into specialized cells responsible for single anatomic or physiological function.) Today, a great deal of investigative focus has revealed multiple mechanisms by which such control of gene function occurs, including regulatory genetic material as well as actions of non-genetic agents such as modifications of the protein histone and the process of DNA methylation which are triggered by extrinsic and environmental stimuli. The latter effects, termed *epigenesis* (factors which influence gene action without altering DNA structure), have received increasing attention as critical factors which establish how genetic information is translated into phenotypic expression. Moreover, some evidence exists that certain early-life effects (nutrition, body composition, locomotor activity), perhaps related to epigenetic mechanisms, may be passed from generation to generation, raising the specter of Lamarckism (26).

These observations have raised awareness that the Watson-Crick models of gene determinism that seemed so attractive may not adequately reflect the complexity by which genes define phenotypic expression. The British biologist Denis Noble has summarized this skepticism in his book *The Music of Life. Biology Beyond the Genome* (47). He claims that the arrows in the "genocentric" model are facing backwards, and that instead of gene → proteins → cells → tissues → organs → organism, the control of expression of genetic information is directed from the interaction of body system functions—often in response to environmental stimuli—in a complex array of interaction, redundancy, and feedback loops. That is, higher complex functions are what really "plays" the gene. "Clearly, the simplistic view that genes 'dictate' the organism is just silly," Noble says. "The greatest challenge of [21st] century biologists is how to account for the phenotype in terms of systems-level interactions of proteins. About this, molecular genetics tells us very little" (p. 47).

If fact, then, the mystery of gene-phenotype relationships remains, to some disillusionment, clouded. Nature, closely guarding her secrets, continues to reveal itself as a set of interactions of complexity on complexity, resisting simplistic, reductionist thinking to which the human brain trying to comprehend it all has been tuned. The bottom line: functions that once were considered to represent pure genetic control must be considered in the light of the potential influences of psychological, social, and environmental factors which may modify gene action.

Genetic Effects of Physical Performance in the Nontrained Individual

It comes as no surprise that the components of traits that compromise "physical fitness" are characterized by a significant influence of genetic factors even in individuals that carry on a sedentary life style. Equally expected is the observation that considering the complexity of the determinants of athletic performance, no single genetic factor has been revealed that accounts for "sports skill." Instead, researchers have focused on assessing the extent of the genetic contribution to the individual physiological and anatomic factors comprising such prowess (48).

A combination of population, twin-twin, and animal studies have indicated that for the principal determinants of endurance and muscular strength performance (VO_2max and explosive strength, respectively), approximately 50% can be accounted for by one's heredity (50). Similar levels of genetic contribution have been described for muscle fiber type, metabolic factors (i.e., aerobic enzyme activity), and body composition (48). The remainder of the variance is assumed to reflect the combination of sampling and technical variability, gene-environment interaction, and environmental influences (such as level of habitual physical activity).

A growing list of candidate genes has accumulated which are associated with different components of physical fitness (50). The effect sizes and levels of association with fitness markers of the genes are generally small. And, as emphasized by Goldspink and Velloso, for these gene loci "a convincing cause and effect relationship has yet to be demonstrated" (28). Still, they "could contribute to the collective account of the genetic component of physical performance" (16).

It might be assumed that these genetic influences on fitness in the untrained individual are static in nature. That is, without a stimulus for change (i.e., athletic training, sustained bed rest) genetic control of aspects such as heart size and muscle volume should remain unchanged. However, it is clear that they, too, are susceptible to control by mechanisms that regulate gene expression. Consider the evolution in the components of physical fitness that occurs in the process of growth and development occurring between infancy and the achievement of the adult state 16 years later. The genetic information at birth residing in one's chromosome complement includes, *de facto*, all that which will direct the mature state, yet its expression is strongly controlled by regulatory factors—genetic and non-genetic (epigenetic)—which dictate not only gene expression but the timing, or *tempo*, of such expression as well.

This field of *developmental genomics* is currently a busy area of research focus. It may well be that such investigations will elucidate the controlling factors which influence the emergence of gene expression that bear on physical fitness as a child grows. It is an intriguing question: could such regulators that control gene expression during normal growth and development reflect those that influence altered gene expression occurring with a period of physical training (see below)?

Genetic Effects on Training-induced Performance Gains

In the previously sedentary adult, a period of structured endurance exercise training typically triggers a 15–25% rise in VO_2max. In a series of training studies in young adults, Bouchard and his colleagues demonstrated a mean gain in VO_2max of approximately 25% above baseline, but with a range of 0–100% increase among individual subjects (8). Similar variability in inter-individual physiological responses to aerobic training has been reported in elderly (35) and childhood (52) populations (ranges of improvement 0–58% and −3–20%, respectively). All of these authors attributed such a wide scatter of responses to individual differences in a genetic-based capacity for metabolic and cardiovascular responses to training.

This conclusion was supported by several experimental studies indicating that the magnitude of response of VO_2max to a period of endurance training is more similar in individuals with identical genotypes (i.e., identical twins) than those with different genotypes (7). Too, Bouchard et al. reported a strong familial aggregation of magnitude of VO_2max response to training (6). In that report, variability in training response was 2.6 times greater between than within families, which provided a calculated heritability estimate of 47%.

Twenty years ago Wesson wrote that

> Philosophically, the holistic approach—the notion of the organism adapting to its surrounding—is attractive. It seems natural. The body, we well know, has remarkable and poorly understood abilities to adapt itself to use and suffers from disuse; the athlete in training gets stronger muscles, the couch potato's muscles weaken; the brain improves with exercise; hikers' feet become callused; bones and tendons get stronger, within limits, as they are stressed. . . . That such responses can be programmed, changing the expression of the genes of the cells involved, suggest the possibility that organisms can be geared to respond genetically to external signals
>
> *(58)*

Research in the years since has supported the logical corollary to these thoughts that *the anatomic, physiological, and metabolic responses to a period of physical training reflect adaptive changes in gene expression.* As outlined above, this signals the potential importance of epigenetic processes which are recognized to alter gene expression, including histone modifications, DNA methylation, and the production of microRNAs. In fact, a growing body of research information indicates that these biochemical activities are triggered by the stress and microdamage of repetitive physical activity and are expected, then, to serve as key modulators of the physical, physiological, and metabolic responses to exercise training. In this way they may serve as models of gene-environment interaction.

The molecular mechanisms underlying these epigenetic processes are just beginning to be revealed (13). In general, they act to influence the availability of DNA sites for transcription to RNA and protein outcomes (16,46). Too, the mechanisms by which muscular stress incurred by exercise serves to trigger these gene-modifying processes remains uncertain. Some evidence exists that the magnitude of such epigenetic responses to exercise are controlled by an individual's genome, thus adding another stratum of gene control of adaptations to training (27,39).

Histone Modification

Histone protein molecules surround base-pairs of DNA as *nucleosomes*. Acetylation of these proteins shifts their position and thereby influences gene expression by exposing new sites for transcription. Single bouts of aerobic as well as resistance exercise have been documented to alter such acetylation and trigger gene transcription (15,41).

DNA Methylation

DNA methylation involves the attachment of a methyl group to a cytosine in the DNA molecule. This effects either an increase or decrease in gene expression, depending on the location of the attachment on the chromosome (14). In their review of the research literature as of the year 2015, Voisin et al. described the findings of 25 studies examining the effect of physical activity on DNA methylation (56). What emerges from these reports, which often suffered from methodological weaknesses, is a picture of considerable complexity and unclear outcomes. In sum, the authors concluded from these compiled data that "both acute and chronic exercises significantly impact DNA methylation, in a highly tissue- and gene-specific manner" (p. 39). A number of observations were made: In most studied genes in muscle tissue exercise interventions reduced DNA methylation (that is, augmented gene expression). However, DNA methylation changes in response to exercise did not always match that expected in gene expression. That is, exercise in some reports, to the contrary, triggered hypermethylation. One study which demonstrated an increased methylation was interpreted as indicating a salutary effect of suppressing pro-inflammatory responses to exercise (45). Some of these reports underscored the problem that the effects of other processes that alter DNA methylation in response to exercise interventions must be appreciated in any such studies.

MicroRNA

MicroRNAs (miRNAs) are small noncoding RNA molecules that bind with messenger RNA and play an integral part of a number of physiological and pathological processes. At least 2,000 miRNAs are known to be coded in the human genome; it has been suggested that as many as 30% of genes are under miRNA regulation. Studies indicate that a period of exercise training—aerobic, interval, and resistance—in animal models promotes adaptive cardiac hypertrophy (22), and miRNAs have also been identified as modulators of skeletal muscle hypertrophy. Baggish et al. demonstrated an increase in circulating miRNAs after both acute exercise and chronic exercise training in adult rowers, some which correlated with peak exercise values and VO_2max (1). Similar findings were reported by Denham and Prestes in adult endurance athletes (14). The authors of both of these articles suggested that levels of miRNA in the blood might serve as a maker of cardiovascular adaptations to exercise training and "would contribute to exercise screening, monitoring, and development of personalized exercise prescriptions" (14).

Other Factors

Additional processes that occur in response to exercise are recognized to trigger adaptive gene function. For instance, alterations in calcium flux during the signaling for muscle contraction can activate alterations in gene transcription (44). And proteins such as AMPK (activated protein kinase) serve as transcriptional regulators of genes responsible for mitochondrial biogenesis in response to aerobic training (34,37).

The concept of genetic determinism of the limits of trainability is expressed in the so-called power law curve (Figure 1.1) (31). The rate of improvement is high at the onset of a training regimen, reflecting the impact of factors altering gene function in response to the stresses of physical exercise. The rate of such improvement gradually wanes as training continues, following a curvilinear path described by a power function of performance vs. training time. In an asymptotic manner performance with continued training approaches a fixed limit, which is defined by the maximum extent of gene-related mechanisms. This, then, forms the basis for the traditional concept that the upper limit of training-induced performance is defined by the limits of one's genetic endowment.

In summary, strong evidence supports a construct whereby repetitive exercise stress triggers the formation of epigenetic and other processes which provide a permissive effect of increasing gene function, resulting in the phenotype expressions that constitutes the physiological, anatomic, and metabolic effects of physical training. But what remains to be firmly established, however, is whether or not there exists a limit, or a ceiling, to this modification of gene expression. Intuitively, the answer might be expected to be "yes." Certainly, one's basic genetic complement is fixed. But does the discrepancy between the number of active genes in this hereditary material and its functional capacity (quantity of transcriptional

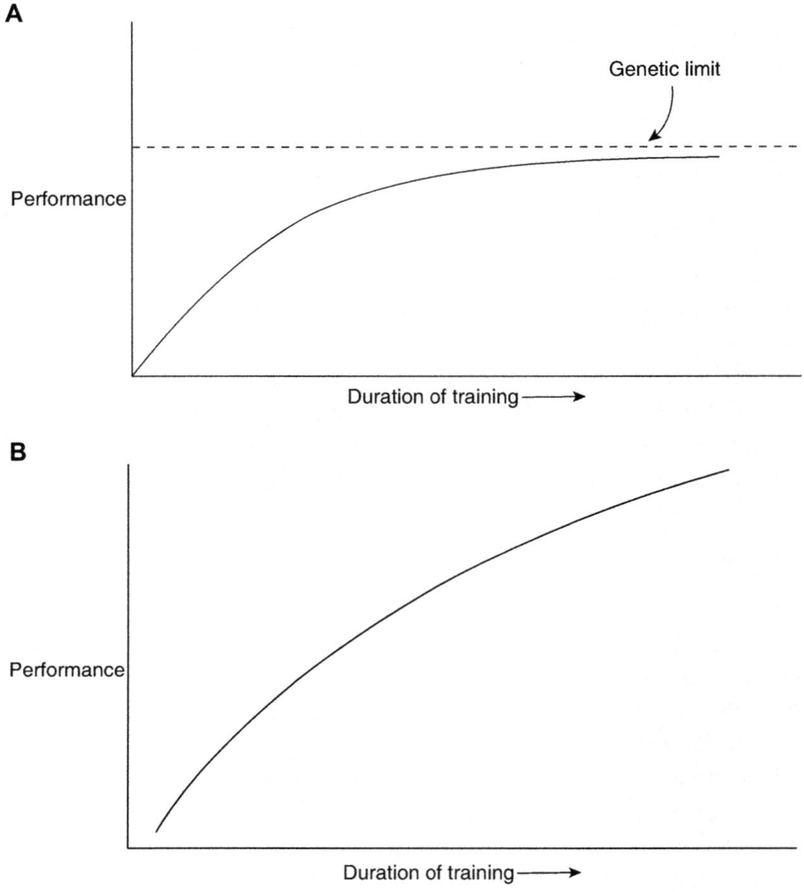

FIGURE 1.1 Performance improvements with training. A. Traditional interpretation that training-induced athletic improvements are ultimately limited by one's genetic endowment. (Reprinted by permission from T.W. Rowland, *Tennisology: Inside the Science of Serves, Nerves, and On-Court Dominance* [Champaign, IL: Human Kinetics Publishers, 2014].), 53,64. B. By the theory of deliberate practice, performance responses to a focused training regimen are not fixed by a genetic limitation.

(Reprinted by permission from T.W. Rowland, *Tennisology: Inside the Science of Serves, Nerves, and On-Court Dominance* [Champaign, IL: Human Kinetics Publishers, 2014.], 53,64.)

proteins produced) imply a certain functional plasticity of genetic determinism? Considering the potential for functions such as alternative gene splicing and the potential latent capacity of 99% of the human genome, the possibility that a true genetic limit does not exist which constrains performance improvements with athletic training cannot be totally discounted.

Theory of Deliberate Practice

Anders Ericsson is a psychologist at Florida State University who has championed, with considerable popular success, the idea that the establishment of sports expertise and the limits of training-induced performance are influenced by engagement in effective training rather than one's genetic endowment. This is termed the *Theory of Deliberate Practice*, which holds that success in athletics is not established by a genetic-imposed ceiling but rather by one's ability to commit to training of sufficient duration, quantity, and focused intensity (21). It takes time to accomplish this—about 10 years and 10,000 hours of training—but it is just this extended focused training regimen, rather than any innate genetic talent, that makes for champion athletes.

The training-performance curve of this theory, then, is altered from the power law of practice defining a genetic ceiling to training improvements over time. Instead it resembles Figure 1.1B, whereby improvement gains in performance can be perpetuated, without a genetically based ceiling, by proper application of focused, sustained practice. It's an idea which has gained considerable acceptance in the athletic world, attractive in that it calls for self-reliance and control over one's athletic destiny rather being constrained by an immutable genetic determinism.

The secret of achieving this success lies in adopting the proper training technique. Normally the early stages of training are accompanied by significant performance gains, but typically such improvement wanes as training progresses. This theory contends that such stagnation is not the effect of approaching genetic-based limits but rather a failure to properly adjust one's training approach. The typical response of the athlete at this point is to simply ratchet up the intensity of the same practice activities, the result of which is failure to progress, since the workout no longer provides any new specific physiological or cognitive challenges. Instead, training regimens must be modified to identify weaknesses and designed to focus progressively on particular components of performance that need improvement.

Deliberate practice, then, is characterized by

- training regimens that focus on a particular aspect of performance and concentrates on solving weaknesses and correcting errors.
- addressing recognized tasks that need challenging.
- hard work, which is not always pleasurable.
- expert feedback from skilled coaches.
- commitment to a long-term training program.

According to this theory, then, expert athletes will continue to demonstrate training improvements as long as continued sports experience is coupled with the principles of deliberate practice. And this involves an active cognitive approach to designing creative, productive training regimens. According to Ericsson

> The key challenge for aspiring expert performers is to avoid the arrested development associated with automaticity and to acquire cognitive skills

> to support their continued learning and improvement. By actively seeking out demanding tasks—often provided by their teachers and coaches—that force the performers to engage in problem solving and to stretch their performance, the expert performers overcome the detrimental effects of automaticity and actively acquire cognitive mechanisms to support continued learning and improvement.
>
> *(18)*

Ericsson first developed these ideas surrounding the plasticity for training improvements from a study in which he found an unexpected ability of human beings to memorize numbers (19). Traditional wisdom held that the average human being could not retain in memory more than seven digits (thus the limit in a telephone number). Ericsson and his colleagues demonstrated, however, that after many practice hours, "unexceptional" college students could be trained to accurately memorize lists of numbers comprising up to over 20 digits. In fact, after several hundred hours of additional practice two students could recite over 80 successive digits from memory (this they accomplished by segmenting numbers into groups and creating novel associations) (17).

The doctrine and principles of deliberate practice were subsequently developed from observational studies of violinists and pianists, comparing groups of different levels of skill levels with their training and practice histories. Among a group of violin students at the Music Academy of West Berlin, Ericsson and his fellow researchers examined three groups, ten musicians in each: those considered sufficiently skilled as to expect their future as international soloists, students who were good violinists but not at an "elite" level, and those involved in music education rather than a performance curriculum (20). By self-estimation, the length of practice time over their careers was directly related to skill level, at age 20 years totaling 10,000, 8,000, and 4,000 hours for the three groups, respectively. Similar findings were observed in young pianists—volume and type of practice were related to their level of performance as adults.

Retrospective reviews have indicated that the training regimens of highly successful athletes have generally conformed to the tenets of deliberate practice (2). Moreover, the link of attainment of athletic expertise and duration of training (i.e., a 10-year commitment) has been largely upheld in a variety of sports, including figure skating, wrestling, soccer, distance running, swimming, and tennis (2). Ericsson warned, however, that despite its adoption as a popular catch-word, the 10,000-hour, 10-year "rule" should not be taken as an absolute guideline: "A closer examination of the evidence for the ten-year rule shows that the number ten is not magical. In fact, the number of years of intense training required to become an internationally acclaimed performer differs across domains" (18).

The value of the principles of deliberate practice in athletic and musical realms have not been lost on other disciplines as well. Indeed, the dogma of concentrated, problem-focused practice under feedback guidance has been employed in such disparate activities as cardiothoracic surgery, performance playing board games, training of suicide prevention professionals, football refereeing, and neonatal resuscitation.

Given these common associations supporting the validity of deliberate practice, the findings of a meta-analysis of 34 studies in a variety of sports by Macnamara et al. are rather surprising (42). Among these studies, which included 52 independent samples and 63 effect sizes, a significant positive correlation was observed between levels of deliberate practice and performance (r = 0.43), with deliberate practice accounting for 18% of the variance in sports performance. This extent of this contribution, however, was related to skill level. Among elite-level athletes deliberate practice accounted for only 1% of the variance.

Indeed, the Theory of Deliberate Practice has not been met without criticisms, not the least of which the contention that this view "requires a blindness to ordinary experience" (25). As noted by Baker and Horton, the descriptions by Ericsson and his colleagues of acquisition of elite musical skills (as well as subsequent similar studies in champion athletes) are entirely retrospective (2). That is, investigators have taken groups of highly talented musicians and athletes and looked at their training characteristics. What is ignored is the set of those who might have followed the same dictates of deliberate practice yet failed to achieve success (or even dropped out altogether). Indeed, as Hambrick et al. put it, "the evidence is quite clear that some people *do* reach an elite level of performance without copious practice, while other people fail to do so *despite* copious practice" (italics theirs) (29). A controlled, prospective study is necessary to support the claims outlined by the proponents of this paradigm in order to provide evidence for causal relationships.

Too, the direction of the arrow of causality—what causes what?—in the studies underpinning the theory of deliberate practice is not clear. Authors have concluded that a relationship between practice hours and duration with elite performance indicates that the former triggers the latter. But it could be equally plausible that it's the other way around (51). Might the inherently talented performer be more likely to seek out a more expert teacher, be more highly motivated, and have access to better facilities and equipment? Also, the dogmas of necessary duration of training represent averages. No assessment of the expected large degree of individual athlete variability in training gains has been provided.

While Ericsson and his colleagues have rejected "any important role" for innate ability in the development of elite performance, they do acknowledge certain potential genetic influences on this process (21). Among the mental characteristics that mark the elite performer (self-confidence, concentration, ability to rebound from mistakes, etc.) the motivational drive to submit to many hours of intense practice over a sustained period of time is essential in the picture of the theory of deliberate practice. Although not well documented, it is reasonable to expect that such motivation is controlled at least in part by genetic factors. For example, polymorphisms of the gene for brain-derived neurotrophic factor (BDNF) have been associated with mood state as well as perception of exercise (10). Too, the determinants of somatotype and anthropometric features (height, weight, muscularity, etc.), which clearly relate to athletic success, are well recognized to be genetically controlled. The 6′ 5″, 250-pound male is unlikely to excel as an elite ballet dancer, no more than the wispy young female would successfully serve as a middle linebacker, regardless of training regimen.

The Theory of Deliberate Practice in explaining athletic success bears importance in the current controversy surrounding the wisdom—or lack of—in early sports specialization in children. Considerable sentiment holds that children in the prepubertal years should avoid early concentration in any one particular sport. Instead, they should opt for a multilateral involvement in a variety of sport activities, a more healthy approach which promotes general fitness and avoids injuries as well as early "burnout" from sports participation (51).

At the same time it is recognized that for many sports, like gymnastics and figure skating, peak performance to achieve levels for international competition must be achieved in the mid to late teen years. A little mathematics reveals that to satisfy the 10-year rule, intense training must commence early, between the ages of 5 and 10 years. Children do not normally possess the level of commitment and motivation required of deliberate practice. Indeed, Ericsson et al. recognized this as a problem that needed to be rectified if elite-level performance was to be based on early sport training: "Consequently, children need help to identify the appropriate training activities, to learn how to concentrate, and to find the optimal training environments" (21).

So, does this mean that any young aspiring athlete, regardless of innate abilities, has the potential for achieving elite status in the future years? Ericsson et al. answer thusly:

> It does not follow from the rejection of innate limits to acquired performance that everyone can easily attain high levels of skill. Contemporary elite performers have overcome a number of constraints. They have obtained early access to instructors, maintained high levels of deliberate practice throughout development, received continued parental and environmental support, and avoided disease and injury. When one considers in addition the prerequisite motivation necessary to engage in deliberate practice every day for years and decades, when most children and adolescents of similar ages engage in play and leisure, the real constraints on the acquisition of expert performance become apparent.
>
> *(20)*

A Compromise Conclusion?

So, is it a matter of nature or nurture? Free will or biological determinism? It's a classic philosophical dilemma made physiological. Regrettably, the answer isn't found in these pages. But some thoughts: that genetic factors largely dictate fitness status and mechanisms for improved performance with training is obvious. Still, no evidence has been brought forward to indicate that the limits of such effects *constrain* one's capacity for these gains. The theory of deliberate practice provides sound training principles, yet the science in its supportive observational studies is weak, and the physiological underpinnings of progressive performance gains remain obscure. Too, both sides of the argument have not adequately addressed in their paradigms the influences of inter-individual variability of training responses.

In their review of both sides of the question, Tucker and Collins provided a conciliatory compromise judgment (55). They concluded that the principles of deliberate practice—hard work, long-term commitment, intelligent and challenging training regimens, supportive coaches, and so forth—are required to achieve elite athletic status, but genetic realities, equally essential, provide the limits to the plasticity of one's training-induced capabilities.

Upon some reflection, though, for the training athlete, does it really matter? There would be no argument on either side of this debate that to achieve elite status in any sport demands commitment to many years of intense training. The precepts of the theory of deliberate practice are solid ones: intelligent training calls for competent coaching, identification of appropriate goals, many hours of hard work over many years' duration, a good deal of self-sacrifice. Whether for any individual athlete there exists a particular limit to performance gains with such a training regimen may be a moot point. The goal is to put forth an effort to fulfill one's potential, to (stealing from the classic advertisement) simply "be all that one can be."

References

1. Baggish AL, Hale A, Weiner RB, et al. Dynamic regulation of circulating microRNA during acute exhaustive exercise and sustained aerobic exercise training. *J. Physiol.* 2011;16:3983–3994.
2. Baker J, Horton S. A review of primary and secondary influences on sport expertise. *High Ability Studies.* 2004;15:211–228.
3. Barrett W. Determinism and novelty. In: Hook S, editor. *Determinism and Freedom in the Age of Modern Science.* New York: New York University Press; 1958. pp. 30–42.
4. Bernard C. *An Introduction to the Study of Experimental Medicine.* New York: Dover Publications; 1957.
5. Blanshard B. The case for determinism. In: Hook S, editor. *Determinism and Freedom in the Age of Modern Science.* New York: New York University Press; 1958. pp. 3–14.
6. Bouchard C, An P, Rice T, et al. Familial aggregation of VO_2 max response to exercise training: results from the HERITAGE Family Study. *J Appl Physiol.* 1999;87:1003–1008.
7. Bouchard C, Malina RM, Perusse L. *Genetics of Fitness and Physical Performance.* Champaign, IL: Human Kinetics; 1997. pp. 311–352.
8. Bouchard C, Rankinen T. Individual differences in response to regular physical activity. *Med Sci Sports Exerc.* 2001;33 Suppl:S446–S451.
9. Bramble DM, Lieberman D. Endurance running and evolution in *Homo. Nature.* 2004;432:345–352.

10. Bryan A, Hutchison KE, Seals DR, et al. A transdisciplinary model integrating genetic, physiological, and psychological correlates of voluntary exercise. *Health Psychol.* 2007;26:30–39.
11. Cannon WB. *The Wisdom of the Body.* New York: W.W. Norton & Company; 1932.
12. Dawkins R. *The Selfish Gene.* Oxford: Oxford University Press; 1989.
13. Denham J, Marques FZ, O'Brien BJ, Charchar FJ. Exercise: putting action into our epigenome. *Sports Med.* 2014;44:189–209.
14. Denham J, Prestes PR. Muscle-enriched microRNAs isolated from whole blood are regulated by exercise and are potential biomarkers of cardiorespiratory fitness. *Front. Genet.* 2016;196. doi: 10.3389/lgene.2016.00196.
15. Drummond MJ, McCarthy JJ, Fry CS, et al. Aging differentially affects human skeletal muscle microRNA expression at rest and after an anabolic stimulus of resistance exercise and essential amino acids. *Am J Physiol Endocrinol Metab.* 2008;295:E1333–E1340.
16. Ehlert T, Simon P, Moser DA. Epigenetics in sports. *Sports Med.* 2013;43:93–110.
17. Ericsson EA. Development of elite performance and deliberate practice. In: Starkes JL, Ericsson KA, editors. *Expert Performance in Sports.* Champaign, IL: Human Kinetics; 2003. pp. 49–83.
18. Ericsson KA. The influence of experience and deliberate practice on the development of superior expert performance. In: Ericsson KA, Charness N, Hoffman RR, editors. *Cambridge Handbook of Expertise and Expert Performance.* Cambridge: Cambridge University Press; 2006. pp. 685–706.
19. Ericsson KA, Chase WG, Faloon S. Acquisition of a memory skill. *Science.* 1980;208:1181–1182.
20. Ericsson KA, Krampe RT, Tesch-Romer C. The role of deliberate practice in the acquisition of expert performance. *Psychol Rev.* 1993;100:363–406.
21. Ericsson EA, Nandagopal K, Roring RW. Toward a science of exceptional achievement. *Ann NY Acad Sci.* 2009;1172:199–217.
22. Fernandes T, Barauna VG, Negrao CE, Phillips MI, Oliveira EM. Aerobic exercise training promotes physiological cardiac remodeling involving a set of microRNAs. *Am J Physiol Heart Circ Physiol.* 2015;309:H543–H552.
23. Finaud J, Lac G, Filaire E. Oxidative stress: relationship with exercise and training. *Sports Med.* 2006;36:327–358.
24. Fulton JF. *Selected Reading in the History of Physiology.* Springfield, IL: Charles C. Thomas; 1930. p. 307.
25. Gardner H. Expert performance: its structure and acquisition. Comment. *American Psychologist.* 1995;50:8020803.
26. Garland T, Cadney MD, Waterland RA. Early-life effects on adult physical activity: concepts, relevance, and experimental approaches. *Physiol Biochem Zool.* 2017; 90:1–14.
27. Gertz J, Varley KE, Reddy TE, et al. Analysis of DNA methylation in a three-generation family reveals widespread genetic influence on epigenetic regulation. *PLoS Genet.* 2011;7:e1002228.
28. Goldspink G, Velloso CP. Genetics and human performance: natural selection and genetic modification. In: Taylor NAS, Groeller H, editors. *Physiological Bases of Human Performance during Work and Exercise.* Philadelphia: Elsevier; 2008. pp. 135–148.
29. Hambrick DZ, Oswald FL, Altmann EM, Meinz EJ, Gobet F, Campitelli G. Deliberate practice: is that all it takes to become an expert? *Intelligence.* 2014;45:34–45.
30. Hamilton MT, Booth FW. Skeletal muscle adaptation to exercise: a century of progress. *J Appl Physiol.* 2000;88:327–331.

31. Heathcote A, Brown S, Mewhort DJK. The power law repeated: the case for an exponential law of practice. *Pschosom Bull Rev*. 2000;7:185–207.
32. Heinrich B. *Why We Run*. New York: Harper Collins; 2001. pp. 166–167.
33. Hospers J. What means this freedom? In: Hook S, editor. *Determinism and Freedom in the Age of Modern Science*. New York: New York University Press; 1958. pp. 113–132.
34. Jorgensen SB, Richer EA, Wojtaszewski JF. Role of AMPK in skeletal muscle metabolic regulation and adaptation in relation to exercise. *J Physiol*. 2006;574:17–31.
35. Kohrt WM, Malley MT, Coggan AR, et al. Effects of gender, age, and fitness level on response of VO_2max to training in 60–71 year olds. *J Appl Physiol*. 1991;71:2004–2011.
36. Komi PV, Nicol C. Neuromuscular adaptation to exercise. In: Taylor NAS, Groeller H, editors. *Physiological Bases of Human Performance During Work and Exercise*. Philadelphia: Elsevier; 2008. pp. 71–90.
37. Lantier L, Fentz J, Mounier R, et al. AMPK controls exercise endurance, mitochondrial oxidative capacity, and skeletal muscle integrity. *FASEB*. 2017;28:3211–3224.
38. Lehrer J. *How We Decide*. Boston: Mariner Books; 2009.
39. Lott SA, Burghardt PR, Burghardt KJ, Grove TB, Ellingrod VL. The influence of metabolic syndrome, physical activity and genotype on catechol-O-methyl transferase promotor-region methylation in schizophrenia. *Pharmacogenetics*. 2012;13:264–271.
40. Mayr E. How biology differs from the physical sciences. In: Depew DJ, Weber BH, editors. *Evolution at a Crossroads: The New Biology and the New Philosophy of Science*. Cambridge, MA: MIT Press; 1985. pp. 43–64.
41. McGee SL, Fairlie E, Garnham AP, et al. Exercise-induced histone modifications in human skeletal muscle. *J Physiol*. 2009;587:5951–5958.
42. Macnamara BN, Moreau D, Hambrick DZ. The relationship between deliberate practice and performance in sports: a meta-analysis. *Perspect Psychol Sci*. 2016:11:333–350.
43. Morton JP, Kayani AC, McArdle A, Drust B. The exercise-induced stress response of skeletal muscle, with specific emphasis on humans. *Sports Med*. 2009;39:643–662.
44. Mukwevho E, Kohn TA, Lang D, et al. Caffeine induces hyperacetylation of histones at the MEF2 site on the Glu4 promotor and increases MEF2A binding to the site via a CaMK-dependent mechanism. *Am J Physiol Endocrinol Metab*. 2008;294:E582–E588.
45. Nakajima K, Takeoka M, Mori M, et al. Exercise effects on methylation of ASC gene. *Int J Sports Med*. 2010;31:671–675.
46. Ntanasis-Stathopoulos J, Tzanninis J-G, Philippou A, Koutsilieris M. Epigenetic regulation on gene expression induced by physical exercise. *J Musculoskelet Neuronal Interact*. 2013;13:133–146.
47. Noble D. *The Music of Life: Biology Beyond the Genome*. Oxford: Oxford University Press; 2006.
48. Puthucheary Z, Skipworth JRA, Rawal J, Loosemore M, Van Someren K, Montgomery HE. Genetic influences in sport and physical performance. *Sports Med*. 2011;41:845–859.
49. Radak Z, Chung HY, Koltai E, Taylor AW, Goto S. Exercise, oxidative stress and hormesis. *Ageing Res Rev*. 2008;7:34–42.
50. Rankinen T, Bouchard C. Genetic differences in the relationships among physical activity, fitness, and health. In: Bouchard C, Blair SN, Haskell WL, editors. *Physical Activity and Health*. Champaign, IL: Human Kinetics; 2007. pp. 337–358.
51. Rowland T. *Tennisology: Inside the Science of Serves, Nerves, and On-Court Dominance*. Champaign, IL: Human Kinetics; 2014. pp. 29–48.

52. Rowland T, Boyajian A. Aerobic response to endurance training in children. *Pediatrics.* 1995;96:654–658.
53. Russell B. *The Problem of Philosophy*. New York: Oxford University Press; 1997.
54. Selye H. *The Stress of Life*. New York: McGraw Hill; 1976. pp. 5–45.
55. Tucker R, Collins M. What makes champions? A review of the relative contribution of genes and training to sporting success. *Br J Sports Med.* 2012;46:555–561.
56. Voisin S, Eynon N, Yan X, Bishop DJ. Exercise training and DNA methylation in humans. *Acta Physiol.* 2015;213:39–59.
57. Waller J. *Heredity. A Very Short Introduction*. Oxford: Oxford University Press; 2017.
58. Wesson R. *Beyond Natural Selection*. Cambridge, MA; MIT Press; 1991.

2

WHY DO PHYSIOLOGICAL AND CHRONOLOGICAL TIME DIFFER?

The question of the nature of time has occupied human thought since antiquity. And still, despite centuries of ideas and debates and arguments and research efforts, the essence of this ephemeral "time" that so dictates the totality of our lives remains shrouded in mystery. Is it "real"? Or just a figment of our cerebral imagination? Is time absolute, or subjective, or relative? What is the meaning of "now"?

A good many have waxed philosophically on the issue:

> The human experience of time is all-pervasive, intimate, and immediate. Life, death, and time combine in an intricate and intriguing manner that is difficult to clarify, yet is recognized in all great philosophies and religions. Time is a constituent of all forms of human knowledge, all modes of expression, and is connected with the functions of the mind. It is also a fundamental feature of the universe. It follows that no single faculty of learning, in itself, is capable of accounting for the nature of time.
>
> *(12)*

To be sure, biological systems run on time. But it turns out to be a very different kind than the one indicated by the clock on the wall, one defined by non-linear relationships to body mass instead of the passage of the heavenly bodies through the sky. What is the basis of this peculiar physiological time? And what does it tell us about the nature of living beings? How is physiological time reflected in human movement? Is physiological time altered by the stresses created on body systems by exercise? More mysteries, difficult questions, all without easy answers.

Chronological Time

> *The clock ticked. The moving instant which, according to Isaac Newton, separates the infinite past from the infinite future advanced inexorably through the dimension of time. Or, if Aristotle was right, a little more of the possible was every instant made real; the present stood still and drew itself into the future as a man might suck forever at an unending piece of macaroni.*
>
> —Aldous Huxley (16)

It may not be define-able, but our common experience tells us what time *is*. Time is an objective, continuous process that proceeds linearly without interruption or influence by outside events. It's an imperturbable progression, always heading in the same direction. "Now" separates this progression into the "past," which is fixed and certain, from the "future," which is undetermined and unpredictable. What is once future becomes, by the constant forward movement of now, the past (8). It is like the forward unrolling of an unending film (or better yet, the flow of a river, to which there has been no shortage of literary allusions).

True, time seems sometimes to vary in its duration, depending on circumstances—a pleasurable activity makes time fly by, while in an onerous one—waiting for a three-hour delayed flight at O'Hare—it barely moves at all. But these would seem to be explained by issues of distraction and over-attentiveness, respectively, rather than any violation of an intrinsic independent progression of time.

That the inexorable progression of time, at least as humans experience it, is unidirectional is in accord with the Second Law of Thermodynamics, which indicates an entropy-dictated universe where all tends to disorder with time. Other physical laws are bidirectional—they are as true when the motion of bodies is observed forward or in reverse, but in the practical world of human experience, no, time just goes forward. On this, Atkins has written (when presumably suffering through not a good day):

> We have looked through the window onto the world provided by the Second Law, and have seen the naked purposelessness of nature. The deep structure of change is decay; the spring of change in all its forms is the corruption of the quality of energy as it spreads chaotically, irreversibly, and purposelessly in time. All change, and time's arrow, point in the direction of corruption. The experience of time is the gearing of the electrochemical processes in our brains to the purposeless drift into chaos as we sink into equilibrium and the grave.
>
> *(2)*

Further evidence of a one-way arrow for time lies in the dictates of cause and effect. If event B follows event A in time, it could be that they are simply linked temporally (like the engine of a train is later followed by the caboose as one watches sitting at a crossing). But if A is the *cause* of B they must occur in that order. B cannot precede A. The explosion caused the building to subsequently to collapse. But, no, the collapse of the building did not cause the explosion. The arrow of causality can temporally only go in one direction. An effect cannot appear in time before its cause (21). Biological support for a unidirectional arrow of time comes also from a consideration of the one-way process of evolution. Structures and functions produced by random genetic variability that offer survival value persist, others are discarded. It can't happen in the reverse direction.

The nature of "now" in this schema has been particularly surrounded by uncertainty and controversy. One of the most intriguing arguments is that "now" does not actually exist. According to this argument, the dividing point between past and future—the marching present—is, like its mathematical counterpart, dimensionless. Indeed, as quickly as one assigns the present as "now," it has become the past. So, we anticipate moments in the future and remember them in the past, but the junction between the two is simply that—an ephemeral interface. "Reality," has written Dainton, "takes the form of a succession of instantaneous (or nearly instantaneous) presents; no sooner has one present come into existence than it will depart from it as it is replaced by another present, and the latter will in turn be immediately annihilated as a new present comes into existence" (8).

It should be noted that the commonplace portrait of the nature of time as absolute, flowing inexorably without external influence, is derived from personal "experience," since in contrast to sensory input of sight, feeling, sounds, and smell, the human brain has no direct means of appreciating any flow of time. That is, there exists no central "time detector." The passage of time is appreciated by the brain only as a *perception* of change. (This idea should not be confused with the sensitive time-keeping by the many biological clocks in the central nervous system which dictate bodily activities such as the coordination of muscular contractions or the 24-hour circadian swings in physiological functions.)

This is the way Isaac Newton saw time. At the opening of his *Principia* he wrote, "Absolute, true, and mathematical time of itself, and from its own nature, flows equably without relation to anything external." And this is the way you and I see it, too—a flow of time providing us with a normal way of interpreting the changes in our lives.

The "True" Nature of Time?

But is this the *reality* of time? Physicists and philosophers alike have long been skeptical. Like the ancient Greek thinker Parmenides, who considered that "time does not pertain to anything that is truly 'real' but only to the logical unsatisfactory world of appearance revealed by our senses" (cited by 48). This objection was echoed over two thousand years later by Davis: "Does our impression of the flow of time, or the division of time into past, present, and future, tell us nothing at all about how time *is* as opposed to how it merely appears to us muddle-headed humans?" (9). That is to say, according to this viewpoint, "the passage of time is to be regarded as merely a feature of our consciousness that has no objective physical significance" (48). This might be a popular concept to scientists and thinkers, perhaps, but one that flies in the face of what is "real" in the life experiences of human beings. Nonetheless, alternative concepts of the nature of time have abounded:

- Leibniz said that instead of an absolute time defining events and experiences, in truth it was the other way around—that time is *defined* by the order that events happen.
- Einstein destroyed Newton's concept of absolute time by indicating that time depends on the velocity of the person making its measurement—that as one approaches the speed of light, time and its clock measurement slow down.
- Einstein's ideas of the relativity of time became incorporated into the concept of a four-dimensional universe, one in which time (the fourth dimension) was on equal footing of reality as length, width, and breadth. In a graphical representation, time and space each has its own axis, creating a space-time continuum. A step further is *string theory*, which holds that gravity (in a nine-dimensional space) can bend the space-time continuum.
- Inspired by Einstein's ideas, many physicists today subscribe to a "block" view of time—so called "spatiotemporal substantialism"—in which "all moments of time (and all events) are equally real, and there is no moving or changing present; the difference between past, present, and future are simply differences in perspective" (8). By this concept, time is not at all like a flowing river, not a series of moments in succession. In fact, the past and present and future exist simultaneously.
- Enter then into the bizarre world of quantum mechanics, the realm of subatomic particles. Here in this non-deterministic world, behavior of particles is based on probabilities, position and velocity cannot be determined at the same time, and events can occur simultaneously instead of in any progression. Time in the quantum domain is something else altogether.

So, Newton—and our everyday concept of time as we view it—may well be wrong. Time is, in all likelihood, not absolute but relative—to velocity, to conditions (subatomic or macroscopic), the effects of gravity, etc. According to the preponderance of contemporary thinking, time as a "flow of moments that make up our life . . . is the ultimate illusion. . . . Our experience of time is an accident of our circumstances as human beings" (40).

But why should our brains be insistent in interpreting Newton's version of the concept of time as the "reality"? It's a particular reality, to be sure, but one which provides us with a basis for conducting our lives, for planning, for providing the possibility for free-will decision-making. It is truly inconceivable to imagine human lives without the direction provided by an obvious, constant current of time. Some have suggested that the answer must lie in some Darwinian-based survival benefit that is proffered by such an interpretation of time (5). And one possibility would be that this construct of time permits the humans brain to make *predictions*, a facility that allows strategy-making—to avoid enemies, devise means of procuring food, and to escape unfavorable environmental conditions.

Measuring Time

To make time real, at least in the daily lives of human beings, it must be measured. Religious ceremonies—not to mention meals, doctor's appointments, and television viewing—need to be scheduled. Basketball game winners must be established, airline flights to Paris reserved, pork roasts cooked—all while blissfully ignoring any nonintuitive metaphysical considerations of the nature of time. And here the course of human history records a remarkable degree of success. For the practical purpose of leading our daily lives we need to measure time, and that means we need to look to *clocks*.

Early attempts to measure time were limited (sundials became inoperable on cloudy days, water clocks froze). In 1657, the Dutch physicist Christiaan Huygens, based on the regularity of swings of pendulums described by Galileo, invented the pendulum clock. The concept here is that time could be measured by any device that counted the changes in a periodic process. From pendulums came vibrations of quartz crystals, and then—most accurately—the electromagnetic radiation being emitted from cesium atoms.

It is important to recognize that all of these measurement tools do not define time. "It is utterly beyond our power to measure the changes of things by time," said the 19th-century physicist Ernst Mach. "Quite the contrary, time is an abstraction, at which we arrive by means of the changes in things" (cited by reference 5). So, chronological or clock time is simply a measure of periodicities of some action.

It has been contended that the development of the clock "dissociated time from natural rhythms" and established time as an independent method for measuring mathematically defined series of events (25). Still, however, it is obvious that the measures of clock time reflect astronomical phenomena, arbitrarily divided into units (i.e., days = rotation of the Earth, month = phases of the moon, year = orbital period of the Earth about the Sun, etc.). In doing so, clocks turn an abstract notion of time into an indispensable standard by which we can conduct our daily lives. But the true nature and meaning of time remain elusive.

We might say (wrongly, it turns out) that a clock measures time. But, then, what is it measuring? Something, in fact, that we cannot see or sense by any objective means (18). Maybe one could argue, as Aristotle did, that the ticking of a clock describes *change* and that change is equivalent to time. But the refutation is not difficult—"change" in what? All of life's events change at a different rate, while time doesn't. To say that the change in a clock (frequency of a pendulum swing, etc.) is a measure of change is circular reasoning. As Richard Morris wrote, "There is no standard by which a flow of time can be measured. At best one can only say that time moves onward at the rate of one second per second, which is about as meaningful as defining the word 'cat' by saying 'a cat is a cat'" (25).

Physiological Time

> Although our perception of time has many subjective and even sociological features, it is based on an objective factor that provides an external control for the timing of our physiological processes.
>
> (48)

Physiological systems are, by their very definition, dynamic—biological machines that operate in respect to a period of time, which we call their *rate*. But when we begin to examine the time frame of this dynamic function, we notice something rather strange. The clock by which physiological functions operate does not tick according to chronological time. We saw from the above that chronological time is measured by the metronomic frequency of oscillations—of pendulums, of vibrations of quartz crystals, of cesium atoms—all of which provide a means of defining the passage of time in respect to astronomical phenomena.

In physiological functions, that periodicity is provided by the regularity of events such as heart beats, milliliters of urine production, and frequency of breaths, which in fact do not at all relate to astronomical time. Instead, quite incomprehensively, when we try to express such function in chronological terms—such as milliliters of flow per hour, or beats per minute—we find that these are mathematically instead related to the mass of the animal in question. The rate of physiological time is inversely related to the size of the animal—the physiological clock ticks slower in large compared to small animals. Not only that, this relationship of function and mass is established by non-linear power equations with allometric exponents. And to further the mystery, the striking consistency of the scaling exponent 0.25 in such equations across all domains of physiological function is a striking mystery yet to be resolved.

What is the basis of this mathematical relationship of physiological function to mass? Surely it must be telling us something about the fundamental nature of living matter. But what? The quote above from Whitrow that opened this section brings home an important point: Certainly there exists strong debate regarding the objective, absolute nature of time versus a broader concept of time that exceeds human perception and experience. Whichever it be, however, in the realm of physiological function, time is mathematical and deterministic. No cerebral perceptual interpretation. No subjective alterations related to state of consciousness. No confounding influence of the speed of light. Just an observable, objective rate of physiological processes in a time frame which are linked to body mass.

Empirical Findings

Mathematics has long been considered the domain of the physical sciences, and biology, being concerned with "softer" issues, could be studied without the requirement of mathematical equations. As Ian Stewart has pointed out in his book *Mathematics of Life*, this perspective is changing (42). "There is mathematics aplenty in today's biology, and it is becoming ever harder to avoid it. It just doesn't mimic the way mathematics is used in physics. It's different, it has its own special quality" (42). And here in dealing with physiological time is a case in point. To understand the vagaries of physiological time, the allometric equation presented by Huxley back in 1932 will be indispensable (16). (The mathephobic may be reassured that this necessary excursion into non-linear equations and fractional exponents is, in fact, easily assimilated):

$$Y = aX^b$$

where the relationship between a variable Y and X is defined by a constant (a) and the exponent b of X. Values of a and b are obtained after log-log transformation from a linear regression equation of

$$\log Y = \log a + b(\log X)$$

The exponent b (sometimes referred to as the "scaling factor") is the key piece of information here, for it indicates how changes in Y are related to changes in X. A value of b of 0.0 means that as X changes, Y remains unchanged. When b is between 0.0 and 1.0, an increase in Y occurs with an increase in X, but Y increases at a proportionately lower rate than X. If b = 1.0, Y increases linearly in direct proportion to X. That is, if X doubles in value, Y also doubles. If b is >1.0, Y increases at a proportionately greater rate than does X. Thus, except in one special case (when b = 1.0), the relationship between Y and X is non-linear, and graphically is manifest in a curvilinear fashion.

Now for the purpose of examining the relationship of changes of physiological time with those of body mass we can substitute C (the rate of the physiological function—a "pendulum" clock) for Y in this equation, and animal mass M for X.

$$C = aM^b$$

In such a mathematical analysis, it is important to recognize that the value of the scaling exponent b for body mass depends on how the physiological clock is expressed. The physiological function can be assigned a rate (frequency F, the number of events over chronological time, equation A), or as a relative rate (the rate expressed per kg body mass) (equation B), or as time (T, our topic of interest) as the duration between two successive events, which is calculated as the reciprocal of rate (equation C).

A) $F \sim M^b$
B) $F/M^{1.0} \sim M^b/M^{1.0}$
C) $T \sim 1/F \sim 1/M^b \sim M^{-b}$

Take heart rate as an example of a periodic, or cyclical, physiologic function. We take warm-blooded animals of disparate size, record their resting heart rate (F) and body mass, and create an allometric equation using the regression equation of one against the other using log-log transformation. Biologists who have done this (i.e., reference 41) have reported that, for mammals at rest,

$$F = 241M^{-0.25}$$

This indicates that the larger the animal, the slower the heart rate. A shrew, which weighs about 3 gm, has a resting heart rate of over 1,000 beats per minute, while that of an elephant is about 30 bpm (36). In humans, the heart rate of a six-year-old in basal conditions is 80 bpm, 30% higher than that of an 18-year-old (23). But we are more interested here in *time*, so if we convert beats per 60 seconds into the time interval between beats (T), the equation turns out to be

$$T = 0.249M^{0.25}$$

which indicates that the time interval between successive heart beats increases, but proportionally slower, as animal size increases. Here, then, is our first example demonstrating that "physiological time is a relative concept, and the size of an animal dictates its time scale.... What 1 day of clock time is for a 10-g mouse may correspond to 2 months of time for a 100-ton blue whale" (36).

It should be emphasized that such allometric relationships established between physiological functions and body mass should not be considered as biological laws but rather as indicators of biological phenomena (19). At the same time, they have, as will become evident, created some yet-unsolved enigmas surrounding the bases for these relationships.

Now let's do the same kind of analysis with something more interesting—animal life span. Sacher (34) found that life span (L) varied with the mass of mammals in captivity by

$$L = 11.8M^{0.20}$$

Two aspects make this equation particularly intriguing. First, on this curve human beings are an outlier (and a good thing, too, since if we complied with the general rule of the equation our average life span would be 28 years) (19). And, second, we observe a value of b of 0.20. In fact, as will be outlined below, a scaling factor for mass approximating one-quarter is observed when such allometrically equations are constructed for a great many physiological processes. This has served as the basis for the notion that all animals are born with a certain fixed amount—like in a bank account—of physiological "events," and those that use them up more quickly (i.e., smaller animals) have correspondingly shorter life spans. True or not, it is evident that all animals, regardless of size, experience about the same duration of physiological life (36). In fact, Stahl estimated that in their lifetimes, all animals, regardless of size, expend a basal energy of 8×10^5 kilojoules per kg body mass (41).

The relationship between body size and resting metabolic rate has received by far the most attention by biological researchers and deserves to be described in a greater detail. Indeed, that smaller animals have a greater resting metabolic rate (oxygen consumption) relative to their body mass has been recognized for over a century, but explaining the mathematical relationship between the two continues to be among the greatest dilemmas facing biologists today.

The story starts in 1883 with Rubner, who reported this inverse relative metabolic rate:mass phenomenon among a small group of dogs (33). The relative resting energy expenditure (VO_2 per kg) in the animal weighing 3 kg was more than twice that of the dog weighing 36 kg. His findings supported earlier ideas of Sarrus and Rameaux, who reasoned that resting metabolic rate per kg should be expected to fall in progressively larger animals since a) body metabolism occurs in respect to body mass, b) the heat generated by that metabolism must be lost through mechanisms related to surface area, and c) the larger animal possesses a smaller ratio of surface area to body mass ratio than a smaller one (35). (In humans, for example, the ratio of estimated body surface area to mass falls from 4.0 at age four years to 2.8 at age 16 [28].)

This was termed the *surface law*: "The relative rate of heat production is higher in the smaller animal [which] has, relative to its mass, larger body surface area. Heat loss takes place from the surface, and in order to [maintain body temperature] an animal must produce heat at a rate equal to the loss" (36). According to dimensionality theory, given two objects of equal density, their surface area should relate to the two-third power of their mass (17). Volume should be proportional to a linear measurement cubed (L^3), while time is expressed as L. Thus the metabolic rate (a volume over time) should relate to L^3/L, or L^2, which is an expression of the body surface area. Consequently, the metabolic rate (oxygen uptake per minute) should be expected to be proportional to $\text{mass}^{0.67}$.

This seemed to make good sense, except that empirically studies across many animal species failed to confirm this. Instead, in 1932, Kleiber's data on adult animals ranging in mass from 0.15 to 679 kg revealed that resting metabolic rate in kilocalories per day (P) was related to mass of the animal by the allometric equation

$$P = 0.19M^{0.75}$$

Since then, abundant research findings have confirmed the consistency of 0.75 as the expected scaling factor for mass in respect to resting metabolic rate in animals of widely diverse size (36). Findings in human beings fit closely to the curve for mammals as a whole (e.g., 20). How to explain this departure from the expected 0.67 value demanded by the surface law? A number of ideas have been offered, ranging from measurement error of body surface area to factors such as the influences of age, elastic similarity, failure to account for circadian variation, and intra-species versus inter-species exponents, all of which Blaxter termed "not particularly convincing" (4).

Some have felt the discrepancy from 0.67 lay in differential organ sizes most responsible for metabolic rate. Others have suggested that the mass exponent should reflect the sum of a cascade of separate scaling exponents for the component functions involved in establishing metabolic rate (15), or that the mass exponent can best be understood in terms of scaling of limitations of oxygen supply (47). In the final analysis, an accepted explanation for the discrepancy between the empirically derived mass exponent of 0.75 and that predicted by dimensionality theory (0.67) remains problematic.

When the resting metabolic rate is expressed per kg body mass, the relation is to $M^{-0.25}$ (i.e., $M^{0.75}/M^{1.0} = M^{-0.25}$). The larger the animal, then, the less the relative (per kg) resting metabolic rate. At rest, a mouse has an oxygen uptake per kg that is 10 times that of a whale (17). Converting resting energy expenditure to time (T), which is the reciprocal of rate, the relationship becomes $T_{met} = aM^{0.25}$, which is the identical mass exponent we found above for heart rate. Schmidt-Nielsen concluded that

> The same relationship holds true for all metabolic processes: physiological time, relative to clock time, increases with increasing body size. . . . It is therefore reasonable to use the metabolic rate as a measure of physiological time and remember that real clock time means very different things in the lives of small and large animals
>
> *(36)*

Allometric equations have been calculated for a host of cyclical biological functions versus body mass. Quite remarkably, when rates are converted to time (as 1/frequency), such periods—as between breaths, heart beats, or gut contractions—all scale to about $M^{0.25}$ (1). In his book *Size, Function, and Life History*, William Calder compiled a list of 18 published allometric equations in mammals relating such biological functions to mass, all with a mass exponent approximating 0.25 or a simple multiple of a quarter-power scaling exponent (6). Some examples:

Animal reproductive maturity (years)	$0.75M^{0.29}$
Gestation period (days)	$65M^{0.25}$
Erythrocyte life span (days)	$23M^{0.18}$
Plasma albumin half life (days)	$5M^{0.32}$
Glomerular filtration rate (sec)	$21M^{0.27}$
Blood circulation time (sec)	$21M^{0.21}$

Concluded the author:

> Physiological time is one of the most significant characteristics of living animals. There are too many time scales that are approximately proportional to body $M^{1/4}$ to deny its importance in repetitive maintenance processes and for stages within the life span devoted to growth, replacement, and decline. Nonetheless, we do not know why the exponent is 1/4 rather than 1/3. It would be fascinating to understand how natural selection or the genome control the physiological time scale [. . .]
>
> *(6)*

Explanations

It is, in fact, difficult to escape the conclusion that the pervasiveness of quarter-power scaling exponents is indicative of some sort of "a common conceptual framework for the function of living matter," an observation that opens "a possible window onto the emergent laws of biology" (45). What that essential principle might be remains uncertain. In this quest, West expressed a note of caution. "Is it conceivable that there are yet-to-be discovered 'Newton's Laws of Biology' that would lead, at least in principle, to precise calculations of any biological processes . . .? This seems very unlikely. After all, life is the complex system par excellence, exhibiting many levels of emergent phenomenon arising from multiple contingent histories. Nevertheless, it may not be unreasonable to conjecture that the generic coarse-grained behavior of living systems might obey quantifiable universal laws that capture their essential features" (45).

Several considerations of the link between physiological function and body mass—particularly the ubiquity of the quarter-power exponent—merit further discussion, each involving physiological time as a determinant factor.

Physiological Time Scale

Lindstedt and Calder presented the interesting argument that the empirically derived mass scaling factor of 0.75 for metabolic rate could be explained by the influence of physiological time (19). They contended that "volumes and organs of capacity have relatively little opportunity to scale except in direct proportion to body mass ($M^{1.0}$) among animals of the same design." Hence, volume-rates must scale as $M^{3/4}$:

$$\text{Volume/time} \sim M^{1.0}/M^{1/4} = M^{3/4}$$

And thus, they concluded, "physiological time scale makes $M^{3/4}$ inevitable" (19).

Effect of Gravity

The researchers whose work has been cited in this chapter have been guilty of a bit of untruth—a *petit mensonge*—in constructing equations involving animal *mass* when instead they have measured animal *weight*. The former represents the amount of material in an object, while the latter is a measure of the force created by influence of gravity on that mass. Could differential effects of gravity on the mass of animals of different size contribute to the relationships between physiologic functions and body size?

A number of authors have felt so (10,26,39). The downward effect of gravity increases metabolic rate, and that influence is directly related to the mass of the animal. Based on studies in rodents, it has been assumed that this gravity-induced increase in metabolic rate relates to $M^{.14}$ (10). If the surface law held true, with a mass exponent of 0.67, and the additional influence of gravity is added, the mass exponent relative to metabolic rate would be expected to approximate 0.75, as observed empirically across a wide range of animal size. Schmidt-Nielsen commented that "the suggestion is intriguing, although difficult to evaluate, because our present understanding of the complexities of metabolic rate is insufficient" (36).

Another influence of gravity should be mentioned briefly for interest's sake. It is well established that gravity affects the passage of chronological time in an inverse fashion, such that time passes faster in tall compared to short animals (the former being farther from the Earth than the latter). The catch is that this influence is infinitesimally tiny. A clock at the top of Mount Everest gains 30 microseconds a year over one at sea level (13). The difference in time experienced by a moderate-sized dog compared to that by a mouse is said to be one part in 10^{17}.

Fractal Scaling

The physicist Geoffrey West has championed the innovative concept that the ubiquity of quarter power-scaling exponents for mass in the animal kingdom reflects geometrical properties linking components of biological systems (45). Hierarchical branching networks that distribute resources (e.g., blood supply via the circulatory system) exhibit fractal properties (they are similar at all scales of size), and the mathematical model expressing this relationship is mass raised to the quarter power. This fractal scaling holds true both within and between organisms; that is, such relationships are fixed and independent of animal size.

West and his colleagues have concluded that "Quarter-power scaling laws are perhaps as universal and as uniquely biological as the biochemical pathways of metabolism, the structure and function of the genetic code, and the process of natural selection, which has exploited variations on this fractal theme to produce the incredible variety of biological form and function. On the other hand, [they] are testimony to the severe geometric and physical constraints on metabolic processes" (46).

By extension of this argument, it can be concluded that physiological time itself is of fractal nature. This might initially be difficult to conceptualize, but consider that time of physiological functions (expressed as the reciprocal of rate) is linked to $M^{0.25}$. Consequently, physiological time is scale-invariant (remains the same at all levels of scale of animal size) when related to the quarter power of animal mass, just as the pattern of branching of a tree is identical regardless of the size of the branches.

Metaphysical Queries (A Short List)

Do these considerations of physiological time bring us any closer to identifying the true nature of time? The physiological clock, our marker of change, varies in its ticking rate according to differences in animal body mass, and that relationship of physiological time to body mass is mathematically defined. So do we here have an objective measure of time? Does it imply that time itself is mathematical? Or are we just changing the measuring device? At least one could suppose that we need not be troubled by the possibility—as has been raised concerning chronological time—that "our perception of the passage of time is an illusion" (5).

In chronological time, the units of time are linked arbitrarily by human device to astronomical events. In physiological time the units of time demarcated by the frequency of the clock are defined instead by nature in a mathematical relationship to body mass. Is this a truer reflection of a reality of time? Or are we engaged still in a circular reasoning where measurement is being confused with an independent nature of time itself?

Physiological Time and Exercise

So far the discussion has addressed the link of physiological time in respect to biological processes with the mammalian machinery on idle—in the basal, or at least resting, state. We turn now to a consideration more to the interest of the exercise physiologist—what happens to physiological time and its relationship to body mass when we take the human machine "out on the road," placing it under the stresses of muscular work. "Real animals were not meant to sit still," argued Schmidt-Nielsen. "The limits on maximal performance are much more informative about animal design . . . than the resting or idling level" (36).

Setting out on one's 3-mile morning run sets into action a vast array of neuromuscular, biochemical, cardiorespiratory, and thermoregulatory processes. The central responses, though, are a) a substantial increase in whole-body metabolic rate and b) a major shift of the tissues responsible for energy expenditure. At a maximal exercise effort, the former might approach a ten-fold increase in oxygen uptake over resting values; the latter is manifest as a shift in the contribution of skeletal muscle to energy expenditure during exercise compared to that in the resting state (90% vs. 18%). Could such perturbations of the physiological status quo provide any insights into the nature of physiological time and its link to body mass?

The answer to that question might be influenced by the dual—and potentially conflicting—Darwinian-based "goals" governing biological responses to a locomotion. As West has noted, evolutionary pressures would favor the persistence of physiological systems that work at optimal efficiency; that is, being partial to the lowest energy expenditure that provides for a given work task (45). On the other hand, abilities to escape enemies and track down food would favor systems with the greatest maximal work capacity. One might reflect on these two disparate issues as allometric relations during exercise are explored in the following sections.

Energy Cost of Locomotion

Biologists have dedicated a good deal of research effort to understanding the relationships between animal locomotion and body size. These have provided insights into such associations in human beings as well. In this section, the theoretical constructs so defined will be examined in respect to those that are observed empirically in nature. This discussion will be limited to information surrounding mammals during level running.

Theoretical Considerations

A conceptual framework regarding the link of dynamics of animal running to body mass can be constructed in a step-wise progression of evidence-based findings:

1. *Stride length is directly related to body size.* The length of a single stride (S) is a reflection of leg length or body height (L). By dimensionality theory, length is a linear function of mass expressed to the one-third power. Thus, $S \sim L \sim M^{0.33}$. Stride frequency (SF), being inversely related to stride length, is then proportional to mass by $SF \sim 1/L \sim M^{-0.33}$.
2. *Energy cost (VO_2 per kg) per stride is independent of animal size.* Studies of basic functional characteristics of mammalian muscle tissue, such as maximal force generated per cross-sectional area and cross-bridges per sarcomere length, reveal no influence of animal size. Consequently, the energy demand relative to body mass for each stride should be expected to be equivalent in large and small animals (as well as human children compared to adults). As a result, VO_2 per stride $\sim M^{1.0}$.
3. *At a given velocity, energy expenditure (per kg) should be greater in small compared to large animals.* $VO_2/kg \sim SF \sim M^{-0.33}$. When running at the same treadmill speed setting, children should be expected to be less energy economical than

adults, which is attributable to the shorter stride length and greater stride frequency of the former (while VO_2/kg per stride is the same).

4. *Energy cost of running (as VO_2/min) a given distance is related to mass raised to the two-thirds power.* That is, over a particular distance, $VO_2/kg \sim M^{0.67}$ is arrived at by multiplying the energy cost of one stride (related to $M^{1.0}$) by the number of strides it will take to cross the distance (related to $M^{-0.33}$).
5. *Energy cost per kg animal mass over a given distance decreases with increasing mass.* VO_2/kg/min per km ~ $(M^{0.67})(M^{-1.0}) = M^{-0.33}$. "This expression says that the work required to move 1 kg of animal over a given distance decreases with increasing body mass. This is a direct consequence of the many more steps required for the small animal to cover the same distance on the ground, each step requiring work in direct proportion to body mass" (36).

Empirical Observations

To the satisfaction of theoretical biologists, the following empirical research observations of such relationships match closely those anticipated from the above hypothetical considerations. Moreover, human beings, although comprised of a relatively narrow dimensional range, conform to the mathematical constructs revealed for mammals as a whole. Corresponding to the numbered theoretical expectations listed above, here are the empiric findings:

1. It is obvious that shorter individuals exhibit greater stride frequencies and shorter stride lengths than taller ones. Confirming the self-evident, Rowland et al. reported stride lengths to be 20% greater in young adult men compared to prepubertal boys at several common treadmill speeds (30).
2. Research findings consistently demonstrate that children demonstrate lower economy than adults when exercising on the treadmill at equivalent velocities to adults. For example, Unnithan and Eston found that 9- to 10-year-old boys demonstrated a 24% greater VO_2/kg when running at a treadmill speed of 9.6 kph compared with 18- to 25-year-old men (43). Too, as children gain in stature and weight through the course of the pediatric years, running economy steadily improves (31,38,44).
3. Running economy, the VO_2/kg measured at a given treadmill speed and elevation setting, is inferior in smaller subjects (i.e., who have greater values) than older ones. But in studies in which stride length is accounted for, such differences disappear. Maliszewski and Freedson reported running economy values in 9- to 11-year-old boys compared to those in 18- to 34-year-old men while running at a common speed (9.6 kph) and again when speed was adjusted for leg length (24). The expected difference in energy economy was observed when the two groups were exercising at the same speed (oxygen uptake for boys 40.6 ± 2.6 and men 34.9 ± 3.2 ml/kg/min), but economy differences became statistically insignificant at the size-adjusted speed (boys

37.7 ± 2.8, men 39.0 ± 3.5 ml/kg/min). In a longitudinal study, Rowland et al. demonstrated that the normal improvements expected in economy during treadmill walking at a common treadmill speed in children between the ages of 9 and 13 years (as leg length increased) were eliminated when values were expressed as VO_2 per kg/min/stride (31) (Figure 2.1A,B).

4. As noted above, a theoretical value of the mass scaling exponent for VO_2 during submaximal exercise is anticipated to be 0.67, which is identical to that indicated by dimensionality theory for resting metabolic rate. In general,

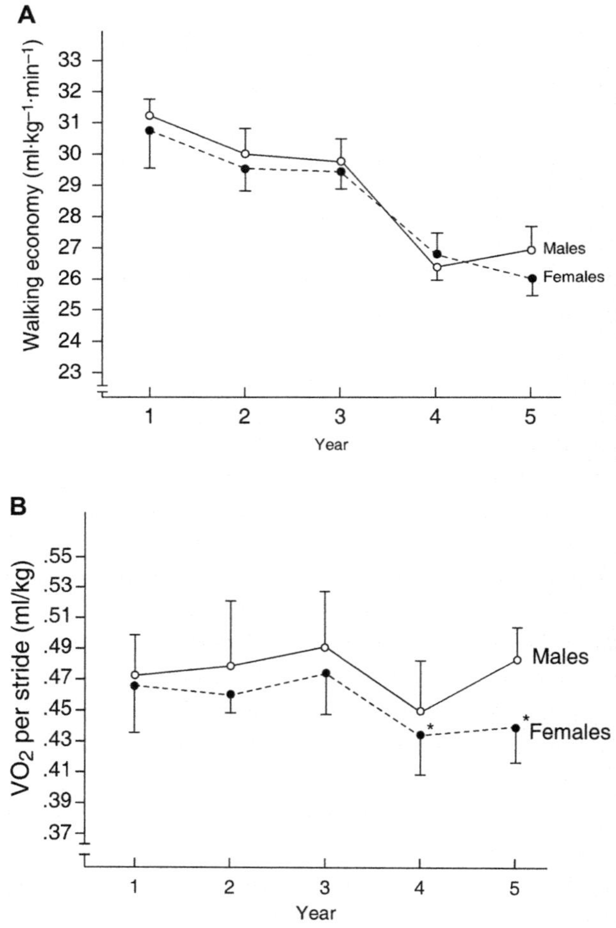

FIGURE 2.1 A, In longitudinal measurements over 5 years, economy (oxygen uptake per kg body mass) at a given walking speed steadily declines with age during childhood. However, B, when expressed as oxygen demand per minute per kg per stride, values remain stable over time.

empirically derived scaling exponents have approximated this value. Some examples: $M^{0.60}$ in 24-year-old men and 14-year-old boys (7), $M^{0.60-0.83}$ in adult endurance athletes (3), $M^{0.75}$ in adolescents (37), and $M^{0.65}$ in prepubertal boys and girls (27). Still, the wide range of values does not preclude a closer approximation to the mass scaling exponent of 0.75 which is empirically observed in respect to resting metabolic rate. One might venture to conclude that resting and submaximal metabolic rate are at least similar. Such a conclusion would be consistent with a desire of Nature to maintain a minimum energy expenditure to perform a given level of metabolic work, at least during non-exhaustive exercise.

Maximal Exercise

When the research question moves on to the link of oxygen uptake and mass at exhaustive exercise, the mystery reappears. For here the mass exponent for VO_2max per kg fails to consistently mimic either the theoretical or empirically observed value (0.67 and 0.75, respectively) for resting metabolic rate. Upon this discrepancy the door is again open for speculation and controversy.

Typical of the recent reports assembling data on VO_2max in mammals is the description by Dlugosz et al. of reported values in 77 species (11). The average allometric scaling exponent for mass was 0.84, with 95% confidence limits between 0.80 and 0.88. As the authors emphasized, this finding is inconsistent with scaling exponents of 0.67, 0.75, or 1.0. That is, the relation between VO_2max and body mass is non-linear, being less in larger compared to smaller animals, with a significantly higher scaling exponent than described for resting metabolic rate or submaximal energy expenditure. In respect to the Darwinian implications of this findings, these authors commented that "the selective factors and sub-organismal mechanisms responsible for whole-body aerobic metabolism seem far more likely to be driven by the maximal demands upon the system represented by VO_2max . . . than by the 'idling' power requirements of basal metabolic rate. Indeed, it is arguable that BMR is largely an epiphenomenon, unlikely to experience direct selection except in unusual circumstances" (11).

Weibel et al. contended that "there is no *a priori* reason why MMR [maximal metabolic rate] should scale the same way as BMR [basal metabolic rate] with body size" (50). The basal rate is an expression of the metabolism of the body to maintain base functional levels, they argued, while with exercise 90% of metabolic rate is contributed by a single tissue—skeletal muscle. In addition, gathered data of VO_2max in animals includes species that are highly athletic with those that are more sedentary. BMR in those two groups are expected to be similar, but VO_2max in the former will be superior. When mass scaling exponents calculated for VO_2max were divided into athletic and non-athletic animals, the value for the former was 0.94 but 0.85 for the latter (50). The greater disparity of scaling exponents for VO_2max versus that for BMR among animals therefore reflects this mixture of athletic versus non-athletic species. Conclusion: VO_2max is dictated by a combination of a) animal size and b) animal athletic prowess, and mass scaling exponents recorded in a mixture of mammals reflect the combined effect of both.

Findings in human beings have been more diverse. Rowland cataloged allometric mass exponents for VO_2max in five studies of youth between 6 and17 years old which ranged from 0.68 to 1.02 (with one outlier of 0.37) (29). These discrepancies were suggested to possibly reflect heterogeneity of subject size, body composition, and athleticism.

The most definite report, though, came from Lolli et al., who performed a meta-analysis of scaling exponents for VO_2max in 36 studies involving over 6,500 human subjects (22). Of the 27 studies that utilized body mass as the scaling denominator, the average allometric exponent was 0.70 with 95% confidence limits of 0.64–0.76. So, according to these data, the scaling exponent for VO_2max in humans encompasses that for *both* resting and submaximal exercise.

At the risk of compounding for the reader the complexity of these issues, it should be pointed out that there are additional considerations here, as well. For example, maximal oxygen uptake, as the measure of peak metabolic rate, should conceptually be most closely linked anthropometrically to the amount of metabolically active tissue. In this case, this is almost exclusively the mass of the skeletal muscle involved in the particular form of exercise. Since this cannot be practically measured, calculated fat-free or lean body mass (FFM) is often used as a surrogate. By this reasoning, VO_2max should be related to FFM raised to an exponent that approximates unity (i.e., 1.0). In other words, theoretically, VO_2max/FFM should be the optimal means of normalizing VO_2max to body size for inter-individual comparisons or when assessing changes within an individual over time. When VO_2 max is expressed to an exponent of mass, body fat content, which is metabolically inert, is included in M; consequently, the scaling factor for M should be less than that of the exponent for FFM.

There are data to support this concept. It will be recalled that in the meta-analysis of scaling exponents for VO_2 by Lolli et al., the average exponent for mass was 0.70. Among the studies which examined this relationship of VO_2max with FFM, however, the average scaling exponent was 0.90 (22). This difference favoring a near-unity scaling for FFM mimics other reports (e.g., 32). In addition, the mass exponent for females averaged 0.52 compared to 0.76 for the males, while the scaling exponent for FFM was similar in both sexes. As per the authors

> Whole body mass is not a robust scaling denominator [for VO_2] as it fails to reflect the real physiological processes during incremental exercise. . . . Fat-free mass, on physiological grounds, is arguably a more appropriate scaling denominator for VO_2, as over 90% of the oxygen passing through the lungs of an exercising mammal is destined for a single sink in the skeletal muscle mitochondria. . . . The main reason for the smaller exponent in females is likely due to their greater amount of adipose tissue than males.
>
> *(22)*

Other constituents of the human body besides fat, such as the bones of the skeleton and blood volume, do not contribute to metabolic rate but are included in measurement of mass. Gunther et al. grouped these together as the *metabolically inactive volume (iV)* in contrast to the *metabolically active volume (aV)*, tissues in which oxygen consumption and oxidative phosphorylation take place to provide energy for locomotion (14). Quantification of aV can be made via measuring mitochondrial volume or density (mtV). The problem here for those examining mass scaling exponents for VO_2max is that the ratio of aV:iV is not invariant and changes with increasing animal size. The authors concluded that "an allometric equation relating mtV and body weight could be tentatively established for interspecies comparisons" (14).

Picking up on that suggestion, Weibel et al. found a close relationship between VO_2max (ml/min) and total muscle mitochondrial volume (V_{mt}) in 11 species ranging in size from a mouse to a steer (49): $VO_2max = 44V_{mt}^{1.01}$ ($r^2 = 0.98$). In that study $VO_2max = 126M^{0.96}$, while $V_{mt} = 25M^{0.96}$, with r^2 values of 0.97 and 0.98, respectively. These observations strongly support the contention that VO_2max is linear related to aV (that is, $VO_2max \sim aV^{1.0}$), a direct reflection of the tissues responsible for metabolic activity at peak exercise.

Concluding Comments

There exists no lack of opinions—sometimes sharply divided—offering to explain the mass scaling exponents for physiological processes obtained by both theoretical and empirical means. Indeed, such controversy reflects one of the most challenging unsolved mysteries confronting the biologic sciences. Beneath all these discussions, though, investigators share in common the strong sense that such relationships offer some essential insights into the nature and behavior of living beings. Eventually resolving this enigma, then, offers to pay significant dividends into the specific and unique features of biological systems.

We entered into this discussion with the hope of gaining an understanding of how physiological time differs from chronological time. Specifically, too, it was anticipated that such an investigation would provide insight into just why physiological time should be related to body size, and why this relationship should be so consistently expressed by quarter-power scaling laws. It was expected, as well, that changes in scaling exponents for mass as they changed with exercise, particularly at maximal levels, might offer some clues to the answers to these questions. On all these scores we can only feel, in a fashion shared by a good many biological scientists, largely frustrated.

Nonetheless, the final section relating how and why scaling exponents for mass (M) differ from those of fat-free mass (FFM) in respect to VO_2max may prove enlightening. It was concluded that the compositional variable whose exponent approached or was equal to 1.0 most accurately reflected the physiological factor(s) that contribute to VO_2max, in this case the volume of metabolically active tissue. It is worth reading back through this section again. For here we see allometric exponents, rather than being indicative of some hidden essential biological principle, as simply reflecting a physiological reality. Perhaps a shift toward considering the potential explanations for anthropometric scaling exponents for biological functions by recognizing the influence of their underlying physiological determinants will serve to gain a greater understanding of their nature (50).

References

1 Adolph EF. Quantitative relations in the physiological constituents of mammals. *Science.* 1949;109:579–585.
2. Atkins PW. Time and dispersal: the second law. In: Flood R, Lockwood M, editors. *The Nature of Time.* Oxford: Blackwell; 1986.
3. Bergh U. Sjodin B, Forsberg A, Svedenhag J. The relationship between body mass and oxygen uptake during running in humans. *Med Sci Sports Exerc.* 1991;23:205–211.
4. Blaxter K. *Energy Metabolism in Animals and Man.* Cambridge: Cambridge University Press; 1989.
5. Buonomano D. *Your Brain is a Time Machine.* New York: W.W. Norton & Company; 2017.
6. Calder WA. *Size, Function, and Life History.* Cambridge, MA: Harvard University Press; 1984.
7. Chamari K, Moussa-Chamari I, Boussaidi L, Hachana Y, Kaouech F, Wisloff U. Appropriate interpretation of aerobic capacity: allometric scaling in adult and young soccer players. *Br J Sports Med.* 2005;39:97–101.
8. Dainton B. *Time and Space. Second Edition.* Montreal: McGill-Queen's University Press; 2010.
9. Davis E. *About Time: Einstein's Unfinished Revolution.* Hammondsworth: Penguin; 1995.
10. Economos AC. Gravity, metabolic rate, and size of mammals. *Physiologist.* 1979;22 Suppl:S71.
11. Dlugosz EM, Chappell MA, Meek TH, et al. Phylogenetic analysis of mammalian maximal oxygen uptake with exercise. *J Experim Biol.* 2013;216:4712–4721,
12. Fraser JT. Introduction. In: Whitrow GJ, editor. *What Is Time?* Oxford: Oxford University Press; 2003. p xi.
13. Gibbs WW. Ultimate clocks. *Sci Amer.* 2002;287:68–75.
14. Gunther B, Morgado E, Gonzalez U. Oxidative metabolism and body weight: inactive, active, and mitochondrial volumes. *Biol Res.* 1993;26:341–356.
15. Hochachka PW, Darveau CA, Andrews RD. Suarez RK. Allometric cascade: a model for resolving body mass effects on metabolism. *Comp Biochem Physiol.* 2003;134A:675–691.
16. Huxley JS. *Problems of Relative Growth.* London: Methuen; 1932.
17. Kleiber M. *The Fire of Life.* New York: Wiley; 1961. pp. 177–225.
18. Le Poidevin R. *Travels in Four Dimensions: The Enigmas of Space and Time.* Oxford: Oxford University Press; 2003. pp. 14–15.
19. Lindstedt SL, Calder WA. Body size, physiological time, and longevity of homeothermic animals. *Quart Rev Biol.* 1981;56:1–16.
20. Lindstedt SL, Schaeffer PJ. Use of allometry in predicting anatomical and physiological parameters of mammals. *Lab Animals.* 2002;36:1–19.
21. Lockwood M. *The Labyrinth of Time.* Oxford: Oxford University Press; 2005.

22. Lolli L, Batterham AM, Weston KL, Atkinson G. Size exponents for scaling maximal oxygen uptake in over 6500 humans: a systematic review and meta-analysis. *Sports Med.* 2017;47:1405–1419.
23. Malina RM, Bouchard C. *Growth, Maturation, and Physical Activity.* Champaign, IL: Human Kinetics; 1991. p. 157.
24. Maliszewski AF, Freedson PS. Is running economy different between adults and children? *Pediatr Exerc Science.* 1996;8:351–360.
25. Morris R. *Time's Arrow.* New York: Simon and Schuster; 1984.
26. Pace N, Smith AH. Gravity and metabolic scale effects in mammals. *Physiologist.* 1981;24 Suppl:S37–S40.
27. Rogers DM, Turley KR, Kujawa KI, Harper KM, Wilmore JH. Allometric scaling factors for oxygen uptake during exercise in children. *Pediatr Exerc Science.* 1995;7:12–25.
28. Rowland T. *Children's Exercise Physiology.* Champaign, IL: Human Kinetics; 2005. p. 15.
29. Rowland T. *Developmental Exercise Physiology.* Champaign, IL: Human Kinetics; 1996. p. 83.
30. Rowland T, Auchinachie JA, Keenan TJ, Green GM. Physiological responses to treadmill running in adult and prepubertal males. *Int J Sports Med.* 1987;8:292–297.
31. Rowland T, Cunningham L, Martel L, Vanderburg P, Manos T, Charkoudian N. Gender effects on submaximal energy expenditure in children. *Int J Sports Med.* 1997;18:420–425.
32. Rowland T, Goff D, Martel L, Ferrone L. Influence of cardiac functional capacity on gender differences in maximal oxygen uptake in children. *Chest.* 2000;117:629–635.
33. Rubner M. Ueber den einfluss der Korpergrosse auf stoffund kraftwechel. *Z Biol.* 1883;19:535–562.
34. Sacher GA. Relation of lifespan to brain weight and body weight in mammals. In: Wolstenholme GEW, editor. *Ciba Foundation Colloquium on Ageing;* 1959. pp. 115–141.
35. Sarrus et Rameaux. Memoire adresse à l'Académie Royale. *Bull Acad Royal Med Belg.* 1839;3:1094.
36. Schmidt-Nielsen K. Scaling. *Why Is Scaling So Important?* Cambridge: Cambridge University Press; 1984.
37. Sjodin B, Svedenhag J. Oxygen uptake during running as related to body mass in circumpubertal boys: a longitudinal study. *Eur J Appl Physiol.* 1992;65:150–157.
38. Skinner JS, Bar-Or O, Bergsteinova V. Comparison of continuous and intermittent tests for determining maximal oxygen uptake in children. *Acta Paediatr Scand.* 1971;Suppl 217:24–28.
39. Smith AH. The roles of body mass and gravity in determining the energy requirements of homeotherms. In: Holmquist R, Stickland AC, editors. *COSPAR: Life Sciences in Space Research 16.* Oxford: Pergamon Press; 1978. pp. 83–88.
40. Smolin L. *Time Reborn.* Boston: Mariner Books; 2013.
41. Stahl WR. Scaling of respiratory variables in mammals. *J Appl Physiol.* 1966;22:453–460.
42. Stewart I. *The Mathematics of Life.* New York: Basic Books; 2011.
43. Unnithan VB, Eston RG. Stride frequency and submaximal running economy in adults and children. *Pediatr Exerc Science.* 1990;2:149–155.
44. Van Mechelen W, Kemper HCG, Twisk J. The development of running economy from 13–27 years of age [abstract]. *Med Sci Sports Exerc.* 1994;26:S205.
45. West G. *Scale. The Universal Laws of Growth, Innovation, Sustainability, and the Pace of Life in Organisms, Cities, Economies, and Companies.* New York: Penguin Press; 2017.

46 West GB, Brown JH, Enquist BJ. The fourth dimension of life: fractal geometry and allomeric scaling of organisms. *Science*. 1999;284:1677–1679.
47. West GB, Savage VM, Gillooly JF, et al. Why does metabolic rate scale with body size? *Nature*. 2003;421:713.
48. Whitlow GJ. *What Is Time?* Oxford: Oxford University Press; 1972.
49. Weibel ER, Bacigalupe LD, Schmitt B, Hoppeler H. Allometric scaling of maximal metabolic rate in mammals: muscle aerobic capacity as determinant factor. *Respir Physiol Neurobiol*. 2004;140:115–132.
50. Weibel ER, Hoppeler H. Exercise-induced maximal metabolic rate scales with muscle aerobic capacity. *J Exper Biol*. 2005;208:1635–1644.

3

WHY WAS ZENO WRONG?

In the 5th century B.C., the Greek philosopher Zeno introduced his Paradox, which goes like this:

> The warrior Achilles is challenged to a 1500-meter race by a tortoise. The sportive Achilles, being a good sport and recognizing his superior speed, agrees and tells the tortoise that he will grant him a 100-meter head start. "In that case," says the tortoise, "there isn't any reason for us to conduct the race, since there is no way that you can win." Incredulous, Achilles listens to the tortoise's explanation.
>
> "When we both start running, you will quickly reach the 100-meter mark where I started. But by that time I will have moved on, maybe to the 110-meter point. Following this, you will reach the 110-meter point, but now by this time I have advanced to the 118-meter mark. Then, when to you arrive at 118-meters, I will be at the 122-meter mark. And so on. There is no way you can catch me. As long as I keep on running, you cannot win the race." Convinced by this logic, Achilles abandons the race.

It is clearly evident, of course, that this is absurd. Common sense dictates that certainly the warrior will easily win the race. In fact, one can easily calculate that if Achilles runs at 100 m per minute and the tortoise at 20 m per minute, the former will win the race in a time of 15:00 compared to that of 75:00 for the tortoise. And the warrior will pass the tortoise sometime about 1:10 minutes into the race.

There is actually a formula, supplied by the mathematician Joseph Mazur, by which one can calculate at what point Achilles will blow by the tortoise (12). If the warrior is running at A kilometers per hour and the tortoise at B kilometers per hour, and the tortoise is provided a head start of H meters, then in time of t hours Achilles will have gone At meters and the tortoise will have covered Bt + H meters. The time t required for the warrior to overtake the tortoise is then given as $t = H/(A - B)$.

Moreover, by this paradox, the race would never end. (This is actually a second of Zeno's paradoxes, this one called the Dichotomy Paradox). That is, both Achilles and tortoise would approach the finish line but neither would ever actually cross it. In each step of Zeno's story the time-distance unit becomes progressively smaller, continuing on in decrements to infinity, but never reaching the finish. And the warrior will progressively close the gap between himself and the shell on the back of his opponent but in this infinitely long competition he can never catch up. Again, one recognizes that this is wrong. So, uncontestably, the conclusion is erroneous. The big question, though, is *why?* Why was Zeno wrong? His story admittedly makes sense but is obviously, for some reason, flawed. A paradox, to be sure: two incompatible outcomes to the race—the warrior wins easily, the warrior can never catch up with the tortoise—both which appear to be correct. What is the explanation?

The answer to this nagging question has troubled philosophers, physicists, and theologians ever since. Indeed, a good many have lost sleep ruminating on the nature of time and reality that would elucidate Zeno's paradox. But attempts to resolve this dilemma have not fully satisfied thinkers even to this day.

What Zeno failed to recognize, one might quickly say, is that the speed of Achilles and that of the tortoise are not the same. We would expect that the winner of any race will be the competitor who can generate the greatest velocity—that is, the first-place finisher will possess a neuromuscular system which can provide the greatest power to cover a particular distance in a given time. But even this is not quite that simple. When the starting gun fires for human beings in the 100-m run, the power driving their legs off the blocks accelerates the sprinters' speed, confirming Newton's Second Law of Motion, and this rise in velocity may continue even as far as half way through the race. There follows a short section of 4–5 seconds of constant peak speed, and, then, as they approach the finish line a few seconds later, their velocity declines—they *slow down*. Often the winner of the race is not the sprinter who can generate the greatest velocity but the one who slows down the least over the final meters (16). It's only an illusion for the spectator that one runner is accelerating to pass another at the finish.

Fundamental Realities

But all this consideration of velocity simply serves to confirm that Zeno was wrong. We already know that, from our common everyday experience. It sheds no light on *why*. No, the answer to that question must involve something more fundamental, some essential aspect regarding the nature of motion and how it is expressed in terms of time and space. But what? It is from this starting point that thinkers for centuries have embarked on a quest for the elusive answer. In this search perhaps Zeno has provided us an opportunity to better understand the nature of reality, be it subjective or objective . . . or even both.

(Not all have been so convinced of the profound implications of Zeno's Paradox. Some, indeed, have insisted that the riddle is "nothing more than picky sophisms of logic with little merit for continued discussion" [10]. For instance, the American philosopher C.S. Peirce contended that "this ridiculous little catch presents no difficulty at all to a mind adequately trained in mathematics and in logic, but is one of those which is very apt to excite minds of a certain class to an obstinate determination to believe a given proposition" [14].)

An Historical Perspective

To start with, it would be useful to understand why Zeno created his Paradox in the first place. What point regarding the nature of reality was he trying to get across? Little is known about the life of this philosopher, for he left no written work. (The lack of documented details regarding his life, in fact, led the mathematician Joseph Mazur to comment that "the absence of Zeno's writings warrants suspicion over whether or not the man actually existed" (12)). According to his contemporary Proclus, Zeno came to Athens in about 450 BC from Elea, a Greek colony situated in modern-day southern Italy. He (Zeno, that is) delved heavily

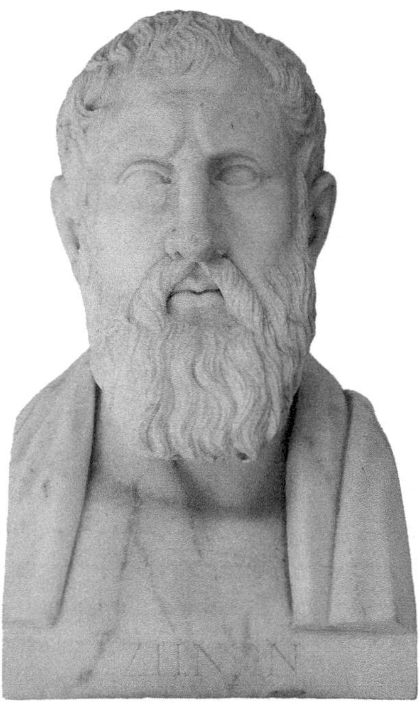

FIGURE 3.1 Zeno.

into paradoxes and, in fact, compiled 40 of them in a book of his philosophies which sadly was either lost or stolen.

(One hardly needs reminding here of the importance of adequate backup of precious manuscripts. That advice was lost on Ernest Hemingway's ex-wife who left a suitcase with all the original and carbon copies of his works to date with a porter on the platform at the Gare de Lyon while she went to obtain some water. As he recounted in *A Moveable Feast*, when she returned, both had disappeared. "I had never seen anyone hurt by a thing other than death or unbearable suffering except Hadley when she told me about the things being gone. She cried and cried and could not tell me" [8]. As for the unfortunate Zeno, having lost his life's work, Mazur could only sympathize: "How devastating his loss must have been, writing day after day on scrolls of papyrus, planning ahead, and anticipating each new thought before cutting the skin and sewing in new patches" [12].)

Zeno was accompanied in his trip to Athens by his close friend and teacher Parmenides, who was very much concerned with questions of metaphysics, the study of the nature of reality. In Athens, Parmenides preached his seemingly doubtful viewpoint, termed *monism*, that reality in the world was an invariable single entity, a unified version of space and time. Change and motion, he said, were simply an illusion. As such, time and space were not continuous nor ultimately divisible, as many of the Greek thinkers at the time contended.

Zeno concocted his paradoxes as a means of supporting his friend's views, aimed at demonstrating that with the alternative opinion—that of a many-faceted or plural existence of reality—one ended up with absurd results. His goal, then, was not to provide a puzzle that would mystify thinkers for centuries but rather to demonstrate that the plurality approach could be falsified. And by demonstrating that falsification, such an argument was, by necessity, invalid. Such an argumentative approach, called the "dialectic," was highly innovative for the ancient Grecian times. By demonstrating the absurdity of one side of an argument it called upon human reasoning in a controversy, not that attributable to heavenly actions or mystical superstition. This technique continues to contribute to philosophical debate to the present day.

Explanations (By Some Accounts)

Mathematical approaches to resolving Zeno's Paradox have satisfied many mathematicians that these have solved the issue. Others—particularly philosophers and physicists—are not so impressed, feeling that the essence of *why* Zeno was wrong has not been adequately revealed. For these thinkers the findings of the Paradox continue to raise difficult questions regarding the nature of space and time. Indeed, recent insights into the nature of both in light of the theories of relativity and the subatomic realm of quantum mechanics have served to complicate rather than clarify any satisfactory interpretation of the Paradox. Consequently, even now, 25 centuries later, the implications of Zeno's paradox as a challenge to the nature of reality continue to evolve, with no clear resolution in sight.

The perplexing nature of Zeno's Paradoxes—both the Achilles and Dichotomy (which are basically identical)—evidently arises in that the Great Race in both is being described in terms of a progressively shortening geometric progression of both time and space. That is, 1 → ½ → ¼ → 1/8 → 1/16 → $1/x^n$, which extends forever and can be measured in infinitely smaller units of measure (i.e., $1/x^n$). It's *because* Zeno described the race in terms of an infinitely divisible continuum of space and time that a) Achilles will never be able to catch up with the tortoise, and b) neither one will ever cross the finish line. And that, of course, is exactly what Zeno was out to show—that by interpreting time and space as occurring in a continuous divisible manner, one ends up with results that defy reality. Thus, his listeners would have to conclude, such an approach is absurd and denies the model of space and time occurring in such a continuous fashion. If one wants to repudiate Zeno's argument—by contending that spacetime is continuous—some flaw must be detected in the construct of these paradoxes. And this is where mathematicians, physicists, and philosophers have sought an answer.

Nature of Space and Time

Attempts to solve the riddle posed by Zeno's Paradox forces one to confront the question of the basic nature of space and time. For just how the absurdity of the outcomes of the Achilles-tortoise race is explainable—or not—must depend on how one views the reality of the passage of time and space (here meaning distance) that define motion. Zeno and Parmenides contended that the nonsensical results of the race as described in the Paradox were accounted for by the fact that time and space are *not* continuous and divisible, that all motion and change are simply an illusion.

The prevailing opinion among scientists at the present time is that, to the contrary, both time and space proceed in a continuum, and that this continuity is infinitely divisible. If one possessed a very large ball of string, it could be unwound such that it would stretch from Chicago to Los Angeles. The string would, without question, be continuous. But at the same time, the string could be divided with a ruler by certain measures, and these measurement units could be progressively made smaller, even to infinity. So one could measure out the string into units of kilometers, and then centimeters, and then millimeters, and so forth to infinity. (Obviously one ignores here that fact that this conceptual model would eventually be limited by an ultimate denouement—a single atom.) This means that the string is also *dense*, meaning that between two points there will always be another point. But when Zeno describes the race between Achilles and the tortoise by using this concept, the outcome is nonsensical.

It is just this density of an infinitely divisible continuum of spacetime that creates the difficulty in explaining away Zeno's paradox. Let's take Z as the race starting point and Z★ as the finish line. Half way through the race Achilles is at Z_1, then at Z_2 he has gone ¼ more, at Z_3 another 1/8, at Z_4 an additional 1/16, etc. Since this series continues to infinity, he cannot actually ever reach Z*. There will always be another Z (call it Z_{n+1}) between Z_n and Z★. The finish line will always be tantalizingly just out of reach. It is the same frustrating dilemma faced by Achilles when he is trying to catch up to the tortoise, because the space between the two is decreasing in progressively smaller distances, but always with *some* gap to close. Concluded Dainton, "the puzzling character of this may be ineliminable: motion through continuous (in the mathematical sense) medium has some radically unfamiliar features, some of which are highly counterintuitive. . . . The real problem is understanding how Zeno can arrive at Z★ at all. To arrive at Z★ he must pass through each of the Z points, but there is an infinite number of these: Z_1, Z_2, Z_3, . . ., Z_n. Since there is no last member of the Z series, it seems Zeno can never reach his destination after all" (4).

Aristotle and the Mathematicians

Aristotle was among the first to weigh in with a proposal for untangling the apparent error in Zeno's Paradox. He argued that there is a difference between a series of events or times which are *potentially* infinite from those that are *actually* infinite (10). So, we may consider the race course to be continuous and infinitely divisible, but actually what we observe, in reality, is that it is smooth, without such demarcations. Zeno's Paradox, he contended, only held if one marks off such divisions in the continuum, which, of course, one does not do. Thus, in the real world, Zeno's Paradox is false. It would only hold true in the hypothetical mind experiment of dividing up the 1,500 m. For Aristotle the paradox of Zeno was an artificial construct, although by itself sensical, that did not conform with the nature of the real world.

More contemporary mathematicians have arrived at what some have considered a resolution to this enigma by different routes. For instance, despite the intuitive difficulty of considering that an infinite series of numbers can actually end in a finite number, this can be shown to be possible via the use of partial sums (12). Still, the difficulty persists. How does Achilles jump from that finite number to Z★ if there is another Z in the way? Others have emphasized that in Zeno's Paradox the time for each step is steadily shortening, and it is evident that time does not slow down in this fashion.

In the 19th century, Georg Cantor described a mathematical proof that many of his colleagues felt definitely resolved the paradox. This is admittedly beyond the full understanding of one not trained in that profession, but basically involves concluding that not all infinite collections of numbers are of the same size. Here Cantor's insights challenge our ideas of just what it means for a number to be "infinite," or for progressively decreasing increments of time and/or distance in a race between a hare and a tortoise to be so (11).

The author and nuclear physicist George Gamow described Cantor's approach to comparing two infinities in his classic book *One Two Three . . . Infinity* (Viking Press, 1947): "If we can pair the objects of two infinite groups so that each object of one infinite collection pairs with each object of another infinite collection, and no objects in either group are left alone, the two infinities are equal. If, however, such arrangement is impossible and in one of the collections some unpaired objects are left, we say that the infinity of objects in this collection is larger, or we can say stronger, than the infinity of objects in the other collection."

As Gamow goes on to point out, such considerations can lead to some rather startling conclusions. For instance, carry out this process by matching up integers in an infinite series of all numbers (one including both odd and even numbers) with an infinite series of just even numbers. That is 1 → 2, 2 → 4, 3 → 6, and so on. In the end, which series would you say holds the greater amount of the numbers, the series including both even and odd numbers or the series of just the even numbers? The first choice seems obvious. But, in fact, a matching of the two series continues to infinity without any numbers "left over," which, according to Cantor means that the two infinities (and the number of integers in the two series) are equal. Counterintuitive, of course, but here "a part may be equal to the whole." What Cantor was saying was that "from any infinite set one may create a new set which actually has more elements than the original set." As Eli Maor has pointed out, "We must realize—and Cantor pointed this out—that we deal here largely with a thought process, with the ability of our mind to *conceive* such sets; whether such sets actually exist (in the physical sense) is quite irrelevant to the issue" (11). (See refs. 4, 11, and 17 for more comprehensive and authoritative descriptions of Cantor's proofs.)

This author must confess to some difficulty in recognizing exactly how Cantor's revolutionary insights into the nature of infinity provide a solution to Zeno's Paradox. Still, thinkers as prominent as David Foster Wallace have been sufficiently impressed with Cantor's proof to call it the "first stroke of incredible, nape-tingling genius" (16). Dainton contended, however, that "The difficulty [of never arriving at the finish line] is more acute in light of Cantor's having established the coherency and consistency—at least in a mathematical sense—of conceiving of the continuum as an actual infinity of points. It can easily seem as though there is an insurmountable gulf separating [Achilles] from his destination" (4).

Robin Le Poidevin, professor of metaphysics at the University of Leeds, agreed: "We have to conclude, then, that Zeno has not uncovered any mathematical impossibility [in his Paradox]. . . . But that is not the end of the story. . . . It is one thing to give a mathematical description of an infinite series, quite another to conceive of a physical realization of that description" (10). "The math is merely a tool," wrote Joseph Mazur. "The underlying reality that the paradox addresses is evaded" (12).

Considering the "Block Universe"

Another perspective on the true nature of time divides arguments for a traditional dynamic concept of time from that of a block, or eternal view. The former, which matches up with our daily experience, holds that time is objective, flowing like a river, independent of outer influences and dividing the fixed past from an undetermined future. The block view, which is that generally accepted by contemporary thinkers, claims, to the contrary, that "all moments of time (and events) are equally real, and there is no moving or changing present; nothing becomes present and then ceases to be present. The differences between past, present and future are simply differences of perspective" (4):

> When first encountering the block view many people find it utterly absurd. That we live our lives in a constantly advancing present, that past and future events are different from those that are present—what could be more obvious? But as block theorists are fond of pointing out, there are plenty of other cases where our everyday experience seems to provide overwhelming support for beliefs that are false. Can you remember how you felt when, as a child, you were told that there are folk in other countries for whom our "down" is their "up"? Even now, are you entirely comfortable with the thought that the Earth is shooting through space at a rate of many miles per second? . . . Our experience does not guarantee that the world is as we normally believe it to be so.
>
> *(4)*

The alert reader has by now recognized that the concept of a block universe, in which all times and events are equally real, is not dissimilar from the stand taken by Parmenides that the world is not in an endless continuous process of change but rather "a single story of a road is left . . . being is ungenerated and undestroyed, whole, of one kind and motionless and balanced . . . nothing is or will be other than what it is—since that has Fate fettered to be whole and motionless" (2). How does one reconcile the accepted idea of a block universe, with its lack of flow of time, with an equally accepted vision of a continuous passage of time and distance in the Achilles-tortoise race? An answer to this question is somehow at the heart of understanding Zeno and his Paradox.

Some have proposed that the explanation exists in a consideration of the means by which memories accumulate (4,13). "Our sense that time is passing is due to the fact that our perceptions and memories combine, not only over the span of a few seconds or minutes but over days, months, and years. . . . [Here is] a plausible account, one that does not require a moving present or the non-existence of times other than the present. All that it requires is for people to have different memories at different stages of their lives" (4).

Is Space-Time (Motion) Discrete?

So far we've been considering the passage of time and space as a constant one—a continuum, if you will—and, as required by Zeno's Paradox, one that is infinitely divisible. But there exists another alternative means of considering the passage of space-time and that would be to think about it as proceeding not continuously but in discrete packages—like pearls on a necklace, or boxcars in a train—which are not divisible. In this case, each point in the race is surrounded by a certain fixed number of other points, and every moment in time has a distinct, unique predecessor and successor (10). In fact, when the 1,500-m race is viewed like this, Zeno's paradox completely falls apart. No more infinity of progressively smaller units of time and space that prevents a competitor from reaching that final step to the finish line. No more Achilles progressively catching up, but not ever quite, to the tortoise. Just take the time it takes to get to the 750-m mark (adjusting for the tortoise's head start), and multiply by two to get the times to finish for each. Now, from this perspective, Achilles wins in a romp. We're back to what we think reality should be, without a paradox to solve. By considering space-time as occurring in fixed non-divisible segments, the winner is obvious. And satisfying to our common-sense expectations.

But is this the way reality works? Could our spacetime, instead of continuous, really be discrete? It takes some courage to even raise the question, given that the usual mathematical constructs surrounding physics are firmly based on the assumption that space and time are continuous. The towering precepts of space-time of Newton and Einstein and a good many other thinkers are continuous, not discrete. Still, new concepts of space-time, particularly in the brave new world of quantum mechanics, offer some support for its discrete nature:

> Time dilation, inconstancy of mass, and special relativity suggest that motion is indeed illusory. Motion changes mass—or is it the other way around? Quantum theory suggests that some motion is not continuous. Electrons cannot just sit anywhere within an atom. They are strictly confined to moving between discrete energy levels around an atom's nucleus.
>
> *(12)*

Certainly, from our (only) frame of reference—our brains, operating on information gathered from our senses—no. When we watch an Olympic 1,500-m race it's continuous, it flows, no herky-jerky parts. It's a continuum. But could we be deceived about this? Could our brain's perception of a continuum of space-time be simply a neurological construct, when it really comes in bits and pieces?

Well, disturbingly, maybe. One only has to consider settling back to view a film at a local theater to raise a cautious flag here. Is the action on the screen continuous? Of course, it is. It mimics real life, a continuum of action, of words, or motion, of time and space. But, of course, this isn't true. The film rolling through the projector (or the computer) is only a progressive series of discrete static images—a set of snapshots, well over 100,000 of them in watching Woody Allen's *Midnight in Paris*—and when they are rolled past our eyes fast enough (around 24 per second) we see the action as continuous.

So, what is "real"—the roll of discrete static images inserted into the projector? Or the continuous motion on the screen, a product of the inability of our nervous system to "keep up"? "Though nature is fantasized as continuous—both by our brains, such as when we are watching a film, and by reason, as argued in Zeno's paradox—she does make jumps. . . . In any event, we must regard that smoothness as an assumption rather than the truth" (12).

This same is true of television. If you're watching the 100-m dash at the World Championships, it all looks to you (and would to Zeno as well) undeniably continuous, but it's not. That TV image is composed of 25 separate pictures, each one shown twice, so that the picture you're seeing on the screen is actually discrete passage of 50 images per second—too fast for your brain to discern (7).

But this is the effect of a mechanism turning discrete into continuous motion. Can the brain do this by itself? Yes, it can, and does. Put yourself on a tennis court, about to return serve. The ball crosses the net and arrives at a speed of, say, 75 mph. Following the admonition of your instructor, you "keep your eye on the ball." You fixate on its smooth trajectory, tracking the ball to that point where the swing of your racket makes contact. A seemingly classic example of continuity of space (that is to say, distance) and time. But, no. What is occurring as you track the ball to that striking point is in reality something entirely different, something that speaks to a discrete, non-continuous progression of space-time.

Here's what really happens: The area in the retina at the back of your eye that provides sharp images, the *foveal region*, is very small, amounting to only about 3 degrees in your visual field. Outside of this, the image is very blurry. You can see motion to some extent in your peripheral vision but no clear details as to its origin or direction. As a consequence, the eye must be in constant motion to give you a clear picture of your surroundings, keeping the image directed on the foveal region, and it does this by shifting its direction in a series of rapid, discrete jumps of vision, called *saccades* (7). If this didn't occur one's vision would be seriously constrained. Moreover, an image that remains focused on the foveal region for even a short period of time rapidly fades. So, the eye roams about the visual field in a series of very rapid saccades, about every 20–30 milliseconds. This series of discrete images in time, being extremely rapid, is perceived by the brain as a continuous picture.

When watching that tennis ball arriving over the net, the eye can move to follow the ball in its flight, keeping the Dunlop image focused on the fovea, at least if the angular velocity across your field of vision is not too fast. But when the ball approaches you, the angular velocity exceeds that which the visual apparatus and brain can process. The eye adjusts for this by again performing saccades, discrete jumps in vision that allow you to predict where to swing the racket. Between these saccades the vision is temporarily shut off, because if it didn't you would see a lot of blurring (7). This will work as long as the ball doesn't take any last-second changes in its trajectory. This explains why you often miss shots that arrive with a good deal of topspin or backspin or when the ball strikes an uneven portion of a clay court. The last piece of information you received from an anticipatory saccade wasn't sufficiently predictive of where it would eventually end up (15). Call it a failed effort to accurately predict a continuous motion by what was in reality a series of discrete visual jumps. (This is particularly problematic for baseball hitters, who must predict the path of curve balls, sliders, and knuckle balls, a challenge which will be addressed in Chapter 7.)

All this raises a bothersome question: Why should we humans perceive motion as continuous when, in reality, at least in certain conditions, it comes in discrete packages? As Mazur queried, "Is there some biological necessity to see continuous movement? . . . Wouldn't staccato motion be enough to protect us from wild beasts and enable us to farm and live as we always have? . . . Perhaps the real world that we live in is truly disjointed, where every movement behaves as though it is a Keystone Comedy. Would we feel discomfort at seeing a disjointed succession of images? . . . Would we know the difference, or would we simply adjust as we did to foods that had bothered us in infancy?" (12). (With no disrespect intended, it might be assumed that Prof. Mazur is not a tennis player, nor has he ever tried to hit a 95-mph fastball. Sometimes an appreciation of continuous motion—even if phony—would seem to be obligatory.)

Trusting the Brain?

This is not the only time we will encounter in this book the idea that the human brain can be "fooled" into certain conceptualizations of the world that are shamelessly concocted and fraudulent—but to our ultimate benefit. Repeatedly we are reminded that our perceptions of the world are only based on an isolated narrow cerebral perspective. The proposed biological explanation for this duplicity in each case is identical—the pragmatic outcome of evolutionary pressures which have created a certain viewpoint of the world from a cerebral perspective that has provided survival value. We "see" the world in the certain fashion as we do because that's what has brought us here. We "see" continuous motion because, well, otherwise how on earth would we ever play tennis?

We are now bumping up against some other classical conundrums that have confounded philosophers since forever. What is reality? Is it out there in the physical world, sharing no regard for human recognition? Or is it just what our senses tell us? Is there an objective reality beyond our senses, one our brains have not been structured to appreciate? Of course, without question, there is. We perceive a very narrow range of sound frequencies and tiny portions of the electromagnetic spectrum. Parallel "worlds" or realities are not just the stuff of science fiction or advanced metaphysical speculation. They truly exist, real objective "things" to which our senses are blind and dumb. And so, it is legitimate to ask if in the real world of any objective reality, is time-space—that is, motion—discrete or continuous? (And, if you are in a particularly contrary mood you are free to ask, as well, does it really matter?)

Let's take a step back and return to the "dialectic" that Parmenides and Zeno engaged in with doubters on the Acropolis. In the late 18th century, the German philosopher Georg Wilhelm Friedrich Hegel formalized this process as "somebody puts forward a thesis, then there's an antithesis, a contradiction of it. And somehow, miraculously, from the clash of these two things, a synthesis emerges" (5). In this to-and-fro, Zeno argued for a particular viewpoint, monism, in which change and motion did not occur, and any perception otherwise was simply an illusion. And to show that the opposing opinion, pluralism, a continuous divisible idea of motion, held no water, Zeno provided a story of a race between Achilles and a tortoise that was, to all evidence of common experience, impossible. Not a bad strategy. To counter the argument offered by this paradox, one would have to show that while, yes, the paradox is absurd, it does not accurately reflect the events that occur in continuous space-time. The reader is free, considering the discussions in this chapter, to decide whether or not that has been achieved.

But we still are faced with yet another troublesome philosophical issue: in making such judgments the nature of space-time, whom do we trust? Another German philosopher, Immanuel Kant, writing at about the same time as Hegel, contended that "we can't really know how the world is, that all we can know is how we perceive it. . . . We only have access to how things appear to us. How things are in themselves is something we cannot know" (5). So, is the human brain free to "create" a reality independent of "how things really are"? And how do we humans formulate an answer to that question, when our only tool for doing so is the brain itself?

The moral of this story is that we cannot assume automatically that the images of the world around us are a just representation of "reality." Indeed, that is just what Parmenides and his sidekick Zeno were arguing on the Acropolis 2,500 years ago—that motion and change are simply an illusion.

What to conclude here? Does one dare challenge the basic principles of physics and claim that Parmenides and Zeno were right, that spacetime is not continuous and divisible, that change and motion are an illusion, that we are victims of a grand deception by our own traitorous brain? Wrote Dainton, "We should not race to any conclusions—other approaches to quantum gravity, such as some versions of string theory, are formulated in terms of orthodox continuous spacetimes. But nor should we rush to rule out the discrete conception simply because history (thus far) has favoured the smooth alternative" (4).

A Dual Nature of Motion?

Any physics-savvy reader is by now conscious of a striking parallel between the arguments regarding the nature of motion in spacetime—continuous or discrete?—and a similar conundrum that confronted physicists a century ago regarding the nature of light. Up until the 1920s, light was generally considered to behave as a wave (although as early as the 18th century, Isaac Newton theorized that light possessed a particulate nature). Albert Einstein established such a particle-like characteristic of light as a *photon* in his studies of the photoelectric effect, and subsequent experiments observing interference patterns of light passing through slits confirmed the duality of light. Light, it was found, can take on the properties of a wave in some experiments, yet as a particle in others.

So here was, indeed, a paradox. How could light act like two distinctly different things—waves and particles—simultaneously? Such duality or "complementarity," became a central feature of quantum mechanics, for such unexplained ambiguity of nature, such "quantum weirdness," was soon observed not just for light but also in the behavior of subatomic particles such as electrons, neutrons, and even entire atoms. The eminent physicist Richard Feynman commented, "Now we know how the electrons and light behave. But what can I call it? If I say they behave like particles I give the wrong impression; also if I say they behave like waves. They behave in their own inimitable way, which technically could be called a quantum mechanical way. They behave in a way that is like nothing that you have ever seen before" (6).

As William Laurence wrote so succinctly in an article in *The New York Times* in 1933, such complementarity is "an inherent essential duality in the nature of things as they relate to man's ability to know them. The paradox of this duality lies in the fact that the Jekyll-Hyde nature of all things is essentially contradictory, with both aspects being true at different times, but with only one aspect being true at any given time. . . . The very process of knowing one aspect of nature makes it impossible for us to know the other aspect. This contradictory duality is inescapable because it lies at the very heart of things" (9).

Today, "the mystery of the two faces of quantum mechanics—wave and particle—is still with us" (3). There is something here that is truly discomforting, an incongruity which escapes our normal conception of the real world—yet must be accepted as one of its authentic features. Whether such a dual nature might extend to that of motion and how it is perceived by the human experience—thereby definitely resolving Zeno's Paradox—remains to be seen.

Summary

We come to the end of this discourse with no clear answer in sight. Why was Zeno wrong? *Was* he wrong? Can the paradox be challenged in respect to the nature of spacetime—continuous or discrete? Is our common experience providing misleading information regarding the true reality of spacetime? Does it matter for our daily existence? As Julian Baggini advised, "Confused? Don't worry—you should be. There is no simple way out . . . Perhaps the real lesson of the tortoise race [is that] armchair theorizing using basic logic is an unreliable guide to the fundamental nature of the universe" (1).

So, the mystery of motion remains:

> Everything in this universe, every atom, every molecule, is in some form of motion, whether it be simple locomotive displacement from one place to another, random molecular bombardments, or complex, astonishingly fast, unavoidable vibrations of energy transfer. And our understanding of that motion remains fundamentally paradoxical.
>
> *(12)*

References

1 Baggini J. *The Pig That Wants to be Eaten. 100 Experiments for the Armchair Philosopher.* New York; Plume; 1995. pp. 46–48.
2. Barnes J. *The Presocratic Philosophers.* London: Routledge; 1982. p. 178.
3. Cropper WH. *The Great Physicists.* Oxford: Oxford University Press; 2001. pp. 275–291.
4. Dainton B. *Time and Space. Second Edition.* Montreal: McGill-Queen's University Press; 2010. pp. 267–312.
5. Edmonds D, Warburton N. *Philosophy Bites Back.* Oxford: Oxford University Press; 2012.
6. Feynman R. *The Character of Physical Law.* Cambridge, MA: MIT Press; 1965. p. 128.
7. Gregory RL. *Eye and Brain. The Psychology of Seeing. Fifth Edition.* Princeton: Princeton University Press; 1997.
8. Hemingway E. *A Moveable Feast.* New York: Scribner; 1996.
9. Laurence WL. Jekyll-Hyde mind attributed to man. *The New York Times.* June 23, 1933. pp. 1, 13.
10. Le Poidevin R. *Travels in Four Dimensions. The Enigmas of Space and Time.* Oxford: Oxford University Press; 2003.
11. Maor E. *To Infinity and Beyond. A Cultural History of the Infinite.* Princeton: Princeton University Press; 1987.
12. Mazur J. *Zeno's Paradox. Unraveling the Ancient Mystery Behind the Science of Space and Time.* New York: Plume; 2007.
13. Mellor DH. *Real Time.* London: Routledge; 1998. p. 122.
14. Peirce C. *The Collected Papers of Charles Saunders Peirce.* Cambridge, MA: Harvard University Press; 1935.
15. Regan D. Visual factors in hitting and catching. *J Sports Sci.* 1997;15:533–558.
16. Rowland T. *The Athlete's Clock.* Champaign, IL: Human Kinetics; 2011. pp. 69–75.
17. Wallace DF. *Everything and More: A Compact History of ∞.* London: Phoenix; 2005.

4

WHAT EXPLAINS THE MYSTERIOUS UBIQUITY OF BIOLOGIC VARIABILITY?

In 1887 the German physician Willem Fliess, a prominent ear, nose, and throat specialist, had an idea. The bodily functions and behaviors of human beings, he said, behaving like those of other natural phenomena—the tides, the motions of the heavenly bodies—fluctuate in regular cycles, or rhythms. Moreover, he proposed that such rhythms in men differed from those in women. According to Dr. Fliess, the male cycle of 23 days in duration featured periodic variations in features such as strength, endurance, and courage, while that in the female occurred with regular swings of sensitivity, intuition, and love every 28 days.

Perhaps not unexpectedly, Fliess advanced in his work *The Rhythm of Life: Foundations of an Exact Biology* the proposal that these cycles were linked with changes in the inner lining of the nose. And disturbing these rhythms, he claimed, spelled trouble. Fortunately, went the message, under his care such difficulties could be resolved by topical applications of cocaine to what he called "genital cells" in the nasal cavity as well as, in more drastic cases—for the more courageous—surgical removal of nasal tissue.

The self-promoting Dr. Fliess gained the confidence and personal friendship of none other than Sigmund Freud, who was so convinced with this idea that he himself underwent two nasal operations in an attempt to cure his own personal neurotic behaviors. The success of these interventions is unknown, but the story goes that one of Freud's own patients suffered severe facial disfigurement at Fliess' surgical hands, thereby bringing Freud's enthusiasm for the idea to an end.

Lest one judge Dr. Fliess too harshly, certain of his ideas were notably prescient, namely that biological rhythms in human beings could be manifest in physical and psychological ways. And he had the insight to place this biological variability into a medical context. Indeed, Dr. Fliess is resuscitated from the dustbin of scientific history by pointing out the critical observation that *disturbing* these rhythms—in interrupting their regularity—the human organism can suffer adverse effects. What's more—and this may be Fliess' most important legacy—he opened the door on a phenomenon that must somehow bear witness to what it means to be "alive." That is, the secret of life, by some means, is tied up in not just helical strands of DNA but needs to in some way be revealed in patterns of an obligatory, constant change over time. As to just what biological rule or principle underlay this variability he remained mute.

Organized variability is an essential property of all living matter. No function remains constant; all biological activity is constantly changing. The interval between successive heart beats, the stride length during a one-mile walk, the filtered volume of the renal glomerulus—they all display continuous variability over time. Such change is not random. Biological variability occurs in patterns—some of it quite rhythmic—and multiple patterns co-exist over the same period of time. It matters not, as well, on which scale of function such change is measured; constant variability is observed from the level of the individual cell to that of the most complex body systems. In short, living beings operate in a constant state of intricate and presumably biologically meaningful physiological flux.

This variability has been recognized since antiquity. The ancients, observing the phasic changes in astronomical events, the seasons, and the tides, were aware that such rhythmic alterations took place in human function as well. To wit: "Everything is in a state of metamorphosis. Thou thyself art in everlasting change" (Marcus Aurelius in his *Meditations*, circa 150 AD), and later Edmund Spencer's description in the 16th century of "The everlasting wheele of change, the which of all mortal things do sway" in *The Faerie Queene*.

In more recent times, the organized variability of physiological function has become recognized as not simply a scientific curiosity but rather one of central importance to human well-being. Indeed, evidence has mounted that such variability is essential to the effectiveness of biological function, and its modification or absence is associated with serious disability and human disease (17,18). This dependence on a constant state of change is so necessarily ubiquitous as to suggest that such variability constitutes or reflects some essential principle of biologic matter, yet to be revealed (3,16). A greater understanding of the characteristics of physiological variability may therefore offer insights into the basic nature of biological function as well as causative mechanisms surrounding disease processes.

Different expressions of variability in physiological function are evident within particular time domains. For example, regular periodicity can occur monthly (or *circalunar*, as observed in the menstrual cycle), daily (*circadian*, regular fluctuations over a 24-hour period), or over seconds of time or less (*time series variability*, as in the fluctuations of time between successive heart beats). These individual patterns often occur simultaneously, such that any particular physiological activity may be observed to exhibit concomitant patterns of variability over time.

Forms of Variability

Circadian rhythms, the most commonly recognized form of biologic variability, are characterized by regular 24-hour phasic swings in bodily processes. Virtually all physiological functions participate in such rhythmic variability, each with its predictable amplitude and particular maximal and minimum daily value. Body temperature peaks in the late afternoon, gastric motility between 8:00 and 10:00 AM, lung airway patency at noon. In isolated environments (caves, experimental chambers) such cycles occur over approximately 24 hours and 15 minutes, the *free-running period*, but are entrained by environmental factors (most particularly exposure to light) to a more precise 24-hour periodicity (13). While this feature implies an astronomical origin, the biological "meaning" of circadian rhythms remains largely obscure. Such rhythms have often been interpreted as evolutionary-based means of "optimizing physiology and behavior to the anticipated environmental alterations that occur across each day and night" (51). Still, within this interpretation it is difficult to explain why joint flexibility in humans is greatest between 4:00 and 6:00 in the afternoon, or that most people concentrate best just before noon.

While the capacity for circadian rhythmicity is possessed by each of the trillion of individual cells in the human body, in a hierarchical manner such patterns in mammals are synchronized on an organism level by a master pacemaker located in the suprachiasmatic nucleus at the base of the brain. Recent investigations have identified particular "clock" genes which command the production of cellular proteins which, in a cyclical feedback fashion, dictate this daily ebb and flow of cellular and tissue function (55).

While Darwinian explanations for the ubiquity of circadian rhythms are often uncertain, it is evident that the presence and stability of these diurnal patterns of function are critical for human well-being. This essential contribution of circadian rhythms to health is most obviously revealed when these rhythms are disturbed or interrupted. The most obvious example, familiar to international travelers, is "jet lag," the unpleasant set of sensations that occurs when one is transported rapidly over multiple time zones. The ensuing disturbance of synchrony of environmental cues (particularly light) with bodily rhythms—a biological dissonance—is typically expressed by fatigue, poor sleep, irritability, and headaches.

While such symptoms may serve as only a temporary inconvenience to travelers, there is growing awareness that long-standing disruption of normal circadian patterns of physiological function may pose a risk for more serious health outcomes (43,81). In this regard, attention has been focused on the mismatch of intrinsic rhythms with dark-light cycles that are habitually experienced by night-time factory shift workers, police and fire personnel, and medical professionals. Accumulating research evidence indicates that shift workers carry a significantly greater risk for a plethora of chronic diseases, including coronary artery disease, breast cancer, obesity, type 2 diabetes, auto-immune illnesses, reproductive problems, and psychiatric disorders (10,11).

That this derangement of normal circadian rhythms can be causal rather than simply the effect of disease is indicated by interventional studies in non-human subjects. For instance, studies demonstrate that animals deprived of circadian rhythmicity by experimental elimination of "clock" genes exhibit cancer growth, obesity, pancreatic dysfunction, heart muscle disease, diminished fertility, and metabolic derangements (11).

Physiological functions such as muscle strength, aerobic capacity, and flexibility that underpin sports performance share in this circadian rhythmicity, and optimal times for participation in particular athletic competitions have been identified. Performance on most endurance events (running, swimming, cycling), for example, tends to peak in the late afternoon (57,61).

The lesson here is that regular diurnal phasic changes in function are essential for effective physiological function. While athletes might reasonably seek to profit from circadian variability by competing and training at recognized peak hours of particular physiological functions, this strategy may have limited practical value to the competitive athlete in light of the large number of variables that influence sports performance (environmental conditions, schedule times of competitions, inter-individual variability).

Heart Rate Variability

The change observed in the time interval between successive heart beats, or heart rate variability (HRV), is a typical example of *time-series variability*. Upon palpating one's pulse or examining the heart's electrical activity on an electrocardiogram (the R-R interval) such rhythm of successive heart beats would seem to be completely regular. When measured more precisely, however, intervals between successive beats vary over time in what would appear to be a completely random, or stochastic, fashion, ranging in a resting individual from approximately 0.75 to 1.10 seconds.

Hidden within this apparent randomness, however, lie specific patterns of variability. Computer analysis of a series of such measurements by Fourier transform of heart beat-to-beat time intervals reveals that there occur four major patterns of sinusoidal oscillations related to distinct frequencies (64,66). A high frequency (HF) band in the range from 0.15 to 0.4 Hz (cycles per second) reflects parasympathetic autonomic activity and is linked to the respiratory cycle. The low frequency (LF) band between 0.04 and 0.15 Hz is related to baroreceptor activity and, in some studies, to sympathetic function. The ratio of LF/HF has thus been considered by some to be a marker of cardiac autonomic balance. However, evidence indicates that multiple physiological influences contribute to this frequency spectrum (68). The nature of the very low frequency band (VLF) between 0.0033 and 0.04 Hz and the ultra-low frequency band (<0.0033 Hz) are less well understood but have been associated with circadian rhythms as well as certain health-related outcomes. Such an analysis, then, provides insight into the relative contributions of these different frequencies to the overall variation in series of heart beat interval measurements.

By frequency domain analysis, HRV has been closely linked to human disease, as alterations of the power spectrum have been described in patients with cardiac, renal, and metabolic disease (64). Total and LF HRV power serve as a favorable prognostic indicator, while a decrease in HF often portends a poor outcome, including mortality (2).

As indicators of autonomic balance, measures of resting HRV may bear importance for athletes (9). Particularly, changes in HRV have been utilized to guide the intensity of training regimens, since autonomic regulation plays a role in such adaptations (52). In this regard, changes in HRV have been associated with athletic overtraining (63).

An acute bout of progressive exercise is accompanied by sympathetic activation and parasympathetic withdrawal, and it might be expected that measures of HRV would reflect this response. Typically, however, during such exercise global amount of variability as well as LF and HF power decrease substantially, and changes in indicators of sympathetic-parasympathetic balance (i.e., LF and HF normalized to total power) have been found to be inconsistent (37). Sandercock and Brodie have pointed out that standard spectral HRV analysis is not accurate during acute exercise due to the marked decrease in overall variability (which may exceed the limits of accuracy of measurement) as well as the increased oscillations of HF which reflect augmented respiratory effort (62).

In sum, HRV defines the co-existence of several regular rhythms that are identified by occurring at different frequencies concomitantly over time in a single, easily measured physiological variable. Such variability largely reflects the separate influences of sympathetic and parasympathetic tone on the sinus node. As with circadian rhythms, HRV is linked to human well-being, and, as well, bears significance for athletic training and performance.

Bounded Variability

While HRV measured by spectral analysis indicates the relative importance of different frequencies to overall heart beat interval fluctuations, analysis of *fine-scale, or bounded variability*, of heart beat intervals and other physiological functions provides insight into the extent that measures within the variability are correlated with each other. This form of variability—a marker of the balance between randomness and deterministic regularity of physiological functions—is likely common to all biological activity, having been documented in not only rate of sinus node discharge but also in such disparate functions as breathing frequency, body temperature, gastrointestinal contraction, and nerve action potentials (75).

As an intrinsic feature of biological systems, bounded variability is characteristic of *complex systems*, which are typified by non-linear relationships, self-organizing functions, hierarchical activities, and emergent qualities. Too, bounded variability is typically *fractal*, or scale-independent, in nature, indicating that the pattern remains similar regardless of the magnification of measurement.

Disturbances of the balance of regularity and randomness in variation of physiological values in a time series are associated with pathologic processes, including chronic leukemia, epilepsy, Parkinson's disease, mental disorders, neurodegenerative disease, and congestive heart failure (75). Direction of the causality arrow in this relationship of variability and disease remains to be clarified. However, the research literature supports the use of changes in variability as a marker of disease change or prognosis.

As will be explored in more detail below, the impact of exercise on bounded variability is just beginning to be explored. These early investigations have largely been restricted to considerations of variability in heart rate. Initial studies suggest that such variability may be "optimized" by a period of resistance training (25). Bounded variability shifts toward greater regularity have been described after single bouts of supra-maximal (Wingate) testing and resistance exercise. Such variability is also altered in response to acute bouts of progressive exercise, but research findings regarding the direction (more randomness or more periodicity) have been conflicting.

Nature of Bounded Variability

Repeated measurements of a particular physiologic function over time reveals a certain range of values, or variability. The possible characteristics of such variability can be defined along a continuum: at one extreme the fluctuation of values could be entirely random. That is, a given measurement would not be connected to or determined by the preceding values. Each would be totally independent, typical of the situation of the repetitive tosses of a coin. Graphically, the distribution of such a collection of random values would describe a normal Gaussian curve, with a mean and ± standard deviation that would include 67% of the values.

At the other extreme the repeated values could conform to a strict pattern of regularity in which each measure is tightly linked to its predecessor. Here the pattern would display a high level of *connectiveness* between its elements, reflected in a clear predictability of future values. The sine wave-like periodicity of a circadian rhythm would serve as a typical example. Just where a given group of data points sits on this continuum of regularity versus randomness can be assessed by a variety of computer-based methods of analysis that will be outlined below.

The regularity and connectiveness of bounded variability lies between these two extremes, reflecting characteristics of both control (periodicity) as well as flexibility (randomness) (Figure 4.1). As will be described below, this compromise or balance offered by the intermediate level of connectiveness of bounded variability may account for its ability to optimize physiological function.

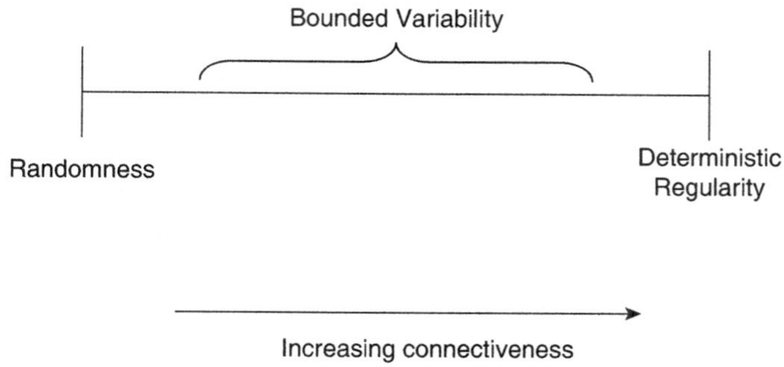

FIGURE 4.1 Bounded variability is a compromise between complete randomness (stochastic variability) and deterministic, predictable variability.

Bounded variability dynamics are characteristically *fractal* in nature, meaning that a magnification of the pattern of fluctuations of physiological values over a short time is similar to that of the larger pattern of change observed over a more extended period. That is, regardless of the scale of measurement, a similar pattern persists (19). As a fractal, the pattern of bounded variability is scale independent and is said to be *self-similar*. As such this form of variability is sometimes referred to as "fractal variability" or "fractal physiology."

Bounded Variability and Complexity

The contemporary literature surrounding bounded variability and its analysis contains unfamiliar concepts such as complex adaptive systems, non-linear dynamics, emergence, scale invariance, and fractals, which not unexpectedly can cause the uninitiated to avoid reading farther. However, these seemingly intimidating terms are easily identifiable within the context of familiar physiological phenomena; indeed, they provide a necessary framework for understanding conceptual shifts from more traditional reductionist interpretations of biological function (1,58,69). Bounded variability is observed in the context of the function of complex systems, and these reflect a "new reality" which has displaced traditional, over-simplistic models of physiological function and grossly complicated narrow arguments for genetic determinism (34,39).

While a universally accepted definition remains elusive, a *complex system* can be considered one in which "relatively simple entities organize themselves, without the benefit of a central controller, into a collective whole that creates patterns, uses information, and in some cases evolves and learns" (41). (Such a designation should not be confused with the colloquial use of "complex," meaning "complicated." A complex system is, to be sure, complicated, but there the similarity ends.) Such systems are termed "adaptive" when they possess the capacity to change or evolve over time based on previous experience and altered environmental conditions.

As a functioning biological machine, the human body is composed of a myriad of such systems. The circulatory system, for example, is composed of discrete functional entities—contractile elements of heart muscle, autonomous generation of electrical pulses from the sinus node, factors controlling vascular tone of resistance blood vessels, reflex baroreceptor control of blood pressure, and determinants of blood volume. As a "collective whole" these provide for the circulation of blood, and the system "uses information" to adjust oxygen supply, carbon dioxide elimination, thermoregulation, and so forth, to conform to extrinsic demands.

A complex system is characterized by a number of descriptive features, including:

- *Self-organization.* As noted in the above definition, a complex system exhibits patterns of behavior with no direction from a central or external controller.
- *Emergent qualities.* The collective behavior of the complex system demonstrates unique qualities which cannot be predicted from the individual elements of the system. That is, "the whole is greater than the sum of its parts." In the example of the circulatory system, the emergent feature—the flow of a viscous liquid through branching vessels—cannot be deduced from the phasic electrical impulses of the sinus node or the sliding of actin-myosin filaments in the myocardium, or, for that matter, any other individual component of the system.
- *Hierarchical organization.* The operation of a complex system involves multiple layers, or tiers, of subsystems. Consider the ascending levels of function from the physico-chemical (such as ion transfer across cell membranes) → cellular → tissue → organ → total body function that permits the circulation of blood, the running of a 5K road race, or the memorization of a Shakespearean sonnet. These "ascending" individual levels of biological function, which in effect perform independent activities, must by necessity communicate with each other, but how this is accomplished remains enigmatic.
- *Non-linear dynamics.* The relationships among components of a complex system are governed by non-linear dynamics such that a change in function X triggers a disproportionate change in function Y, and that effect is defined mathematically as X raised to the exponent b (the so-called power law, expressed as an *allometric* equation): $\Delta Y \sim \Delta X^b$ (76). In non-linear relationships, then, "small effects can have very large and unexpected consequences" (7). (If a non-linear association exists between variables X and Y, b cannot equal 1.0. A value of b of 1.0 would indicate instead a linear relationship between the two, meaning that the magnitude of change in one would be directly proportional and predictable by the amount of change of the other.)
- *Bounded variability.* "By anyone's measure, living systems are complex—they exist somewhere in the middle ground between order and disorder" (41).

Bounded variability reflects this "middle ground" as defined by fluctuations over time that are at once random and deterministic (58).

Measurement of Bounded Variability

Bounded variability reflects underlying fractal, non-linear relationships in biological processes which are manifest as a balance of regularity (connectiveness) and randomness (non-connectiveness) in measurement variability. To utilize the characteristics and changes of such variability as markers of health and well-being (and, as will be discussed later, exercise) it is important to quantify the degree of connectiveness of the variable measures obtained in any given data set. A number of techniques for doing so are briefly outlined below. All possess the ability to place the nature of the variability of a set of measurements on the continuum of total randomness and uncorrelated values (so-called "white noise") to that of strong regularity and predictable periodicity ("Brownian noise"). Constraints of space preclude an in-depth discussion each, and the reader is referred to other publications for a more extensive review of these analytical methods (46,50,64).

Poincaré plot is a graphical technique in which individual measures (m) are plotted against the next measure in the series (m + 1). If the variability is random in nature, no correlation should be expected between the two, and the graph resembles a "snowball." In a highly regular series of measures, on the other hand, a tight correlation will occur, with little deviation from a linear relationship (i.e., straight line). With fractal behavior an intermediate degree of correlation is expected, producing an ellipsoid spread of values.

The amount of the variability surrounding the line of identity on the graph provides, then, a means of estimating degree of connectiveness in the set of measures. This can be quantified by assessing the variability by SD1, the instantaneous standard deviation of values, and SD2, the standard deviation of long-term variability (reflecting the total amount of variability), which represent the minor and major axes of the ellipse, respectively. The ratio of SD1:SD2 is then a marker of the randomness of the variability of the measures. While elevated values indicate high randomness and low values regularity, the particular value of the SD1:SD2 ratio signifying healthy fractal behavior remains to be clarified and may depend on the physiological function under study.

Detrended fluctuation analysis (DFA) characterizes the pattern of variation in a data set across different scales of measurement, calculated with a computer algorithm. In a series of steps, the data are trended (summing the difference between the mean and individual values), and then analyzed for variability. Variability is then repeated for different group sizes, and variability is plotted as a function of the size of the group. On a log-log plot, this approach provides short- and long-term scaling exponents (the slope of the regression line) as α_1 and α_2, respectively. A value of 0.5 indicates random variability, while 1.5 reflects complete regularity. A scaling exponent of 1.0 is considered to signify bounded variability behavior.

Entropy analysis (by several different methods) defines the degree of irregularity or randomness of variability. This approach measures the frequency of occurrence of patterns in repetitive series, then identifies the differences in such frequencies in runs of values of length m with that of runs of length $m + 1$. By approximate entropy, for example, the similarity of repeated patterns of length m and $m + 1$ should be high in the presence of regularity, and this would result in smaller values. Higher values of approximate entropy therefore are consistent with randomness and disorder.

While not strictly speaking a measure of bounded variability, the *fractal dimension* is a calculated marker of the extent of the fractal nature (scale independence) of any series of measurements over time. Since the fractal characteristics of such a set of measurements is reflected in the degree of "connectives" in its values, the fractal dimension is also considered to serve as an indicator of bounded variability as well (19). A fractal dimension of 1.0 indicates a totally regular process, while 1.5 characterizes uncorrelated randomness. Bounded variability, then, should be expected to demonstrate a value between these two extremes.

Biological "Meaning" of Bounded Variability

But *why* this bounded variability of biological function? What is the explanation for the constant state of change that appears to be so essential for the effective function of biological activities? What is its "meaning"? Biologists have traditionally sought answers to these types of questions in the context of Darwinian natural selection. That is, functions which provide the opportunity for reproductive fitness persist, while those that fail to do so are "discarded" in the evolutionary process. But by what explanation—what evolutionary pressure—can this ubiquitous form of biological variability be viewed as a selective advantage for living beings?

No clear-cut answer to these queries has been forthcoming, but a number of concepts have been proposed. Many have concluded, for instance, that functional variability is an expression of the means by which such systems communicate and relate both within the individual elements of the system and in the coordination between systems (7,17,51). Consider the importance—indeed the necessity—that elements of the circulatory system (heart rate, myocardial function, vascular tone) communicate with each other to permit appropriate blood flow. Each of these elements must also communicate "vertically" with hierarchical subsystems (cellular energy systems, transmission of electrical signals) as well as "horizontally" with other systems (pulmonary, thermoregulatory) for essential physiological control (6).

Considering the "mind-numbing number" of such interactions within and between the cellular, tissue, organ, and whole-body levels (in fact, hundreds of billions), such communication represents a critical challenge for living beings (76). It has been suggested that functional variability by some means facilitates such "talk" within and between systems, providing the capacity to maintain regularity and physiological stability while permitting sufficient adaptability to respond effectively to the challenges of environmental insults. Coffey (7) summarized this concept:

> Living systems usually evolve towards a boundary between order and randomness [and] organisms and cells modulate the strength of the interaction with neighboring units to maximize their fitness. . . . If the interactions between the individual units are too strong, the network is ordered and rigid and contains little diversity in its ability to respond to changing states and to the environment. If the interactions are too weak, the system tends to disperse and becomes disorganized in behavior because of the lack of feedback between units. Dynamic variations in the degree of interaction between the individual units gives diversity to the collective network, which in turn provides the system with plasticity to rapidly adapt to changing environmental situations.

Alternatively, "fractal fluctuations have been explained in the context of so-called critical systems—systems undergoing a transition from one stable state to another" (51). As proposed by Pittman-Polletta et al.

> Fractal fluctuations are thus "the sound of the engine" of a healthy person. It is widely believed the rumble of the human engine represented by fractal fluctuations does not correspond to a single gear but rather a characteristic pattern of "gear shifts." When the physiological system "switches gears" dramatically—entering an entirely different control regime such as sleep or exercise—we can expect the pattern of fluctuations to change as well, as a different linkage of neurophysiological systems is put into play. . . . The pattern of changes is an indication of the underlying mechanisms—the pushes and pulls—that constitute the physiological system.
>
> *(51)*

Mitchell offered an explanation of bounded variability based on a necessary balance between random and deterministic fluctuations (41). The former, she proposed, represent stochastic physiological activity which serve as "trial balloons," while the latter reflect deterministic factors, presumably of genetic origin, that "select" the most appropriate functional activity for a given external or internal condition. So both randomness (to provide options) and determinism (to select the most appropriate to environmental conditions) are necessary. "Randomness must be balanced with determinism . . . maintaining a correct balance between these two modes of exploring is essential" (41).

Moreover, she has suggested that the balance between the two changes over time as the system "learns" from experience. "Early explorations, based on little or no information, are largely random and unfocused. As information is obtained and acted on, explorations gradually become more deterministic and focus in response to what has been perceived by the system" (41).

It is difficult to escape the conclusion that the nature of bounded variability is providing some important clues regarding the essence of living matter, reflected in its impact on human well-being. Still, just what that message entails remains obscure.

New Perspectives on Homeostasis

The reader with even a glancing knowledge of biology has by now recognized that the role of bounded variability in maintaining the efficiency of biological systems runs counter to the traditional concepts of *homeostasis* in supporting physiological equilibrium (5). According to the long-established viewpoint, the *milieu intérieur* is maintained by a multitude of controlling centers operating in feedback loops, whereby afferent signals provide incoming information on physiological variability which in a linear fashion trigger efferent signals to adjust the variable to an optimal level. As a consequence, body temperature, blood oxygen content, cellular pH, body water content, caloric intake, and the like are all maintained within very narrow ranges which are critical for body function. By this concept a minimization of variability to establish physiological stability is a central goal.

The recognition of the role of functional variability in maintaining physiological well-being has necessitated a re-appraisal of this traditional view of homeostatic control. In effect, in the non-linear real world of complex adaptive systems, fluctuations of physiological variables reflect a salutary influence rather than a threat to functional stability. In this way, the traditional homeostasis model is not consistent with contemporary views of physiological function, which are highly hierarchical, driven by fractal relationships, and correlated by non-linear rather than linear dynamics.

Vodovitz et al. have emphasized that "the concept of constancy of the internal environment is not meant to imply invariability. . . . Rather constancy implies dynamic characteristics, manifesting themselves in the form of 'homeostatic rhythms' rather than a 'homeostatic flat line'" (74). By this viewpoint, then, bounded time series variability reflects an expression of this dynamic homeostasis, which assumedly bears adaptive advantages of physiological resiliency and, by extension, optimizes human health and well-being.

West proposed that such variability permits "allometric control" of physiological function by responding to long-range changes or "memory" as manifest by its power law features (75). That is, such control works by superimposing the pattern of change in measures from the past onto present fluctuations in order to maintain physiological stability. By this interpretation, then, variability becomes a "friend" rather than a "foe," a form of physiological control which accommodates the need for coordination of the myriad of participating physiological networks involved in any particular biologic function (74).

Bounded Variability and Health

The driving factor in the growing interest in bounded variability derives from its recognized association with human disease. Early studies revealed that patients with heart disease demonstrated abnormal shifts in such variability as measured by fractal dimension (18). While the normal heart exhibits fractal variability in heart rate with a fractal dimension of 1.1–1.3, a patient with congestive heart failure has a value of approximately 1.0, indicating a high degree of regularity. On the other hand, an individual with atrial fibrillation was found to have a value of 1.5, typical of a shift to complete randomness. Such observations indicated that human disease can be associated with breakdown in normal bounded variability by shifts in opposite directions, that is, both toward complete loss of randomness or in the opposite extreme toward total regularity (75).

There followed, as West colorfully described it, a "parade of pathological phenomena" which exhibited loss of normal bounded variability (75). Depressed values of DFA (indicating increased randomness) have been reported with Huntington's disease (22), aging (18), Alzheimer's disease (29), and asthma (14). On the other hand, shifts toward greater regularity have been described with obstructive sleep apnea (47), Parkinson's disease (21), and epilepsy (56).

Among the many mysteries surrounding the nature and implications of physiological variability rests the question: How can such disturbances be associated with such a wide diversity of pathophysiologic processes (plaque formation in coronary artery disease, glucose intolerance with diabetes, etc.)? Assumedly the answer lies somewhere in its link to a base-level "common denominator" existing between these various disease processes—perhaps abnormal functional connectivity and communication, either "vertical" (between elements in a given system) and/or "horizontal" (between systems), mitochondrial dysfunction, or disturbed immunological function (44).

The extent that changes of bounded variability characteristics shift away from the expected intrinsic dynamics of healthy individuals simply reflects or, to the contrary, contributes to physiological dysfunction and human disease is unclear. The clinical importance of measures of variability may lie principally in their prognostic value. Changes in time series variability have proven predictive of serious heart arrhythmias (35), cardiac mortality (36), and deterioration of lung function in patients with pulmonary disease (14).

In summary, bounded variability is a form of time series variability which is characteristic of complex systems, sharing features of non-linear relationships and fractal scale independence. Bounded variability exhibits features of both random and regular (deterministic) fluctuations over time; its importance to healthy physiological function is evidenced by shifts of this balance observed in individuals with human disease. Current concepts of the nature and function of such variability challenge traditional models of homeostatic control which instead focus on minimization of variability. While many mysteries surround bounded variability, current research has provided sufficient clues to suggest that an understanding of physiologic variability may offer key insights into the nature and optimization of human health.

With these concepts in mind, the current empiric research observations of responses of bounded variability to both acute exercise and exercise training can be considered. Such exercise responses may serve as a useful model for extrinsic perturbation to biological systems, providing insights into the essential function of physiological variability as well as its role in optimizing physical performance.

Acute Exercise

Burggren and Monticino suggested that complex systems might possess the capability to alter their level of complexity in differing conditions of function, thereby distinguishing *kinetic* from *potential* physiological complexity (4):

> One might ask, is an automobile sitting silently in a garage only "potentially" complex until its engine is started and it is driven down the street? . . . If we fail to acknowledge the potential complexity of a poorly understood system, we then mistakenly view all physiological observations as reflecting the maximum complexity of that system. Not acknowledging the potential complexity of the system leads us to underestimate the complexity of its ultimate emergent behaviors. . . . Thus, while the complexity of well-understood systems seems obvious, how much potential complexity remains undiscovered until we make observations under new configurations of physiologically relevant conditions?

An examination of potential changes in bounded variability during exercise as a measurable "window" on the nature of complex systems may provide an opportunity to address this issue. Specifically, are the relative contributions of stochastic and deterministic variability altered when the intensity dial on the activity of biologic systems is turned up?

A second aspect of interest in responses of variability with exercise relates to mechanisms by which inherent fluctuations are linked to stability of physiological function. As reviewed above, by the traditional concept, physiological constancy critical to a stable *milieu intérieur* in matters such as body temperature, acid-base balance, and blood glucose levels is maintained by a central controller which detects external variation and adjusts levels to an optimal target value in a linear, feedback fashion. Such a model, however, is inconsistent with the current understanding of how complex biological systems work, which instead involves an intrinsic dynamic variability linked to physiological function by non-linear relationships. By this latter interpretation, then, there exists no fixed set point for particular physiological function but rather a dynamic variability that serves, by a means not yet well understood, to maintain a non-linear intra- and inter-coordination of complex adaptive systems. As West et al. have commented, "in this paradigm, the single scale steady state of homeostasis is replaced by a multiplicity of nonequilibrium states correlated over many scales" (77).

There exist, in fact, few events that create as great a global challenge to physiologic stability than a bout of progressive exercise to exhaustion. Rise in body temperature, fall in cellular pH, shifts in blood distribution, provisions for augmented cellular metabolism, hypoxemia, hypercarbia—these challenges must all be met by mechanisms to maintain physiological stability. Acute exercise therefore serves as an ideal model to examine changes in bounded variability which might prove insightful in deciphering the mechanisms by which these intrinsic biological fluctuations serve to maintain human well-being. It is not, then, without considerable interest that one examines studies which have demonstrated responses of bounded variability to exercise interventions.

West et al. measured heart rate and breathing interval variability during rest, moderate exercise, and exhaustive exercise on a cycle ergometer in 18 healthy adults (mean age 42 years), calculating the fractal dimension from the allometric relationship of mean and variability of aggregated values (77). Mean fractal dimension fell with increasing exercise intensity for heart beat interval (1.19 at rest $\rightarrow$ 1.05 $\rightarrow$ peak 1.02), breathing interval (1.33 $\rightarrow$ 1.29 $\rightarrow$ 1.19) and tidal volume (1.36 $\rightarrow$ 1.20 $\rightarrow$1.14).

These findings are consistent with an increased physiological regularity effected by progressively intense exercise work. Indeed, the fractal dimension of the heart beat interval reached unity at peak exercise, indicating a completely periodic activity. Noting that such a change is observed in pathological conditions (i.e., congestive heart failure) (18), the authors commented that "it remains to be seen whether the loss of variability seen here during exercise implies a similar adverse risk" (p. 231). As an alternative explanation, they suggested that "increased physiological demands at higher exercise rates reduce the individual's tolerance for it [and] in order to achieve the required increases in minute ventilation and cardiac output [during high intensity exercise], the organism may not be able to 'afford' the variability."

Other interpretations are possible. As will be discussed below, the shift toward regularity of variability in heart beat intervals with acute exercise might reflect the increase in sympathetic drive and circulating norepinephrine levels which accompany progressive exercise. Or, alternatively, an increased regularity with exercise might imply that the traditional linear model of homeostasis supersedes bounded variability when systems are assaulted by such an abundance of physiological perturbations.

Other reports have supported an effect of increased regularity in physiological variability of heart beat intervals in response to acute exercise. Mourot et al.

compared Poincaré plot findings in eight adult males at supine rest and during submaximal cycle exercise at a moderate work intensity (50% peak work rate) (42). With exercise, overall heart rate interval variability diminished, with a fall in SD1 from 30 to 9 and SD2 from 61 to 32, consistent with the dramatic decline observed in total power by HRV spectral analysis from 930 to 37. SD1/SD2 fell from 0.49 to 0.28, consistent with a shift of variability toward greater regularity.

In a similar study, Tulppo et al. examined Poincaré plots in response to maximal cycle exercise in 31 healthy subjects (73). Again, total power by HRV spectral analysis plummeted with exercise, falling from 1,700 and 500 at rest to barely measurable values in HF and LF power, respectively, with exercise. SD1 fell from 27 to 3 and SD2 from 85 to 3. In this study, however, SD1/SD2 rose, from 0.3 to 1.0.

Studies of bounded variability changes of heart beat interval in response to 30-second bouts of supra-maximal exercise (Wingate test), as well as single sessions of resistance exercise, have also indicated shifts toward greater predictability and periodicity. Mendonca et al. reported average increases of short-term DFA (α_1) on heart rate interval series immediately following a Wingate test from 0.84 to 1.26 in males and from 0.77 to 1.37 in females (38), mimicking similar changes described by Millar et al. (40) and Perkins et al. (48). In those two studies, in addition, average sample entropy fell from an average of 1.66 to 0.91 and from 1.49 to 0.70, respectively, following Wingate testing, indicative of increased regularity. Also, Heffernan et al. described a decline of values of sample entropy for heart rate from 1.56 pre-exercise to 1.37 in the immediate period following a bout of resistance exercise (15 sets of 10 repetitions at 75% 1-RM) (26).

On the other hand, other studies utilizing measures of DFA have demonstrated trends toward diminished regularity and greater randomness with increasing exercise intensity. Perkins et al. described a significant fall in α_1 after 45 minutes of cycle exercise at 63% of maximal heart rate, while α_2 showed no significant change (48). Values of sample entropy, however, declined from an average of 1.15 to 0.93, indicating increased regularity. Other studies utilizing a model of progressive exercise have reported a fall in α_1 (31,32). Karavita et al. described mean values of 1.37 at 30% of maximal work falling to 0.54 at 90% peak work (32).

In addition, other authors have described a biphasic response of bounded variability during a bout of progressive exercise (24,49,78). For example, Hautala et al. found that DFA α_1 rose from a mean value of 1.07 at rest to 1.50 at a cycle exercise intensity equivalent to 40% VO_2max, consistent with increasing periodicity and regularity (24). As workload further increased, however, α_1 steadily declined, reaching 0.58 at maximal exercise (heart rate averaging 160 bpm), a value associated with a high degree of randomness. Sandercock and Brodie hypothesized that "the biphasic responses of certain non-linear measures may indeed represent the number of inputs impinging on the SA node" (62).

Perhaps the only reasonable conclusions one can draw from these studies is that an episode of progressive exercise can be expected to a) diminish significantly the overall quantity of biological variability and b) alter the pattern of heart rate time series variability. Just how these two observations can be interpreted in light of the contrast of new concepts of allometric versus that of traditional homeostasis is not immediately obvious.

The observation that an acute bout of exercise can shift the nature of bounded variability in opposite directions—toward both increased randomness as well as greater regularity—mimics the same finding in pathological states. As described above, findings in the research literature are mixed with a shift to increased regularity of variability in some chronic illnesses (Parkinson's disease, congestive heart failure) but change toward increased randomness in others (asthma, Alzheimer's disease).

One hesitates to label acute exercise as "pathologic," but, in fact, such exercise does create stresses that involve tissue microdamage, particularly of the musculo-skeletal system. In essence, an acute bout of exercise is a *catabolic* event, with disruption of structural and functional protein as well as reduction of energy stores (65). Adaptive changes in response to such stress serve as the traditional model for physiological and performance improvements resulting from a period of athletic training. Excessive exercise, on the other hand, can cause more significant damage in the form of overuse injuries. The alternative directional changes in bounded variability reported with exercise may reflect—as they do with disease states—a generic reaction of such variability to stress or malfunction.

In examining the outcomes of the studies reviewed above it is difficult to ignore the possibility that such findings might reflect the metric in any particular investigation utilized to assess bounded variability. Indeed, each form of analysis is subject to certain conditions, including *stationarity* (stability of the function over the measurement period), size of data set, sampling frequency, elimination of artifact, and effect of respirations and body position, the violation of which can compromise accuracy in defining connectiveness in time series measurements (64). Certain inconsistencies evidence the empirically derived responses of measures of such variability to acute bouts of physical exercise.

Autonomic Influence on Bounded Variability

Based on sympathetic/parasympathetic blocking studies, some have considered these changes in bounded variability outlined above as reflections of the changing balance of autonomic influences on the sinus node during increasing work intensity (73,80). Effects of atropine on non-linear heart rate variability indicate that parasympathetic activity is associated with increasing randomness of time series variability (73,80). On the other hand, no link appears to exist with sympathetic activity, since beta-blockade has no effect of variability (79), and no relationship has been observed with indicators of bounded variability and direct measurement of sympathetic nervous activity (72).

Porta et al. (53) examined the influence of autonomic tone on measures of bounded variability by placing subjects in a head-up tilt position, a maneuver which triggers sympathetic activity. Approximate entropy and sample entropy measures of time series heart beat intervals were recorded at supine rest in 17 healthy subjects ages 21–54 years and then at progressive tilts of 15, 30, 45, 60, 75, and 90 degrees. "Corrected" approximate entropy and sample entropy fell progressively as a function of the tilt angle, indicating an increased regularity of variability. This the authors attributed "a progressive shift of the sympathovagal balance toward sympathetic prominence" as evidence that bounded variability is under the control of the autonomic nervous system.

As noted previously, the high frequency band identified by standard HRV spectral analysis is linked to respirations (sinus arrhythmia), supporting a role of vagal (parasympathetic) influence on both variables. In respect to bounded variability, however, Yamamoto et al. (78) could find no statistically significant correlation between fractal measures of respiratory and heart beat interval fluctuations in resting subjects. Similarly, in the report of West et al. (77) noted above, in which fractal dimension decreased in both respiratory and heart beat intervals with progressive exercise, no correlation was observed between the two. These findings suggest that factors other than autonomic balance are important in establishing patterns of bounded variability in such measures at rest and during exercise.

Other Measures

The responses of fractal variability to these different modes of exercise has involved almost entirely heart beat (R-R wave electrocardiographic) intervals. Few other parameters have yet been described. In an unpublished study Biltz et al. performed a sample entropy analysis comparing responses of respiratory exchange ratio (RER, calculated as VCO_2/VO_2, a measure of the relative contributions of fat and carbohydrate to energy substrate utilization) over five minutes of cycling at an intensity of 50W in groups of lean and obese children. When matched for RER, sample entropy values were 2.19 and 1.42 for the lean and obese subjects, respectively, and sample entropy score correlated with percent body fat ($r = -0.42$, $p = 0.049$). These findings suggest that the variability pattern of RER can provide information regarding metabolic state, and in this study revealed a relative inflexibility of this measure in young obese subjects.

Responses to Exercise Training

According to the stress adaptation syndrome model of Selye (65), training-induced improvements in physiological function and physical performance occur consequent to positive adaptive responses to the repetitive stresses of acute bouts of exercise. Given the above observations of measures of bounded variability to the latter, it is of interest to examine similar metrics following a period of exercise training.

Information regarding alterations of bounded variability heart beat intervals in response to exercise training is limited. Heffernan et al. measured DFA α_1 at rest in 34 healthy men ages 18–30 years before and after a six-week program of resistance training (25). Following a control period and training, no significant changes in mean values were observed (1.01 ± 0.06 → 0.98 ± 0.06 → 0.93 ± 0.04, respectively). However, when the subjects were clustered retrospectively into groups with initial high and low values, α_1 decreased as a result of the training in the former and increased in the latter, both approximating 1.0 as an indication of optimal fractal variability.

Given these findings, the authors suggested that resistance training might possibly be utilized as a means of "improving clinical outcomes in select patient populations" (25). Extending such speculation, could optimizing the balance in variability between connectiveness and flexibility serve as a mechanism by which physical activity contributes to human health (44)? Future research efforts might well be directed to answer this question.

Karavirta et al. randomized older men (ages 40–67 years) into endurance training, strength training, combined endurance and strength training, and control non-training groups (32). Following a 21-week training period, no significant change in DFA α_1 was observed in any of the groups except for a decrease in those who underwent combined strength and resistance training (1.18 ± 0.20 → 1.11 ± 0.21). The authors suggested that discrepancies in these findings compared to those of Heffernan et al. might be explained by the differences in subject ages.

Mourot et al. described Poincaré plots in eight subjects after a short-term period of endurance training (42). Patterns post-training resembled those before training, but an increased scatter was evident as a training outcome, interpreted by the authors as a manifestation of enhanced parasympathetic activity. That conclusion was supported by an additional cross-sectional comparison of eight highly trained subjects which disclosed a similar wide scatter. SD1/SD2 values at rest were 0.49, 0.59, and 0.66 for the pre-training, post-training, and highly trained subjects, respectively.

In an unpublished study, researchers at the University of Minnesota measured sample entropy for RER as well as respiratory tidal volume in 25 college-age subjects who were training for participation in a marathon race. Average maximal oxygen uptake (VO_2max) rose from 49.5 ± 6.8 to 53.6 ± 6.7 ml kg^{-1} min^{-1} with training. Sample entropy for RER at rest increased from 0.79 ± 0.38 to 1.01 ± 0.27 ($p = 0.03$) and for tidal volume from 1.17 ± 0.25 to 1.29 ± 0.23 ($p = 0.03$), indicating a trend toward greater regularity as an outcome of endurance training.

It should be emphasized that all these studies have assessed responses of bounded variability to exercise training with subjects at rest (as in the analogy of Burggren and Monticino, "sitting silently in a garage" rather than "driven down the street" [4]). More insightful would be studies in which responses of bounded variability are recorded to the stresses imposed by a bout of acute exercise before and following a period of exercise training.

Gait Dynamics

During a walk or run at a constant speed the interval between one's strides, as well as the stride length, would appear to remain entirely regular, or metronomic. The amount of variation among strides is very small, with coefficients of variation from 1% to 4% (30), and biomechanists have considered models of such rhythmic motor behavior as that of a harmonic oscillator conforming to the regularity of pendular motion (28). In fact, however, close analysis reveals a constant fluctuation of these measures over time which exhibit long-range correlations characteristic of bounded variability. These observations have prompted interest in such variability in gait dynamics as a means of better understanding neurological disturbances of gait in the elderly and in patients with degenerative diseases (18).

Hausdorff et al. (23) found mean values of the DFA scaling exponent *a* to be 0.98 ± 0.07, 0.90 ± 0.04, and 0.97 ± 0.05 for stride interval when healthy subjects walked at slow, normal, and fast walking speeds, respectively. The smaller value at the normal walking rate was significantly different, indicating a trend toward decreased regularity when pace was self-selected.

Jordan et al. extended these observations to stride interval dynamics during treadmill running in eight young adults (30). Subjects ran at speeds of 80%, 90%, 100%, 110%, and 120% of a preferred running speed (PRS). Measures of *a* by DFA in respect to speed approximated a U-shaped curve, with values falling from 0.86 at 80% PRS to a nadir of 0.73 at 100% PRS and then a small statistically insignificant rise to 0.76 at faster speeds. That is, variability was most random at PRS and demonstrated trends toward greater regularity when speeds deviated from the PRS.

West interpreted such findings as indicating that speeds of locomotion slower or faster than self-selected, "most comfortable" speeds constitute a "biological stress" which increases strength of long-range correlations and produces greater regularity in physiological variability (75). Such observations might be considered consistent with findings that preferred running or walking speeds correspond to that of greatest energy efficiency (59). Too, such explanations resemble those which would interpret greater regularity of variability with increasing work intensity during acute exercise (as noted above) as an expression of augmented physiological stress.

Bounded variability in gait dynamics is altered when neuromuscular function is deranged. Hausdorff et al. (22) reported that a group of patients with Huntington's disease (a degenerative central nervous system disorder) demonstrated a scaling exponent α of 0.60 ± 0.24 for gait interval compared to an average of 0.88 ± 0.17 in healthy control individuals. Moreover, these authors found that the severity of the disease increased inversely with the scaling exponent, suggesting that disease progression is reflected in a reduction in regularity of variability of stride interval.

Analysis of gait variability from a dynamic systems perspective may provide practical information for competitive athletes (8,20,54). For example, Fuller et al. (15) found a reduction in DFA α among runners wearing minimalist compared to conventional footwear. They proposed that "the reduced variability and self-similarity observed for runners in the minimalist shoe may be suggestive of a system that is less flexible and more prone to injury."

Complex Systems and Exercise Fatigue

Despite decades of research efforts, the specific factor(s) which determines exercise-limiting fatigue remains elusive. Many candidate variables have been identified—each supported by research findings—yet how these might fit into a cohesive explanatory picture remains the "holy grail" for exercise scientists. There are indications that exercise fatigue is most appropriately viewed in the context of complex systems. As such, fatigue may be best regarded as an emergent quality arising from the interactions of metabolic, biochemical, and musculoskeletal systems.

Such a conclusion is supported by the observation that the relationship between work intensity and time to exhaustion on a physical task is a non-linear one. That is, a plot of the length of time that a bout of exercise can be tolerated to the point of exhaustion against work intensity describes a hyperbolic curve which, for example, is allometrically expressed for road racing as

$$V = aD^b$$

Where V is run velocity, D is the race distance, b is the scaling exponent, and a is a constant (60). Shorter races are run at a greater speed, but the relationship between the two is not linear, and the hyperbolic curve describing this link is "created by the factor or factors that constrain and define exercise performance" (60). This non-linear relationship has been reported in other domains of exercise performance as well, including swimming (27), cycling (12), and isometric exercise (70).

Variability in complex systems has been considered in the model of exercise fatigue based on the *central governor hypothesis*. The latter holds that within the central nervous system exists a controlling mechanism which subconsciously limits physical exercise with the goal of preventing catastrophic consequences (hyperthermia, myocardial failure, cardiac arrhythmias, skeletal muscle tetany, bone fractures) which would pose risk to excessive physical exertion (45). According to this model, the brain imposes this safety limit by a) reducing central command—decreasing signals descending in the spinal cord which control strength of skeletal muscle contractions, and b) creating the familiar unpleasant sensations of fatigue—breathlessness, dizziness, nausea, muscle weakness—which make further exercise effort intolerable. In this way, exercise-limiting fatigue is viewed as a *sensation* created by a guardian central nervous system, rather than entirely as a physiological state.

Still, physiological and metabolic factors (such as respiratory rate, blood pH, core temperature) remain critical determinants of performance in this model as providing the information basis by which the brain regulates safe level of muscular work. This regulation comes into play, for example, during competitive distance events. The central governor, based on past experience, physiological input, and environmental conditions "selects" the proper pace to deliver the athlete to the finish line with the greatest amount of muscular work over time that is safe for that particular distance (61). St. Clair Gibson and Noakes (67) have viewed bounded variability within this process as an expression of the interaction of complex adaptive systems:

> A complex non-linear dynamic system therefore requires a deterministic control mechanism and a fluctuating environment in order to generate alternating or oscillatory changes in physiological variables. During exercise the desire to reach the end point in the fastest time would be the deterministic control, and the fluctuating environment would be provided by changes in both the external environment and the internal physiological milieu.

These authors point to studies indicating variability of muscular work during the course of exercise as evidence of "non-linear oscillations of exercise intensity caused by oscillations in the number of motor units that are allowed to be recruited by the central regulator in the subconscious brain" (67). For example, Tucker et al. recorded the power output every 200 m in 11 trained cyclists performing a self-paced 20-km time trial (71). The fractal characteristic of the bounded variability exhibited by these measures was demonstrated by a calculated fractal dimension ranging from 1.5 to 1.9.

Such fluctuations in power output could also reflect a) the interaction of the multiple complex systems involved in physical effort, especially as they communicate with a central controller, and/or b) the changing afferent information being received by the central governor from the physiologic and metabolic alterations occurring with exercise. The latter, it has been proposed, may cause oscillations as an expression of a time lag before effective efferent actions to maintain homeostasis can be effected during exercise (33).

Concluding Comments

Variability of physiologic function is intrinsic to biological systems. The biologic basis and implications of these fluctuations—and how to best measure them—remain to be fully deciphered. However, current research data suggest that within the nature of this variability lie important insights into the essential nature of living matter as well as specific mechanisms which sustain human physiological well-being.

The current understanding of the effects of exercise on bounded variability can be best characterized as embryonic. Still, sufficient clues are evident in the extant research literature to suggest that much may be gained from greater insights into how the stresses of exercise—as a key model of challenge to physiological stability—impact fluctuations in biological processes.

Bounded variability is an expression of the reality of complex systems, typified by fractal relationships, hierarchical structure, and non-linear dynamics. Disturbances of physiological function (human disease) and response of these functions to external perturbation (exercise) must be sought within the context of this "new reality." Much remains to be learned:

- How do alterations observed in bounded variability in response to perturbations created by exercise reflect the function of homeostatic mechanisms aimed at maintaining physiologic stability?
- What metrics are most appropriate for examining changes in variability occurring with exercise?
- To what extent do such changes in variability under the stresses of exercise reflect cause or effect of functional responses of complex adaptive systems?
- To what utility can an understanding of variability and its responses to exercise serve health care providers, athletes, and exercise scientists?

References

1. Bassingthwaighte JB, Liebovitch LS, West BJ. *Fractal Physiology*. Oxford: Oxford University Press; 1994.
2. Bigger JT, Fleiss JL, Steinman RC, Rolnitzky LM, Kleiger RE, Rottman JN. Frequency domain measures of heart period variability and mortality after myocardial infarction. *Circulation*. 1992;85:164–171.
3. Brown JH, Gupta VJ, Li B-L, Milne BT, Restrepo C, West GB. The fractal nature of nature: power laws, ecological complexity, and biodiversity. *Phil Trans R Soc Lond*. 2002;357:619–626.
4. Burggren WW, Monticino MG. Assessing physiological complexity. *J Exp Biol*. 2005;208:3221–3232.
5. Cannon WB. Organization for physiological homeostasis. *Physiol Rev*. 1929;9:399–431.
6. Cerutti S, Hoyer D, Voss A. Multiscale, multiorgan and multivariate complexity analyses of cardiovascular regulation. *Phil Trans R Soc*. 2009;367:1337–1358.
7. Coffey DS. Self-organization, complexity and chaos: the new biology for medicine. *Nature Med*. 1998;4:882–885.
8. Davids K, Glazier P, Araujo D, Bartlett R. Movement systems as dynamical systems. *Sports Med*. 2003;33:245–260.
9. Dong J-G. The role of heart rate variability in sports physiology. *Exper Ther Med*. 2016;11:1531–1536.

10. Esquirol Y, Perret B, Ruidavets JB, et al. Shift work and cardiovascular risk factors: new knowledge form the past decade. *Arch Cardiovasc Dis.* 2011;104:636–668.
11. Evans JA, Davidson AJ. Health consequences of circadian disruption in humans and animal models. *Prog Molec Biol Transplant Science.* 2013;119:283–323.
12. Fawkner SJ, Armstrong NA. Assessment of critical power with children. *Pediatr Exerc Science.* 2002;14:259–268.
13. Foster RG, Kreitzman G. *The Rhythm of Life.* New Haven, CT: Yale University Press; 2004.
14. Frey U, Brodbeck T, Majumdar A, et al. Risk of severe asthma episodes predicated from fluctuation analysis of airway function. *Nature.* 2005;438:667–670.
15, Fuller JT, Amado A, van Emmerik RE, et al. The effect of footwear and footfall pattern on running stride interval long-range correlations and distributional variability. *Gait Posture.* 2016;44:137–142.
16. Gisiger T. Scale invariance in biology: coincidence or footprint of a universal mechanism? *Biol Rev.* 2001;76:161–209.
17. Glass L. Synchronization and rhythmic processes in physiology. *Nature.* 2001; 410:277–284.
18. Goldberger AL, Amaral LAN, Haussdorff JM, Ivanov PC, Peng C-K, Stanley HE. Fractal dynamics in physiology: alterations with disease and aging. *PNAS.* 2002;99 Suppl 1:2466–2472.
19. Goldberger AL, Rigney, West BJ. Chaos and fractals in human physiology. *Scientific American.* 1990; February:43–49.
20. Hamill J, Van Emmerik REA, Heiderscheit BC, Li L. A dynamical approach to lower extremity running injuries. *Clin Biomech.* 199;14:297–308.
21. Hausdorff JM. Gait dynamics in Parkinson's disease: common and distinct behavior among stride length, gait variability, and fractal-like scaling. *Chaos.* 2009;19:026113.
22. Hausdorff JM, Mitchell SL, Firtion R, et al. Altered fractal dynamics of gait: reduced stride interval correlations with aging and Huntington's disease. *J Appl Physiol.* 1997;82:262–269.
23. Hausdorff JM, Purdon PL, Peng C-K, Ladin Z, Wei JY, Goldberger AL. Fractal dynamics of human gait: stability of long-range correlations in stride interval fluctuations. *J Appl Physiol.* 1996;80:1448–1457.
24. Hautala AJ, Makikallio TH, Seppanen T, Huikuri HV, Tulppo MP. Short-term correlation properties of R-R interval dynamics at different exercise intensity levels. *Clin Physiol Func Imaging.* 2003;23:215–223.
25. Heffernan KS, Sosnoff JJ, Fahs CA, Shinsako KK, Jae SY, Fernhall B. Fractal scaling properties of heart rate dynamics following resistance exercise training. *J Appl Physiol.* 2008;105:109–113.
26. Heffernan KS, Sosnoff JJ, Jae SY, Gates CJ, Fernhall B. Acute resistance exercise reduces heart rate complexity and increases QTc interval. *Int J Sports Med.* 2008;29:289–293.
27. Hill DW, Steward RP, Lane CJ. Application of the critical power concept to young swimmers. *Pediatr Exerc Science.* 1995;7:281–293.
28. Holt KG, Hamill J, Andres RO. The force-driven harmonic oscillator as a model for human locomotion. *Hum Movement Science.* 1990;9:55–68.
29. Hu K, VanHu K, Van Someren EJW, Shea SA, Scheer FAJL. Reduction of scale invariance of activity fluctuation with aging and Alzheimer's disease: involvement of the circadian pacemaker. *Proc Nat Acad Sci USA.* 2009;106:2490–2494.
30. Jordan K, Challis JH, Newell KM. Long range correlations in the stride interval of running. *Gait Posture.* 2006;24:120–125.

31. Karasik R, Sapir N, Ashkenazy Y, et al. Correlation differences in heartbeat fluctuations during rest and exercise. *Phys Rev*. 2002;66:e062902.
32. Karavirta L, Tulppo, Laaksonen DE, et al. Heart rate dynamics after combined endurance and strength training in older men. *Med Sci Sports Exerc*. 2009;41:1436–1443.
33. Lambert EV, St Clair Gibson A, Noakes TD. Complex systems model of fatigue: integrative homeostatic control of peripheral physiological systems during exercise in humans. *Br J Sports Med*. 2005;39:52–62.
34. Liebovitch LS, Scheurle D. Two lessons from fractals and chaos. *Complexity*. 2000;5:34–43.
35. Makikallio TH, Koistinen J, Jordeans L, Tulpollo MP, Wood N, Golosarsky B. Heart rate dynamics before spontaneous onset of ventricular fibrillation in patients with healed myocardial infarcts. *Am J Cardiol*. 1999;83:880–884.
36. Makikallio TH, Hoiber S, Kober L, Torp-Petersen C, Peng C-K, Goldberger AL. Fractal analysis of heart rate dynamics as a predictor of mortality in patients with depressed left ventricular function after acute myocardial infarction. *Am J Cardiol*. 1999;83:836–839.
37. Mendonca GV, Fernhall B, Heffernan KS, Pereira FD. Spectral methods of heart rate variability analysis during dynamic exercise. *Clin Auton Res*. 2009;19:237–245.
38. Mendonca GV, Heffernan KS, Rossow L, Guerra M, Pereira FD, Fernhall B. Sex differences in linear and nonlinear heart rate variability during early recovery from supramaximal exercise. *Appl Physiol Nutr Metab*. 2010;35:439–446.
39. Mesarovic MD, Sreenath SN, Keene JD. Search for organising principles: understanding in systems biology. *Sys Biol*. 2004;1:19–27.
40. Millar PJ, Rakobowchuk M, McCartney N, MacDonald MJ. Heart rate variability and nonlinear analysis of heart rate dynamics following single and multiple Wingate bouts. *Appl Physiol Nutr Metab*. 2009;34:875–883.
41. Mitchell M. *Complexity: A Guided Tour*. Oxford: Oxford University Press; 2009.
42. Mourot L, Bouhaddi M, Perry S, Roullon J-D, Regnard J. Quantitative Poincaré plot analysis of heart rate variability: effect of endurance training. *Eur J Appl Physiol*. 2004;91:79–87.
43. Nagy AD, Reddy AB. Time dictates: emerging clinical analyses of the impact of circadian rhythms on diagnosis, prognosis and treatment of disease. *Clin Med*. 2015;15:s50–s53.
44. Neufer PD, Bamman MM, Muoio DM, et al. Understanding the cellular and molecular mechanisms of physical activity-induced health benefits. *Cell Metab*. 2015;224–211.
45. Noakes TD, St Clair Gibson A, Lambert EV. From catastrophe to complexity: a novel model of integrative central neural regulation of effort and fatigue during exercise in humans. *Br J Sports Med*. 2004;38:511–514.
46. Peng CK, Havlin S, Stanley HE, Goldberger AL. Quantification of scaling exponents and crossover phenomena in nonstationary heartbeat time series. *Chaos*. 1995;5:82–87.
47. Penzel T, Kantelhardt JW, Grote L, Peter JH, Bunde A. Comparison of detrended fluctuation analysis and spectral analysis for heart rate variability in sleep and sleep apnea. *IEE Eng Med Biol Soc*. 2003;50:1143–1151.
48. Perkins SE, Jelinek HF, Al-Aubaidy HA, de Jong B. Immediate and long term effects of endurance and high intensity interval exercise on linear and nonlinear heart rate variability. *J Sci Med Sport*. 2017;20:312–316.
49. Perkiomaki JS, Zareba W, Badilini F, Moss AJ. Influence of atropine on fractal and complexity measures of heart rate variability. *Ann Noninvasive Electrocardiol*. 2002;7:326–331.
50. Pincus SM. Approximate entropy as a measure of system complexity. *Proc Natl Acad Sci*. 1991;88:2297–2301.

51. Pittman-Polleta BR, Scheer FAJL, Butler MP, Shea SA, Hu K. The role of the circadian system in fractal neurophysiological control. *Biol Rev Camb Philos Soc.* 2013;88:873–894.
52. Plews DJ, Laursen PB, Stanly J, Kilding AE, Buchheit M. Training adaptation and heart rate variability in elite endurance athletes: opening the door to effective monitoring. *Sports Med.* 2013;43:773–781.
53. Porta A, Gnecchi-Ruscone T, Tobaldini E, Guzzetti S, Furlan R, Montano N. Progressive decrease of heart period variability entropy-based complexity during graded head-up tilt. *J Appl Physiol.* 2007;103:1143–1149.
54. Preatoni E, Hamill J, Harrison AJ, et al. Movement variability and skills monitoring in sports. *Sports Biomech.* 2013;12:69–92.
55. Preuβner M, Heyd F. Post-translational control of the mammalian circadian clock: implications for health and disease. *Pflugers Arch.* 2016;468:983–991.
56. Ramon C, Holmes MD, Freeman WJ, McElroy R, Rezvanian E. Comparative analysis of temporal dynamics of EEG and phase synchronization of EEG to localize epileptic sites from high density sleep EEG interictal recordings. *Conf Proc IEEE Eng Biol Soc.* 2008;45:48–50.
57. Reilly T, Atkinson G, Gregson W, Forsyth J, Edwards B, Waterhouse J. Some chronological considerations related to physical exercise. *Clin Ther.* 2006;157:249–264.
58. Rickles D, Hawe P, Shiell A. A simple guide to chaos and complexity. *J Epidemiol Comm Health.* 2007;61:933–937.
59. Rowland T. *Children's Exercise Physiology.* Champaign, IL: Human Kinetics; 2005. p. 153.
60. Rowland T. Thoughts on a hyperbolic curve. *Pediatr Exerc Science.* 2007;19:1–5.
61. Rowland T. *The Athlete's Clock.* Champaign, IL: Human Kinetics; 2011. pp. 95–125.
62. Sandercock GRH, Brodie DA. The use of heart rate variability measures to assess autonomic control during exercise. *Scand J Med Sci Sports.* 2006;16:302–313.
63. Schmitt L, Regnard J, Desmares M, et al. Fatigue shifts and scatters heart rate variability in elite endurance athletes. *PLoS ONE.* 2013;8:e71588.
64. Seely AJE, Macklem PT. Complex systems and the technology of variability analysis. *Crit Care.* 2004;8:R367–R384.
65. Selye H. *The Stress of Life.* New York: McGraw Hill; 1976. pp. 5–45.
66. Shaffer F, McCraty R, Zerr CL. A healthy heart is not a metronome: an integrative review of the heart's anatomy and heart rate variability. *Front Psychol.* 2014;5:1040.
67. St. Clair Gibson A, Noakes TD. Evidence for complex system integration and dynamic neural regulation of skeletal muscle recruitment during exercise in humans. *Br J Sports Med.*
68. Strauss HM. Heart rate variability. *Am J Physiol Regul Integr Comp Physiol.* 2003; 285:R927–R931.
69. Thamrin C, Stern G, Frey U. Fractals for physicians. *Paediatr Resp Rev.* 2010;11:123–131.
70. Townsend MS. *Mathematics in Sports.* Chichester: Ellis Horwood Ltd.; 1984. pp. 84–85.
71. Tucker R, Bester A, Lambert EV, Noakes TD, Vaughan CL, St. Clair Gibson A. Non-random fluctuations in power output during self-paced exercise. *Br J Sports Med.* 2006;40:912–917.
72. Tulppo MP, Kiviniemi AM, Hautala AJ, et al. Physiological background of the loss of fractal heart rate dynamics. *Circulation.* 2005;112:314–319.
73. Tulppo MP, Makikallio TH, Takala TE, Seppanen T, Huikuri HV. Quantitative beat-to-beat analysis of heart rate dynamics during exercise. *Am J Physiol.* 1996;271:H244–H252.
74. Vodovitz Y, An G, Androulaskis IP. A systems engineering perspective on homeostasis and disease. *Front Bioeng Biotech.* 2013;1:1–8.

75. West BJ. *Where Medicine Went Wrong: Rediscovering the Path to Complexity*. Singapore: World Scientific; 2006.
76. West BJ. Fractal physiology and the fractional calculus: a perspective. *Front Physiol.* 2010;1:1–17.
77. West BJ, Griffin LA, Frederick HJ, Moon RE. The independently fractal nature of respiration and heart rate during exercise under normobaric and hyperbaric conditions. *Resp Physiol Neurobiol.* 2005;145:219–233.
78. Yamamoto Y, Fortrat JO, Hughson RL. On the fractal nature of heart rate variability in humans: effects of respiratory sinus arrhythmia. *Am J Physiol.* 1995;269:H480–H486.
79. Yamamoto Y, Hughson RL. On the fractal nature of heart rate variability in humans: effects of data length and beta-adrenergic blockade. *Am J Physiol.* 1994;266:R40–R49.
80. Yamamoto Y, Nakamura Y, Sato H, Yamamoto M, Kato K, Hughson RL. On the fractal nature of heart rate variability in humans: effects of vagal blockade. *Am J Physiol.* 1995;269:R830–R837.
81. Zuurbier LA, Luik AI, Hofman A, et al. Fragmentation of circadian activity rhythms predicts mortality: the Rotterdam Study. *Am J Epidemiol.* 2015;181:54–63.

5

WHAT CAUSED THE DISTURBING COLLAPSE OF THIS YOUNG ATHLETE?

We sat together in my office and watched the video that his parents had taken at the finish line. For the Western Massachusetts high school cross-country championships there was quite a large crowd of spectators, presumably due to the unusually warm New England November afternoon. As the winner approached the finish line we could see Scott closing rapidly in second place under a full head of steam. He looked strong, I thought, with powerful strides and a look of grim determination on his face. But then, about 30 yards from the finish, he suddenly began to stagger, side to side, and crumpled to the ground, his arms flying out to the side. After what seemed like a rather long pause, his coach ran out to Scott's prone, apparently lifeless body. Here the video ended, as his father had obviously dropped the camera in his alarm.

"Scott," I asked. "What were you feeling when this happened?"

"I don't know. The last thing I remember is chasing the back of that Amherst runner as we neared the finish."

I turned to his parents. "What did the coach tell you he was like when he reached him?"

"He said he was very groggy and dazed, and that he was speaking incoherently."

"So, we don't actually know if he lost consciousness or not. What happened then?"

"They called an ambulance and took him to the hospital emergency room in Greenfield."

"What was he like when you saw him there?"

"He seemed very tired, but other than that he was fully conscious and speaking normally, although very slowly. They couldn't find anything wrong with him."

I could read the torment of the parents' anxiety in their eyes.

"We just don't understand. This kind of thing never happened to him before. He's played all sorts of sports—he's very talented that way—and he had been running cross-country for four years. At first when he was a freshman he didn't do so well, but now in his senior year he really had blossomed. We thought he had a good chance to win the championship that day. And he's always been in good health. In fact, he had been cleared to run after his usual pre-participation evaluation that you performed last summer."

This was true. His visit at that time had revealed no problems by my history or physical examination. To be safe, I had even performed an electrocardiogram, which was completely normal. "I seem to remember that it was really quite warm that day. Had Scott hydrated before the race?"

"Yes, it was about 70 degrees, which was unusual, but he had been used to running in the heat. And we had Scott drink a bottle of sports drink just before the start."

"Scott, did you feel anything just before this collapse? Like chest pain, dizziness, tingling of your fingers, or difficulty breathing? And had you been feeling unwell at all that day, like a cold or upset stomach, something like that? Were you taking medications for anything?"

"The answer is 'no' to all those questions."

"So, Doctor, Scott has basketball tryouts next week. Is he going to be able to play?"

There is probably not a primary care physician who at some point in their career will not be confronted with a story like this one—a vigorous, ostensibly healthy young athlete who collapses during competition or practice, surrounded by uncertain details beyond the subjective observations of stunned on-lookers. The physician charged with untangling this mystery recognizes that by far most such events are caused by factors that are benign and readily remedied—dehydration from insufficient fluid intake, hyperthermia, "vagal" responses, post-exercise venous pooling of blood in the legs. Yet, the disturbing point is that such episodes of collapse can signal—in a very small percentage of cases—the existence of cardiac conditions which can serve as a substrate for sudden death, conditions which, when identified, would preclude future sports participation. And, unhappily, in not a small percentage of cases no clear-cut etiology for an athlete's collapse is uncovered despite an extensive clinical evaluation. And that leaves some important questions unanswered. Certainly, *something* led to the collapse. Was a cardiac risk factor for sudden death missed in the evaluation? Were the laboratory tests misleading or misinterpreted? Should the evaluation be repeated? And—bottom line—is it safe for the athlete to resume sports play?

Traditionally, the diagnostic approach to such events is based on an *algorithmic* approach, a decision-making tree whose branch points are determined by the information gathered regarding a) the history of the episode (i.e., what happened), b) findings on the physical examination by the physician, and c) the outcomes of any laboratory and diagnostic tests subsequently ordered. To start with, the first decision point involves an appraisal of the apparent seriousness of the episode. A linebacker complaining of transient dizziness during two-a-day drills in August practice sessions is not likely to warrant much diagnostic attention. On the other hand, an overt syncopal collapse with accompanying seizure activity during a basketball game would clearly deserve a comprehensive assessment. The case of Scott's collapse would probably fit in the latter category. Still, he might have simply stumbled while driving hard to the finish, causing him to strike his head on falling, this being responsible for his concussion-like signs and symptoms (confusion, incoherence, fatigue, etc.).

In the decision-making tree, certain pieces of information can be highly insightful. For instance, many of the cardiac causes of sudden collapse are inherited; thus, recognizing that a first-degree family member suffers from such a condition would obviously prompt a full cardiac evaluation. If the collapse occurred before the finish (as in Scott's case) one can eliminate benign venous pooling that occurs in the legs following immediate cessation of running as a possibility. A report of tingling of the fingers in a highly competitive situation raises the possibility of syncope secondary to hyperventilation (more on this later).

Following an algorithm thus provides a formal, orderly, seemingly objective means of establishing a diagnosis. So much so that, in fact, one could conclude that this is a process that could be readily conducted by a well-informed computer. Unfortunately, as every physician knows, life is not that simple. In the real world of the practice of medicine such an organized approach to diagnosis is not infrequently complicated by ambiguities, uncertainties, and problematic outcomes that cloud a confident concluding diagnosis and clinical outcomes. A number of examples will become obvious in the discussion of diagnostic possibilities for collapse in the sections that follow.

Now what was once a reasonably objective assessment of possible causes for collapse becomes a more subjective matter of individual physician judgment. How important can information be considered from the events and conditions surrounding the collapse? How much of a diagnostic workup should be performed? How should ambiguous laboratory findings be interpreted? And, ultimately, can this athlete safely return to play?

Physicians are, in fact, human beings, and such judgments can be strongly colored by their individual experience and personality characteristics (53). Consider how such an evaluation and decision-making would be altered by a young physician who just last month had a young patient, cleared for sports play, who died suddenly on the football field from occult heart disease, compared to the judgments of a 65-year-old experienced practitioner who has never had such an unfortunate experience. Likewise, how aggressive would be the diagnostic workup and return-to-play decision by a self-confident, risk-taking physician who played linebacker in college compared to that of a physician who is sports-averse and risk-avoiding by nature? If the diagnostic evaluation of Scott failed to disclose any abnormalities, how might the advice offered by these two physicians differ?

One of the basic tenets of the practice of medicine is "First do no harm." And there exists the potential for serious "harm" here on both sides of the decision-making tree: disallowing a young athlete from sports play by the erroneous, conservative decision that the collapse event might have reflected some occult, unidentified anomaly posing risk for sudden death when no such condition actually exists, or, conversely, an overly liberal decision to permit play when an inadequate evaluation fails to reveal a serious disorder, placing the athlete at peril for tragic consequences. The fate of the young athlete whose major enjoyment in life may lie in sports play hangs in the balance. The decisions of the physician are not always easy, particularly when episodes of collapse during sports play remain unexplained after a thorough medical assessment or when such an evaluation reveals results which are ambiguous or borderline abnormal.

Sudden Cardiac Death in Young Athletes

Occurrences of sudden unexpected death in young athletes during sports play—often in front of horrified spectators or on national television—have created a worried public. And when an athlete collapses—and quickly recovers—the fear on the part of parents, coaches, and sport administrators that such events signal a risk for subsequent death is magnified. Any evaluation of an athlete who "goes down" during competition or training needs to be considered in the context of this underlying dread. Fortunately, however, only a tiny percentage of cases of collapse in athletes are signals of serious underlying cardiac disease.

The occurrence of sudden unexpected demise in a young athlete is a particularly poignant tragedy, given a) the ostensible health and vigor of the athlete and b) his or her participation in an activity deemed to contribute to a healthy life style. Fortunately, despite their highly publicized nature, the incidence of sudden death in the young athlete is extremely low. Among the mysteries surrounding this topic, in fact, is uncertainty surrounding the true incidence of cardiac-related deaths during sports play. In the 1990s, early reports indicated 10–13 such occurrences annually in the United States, suggesting a statistical chance of a young adolescent athlete dying suddenly from underlying heart disease in the order of 1:250,000 (38). Since that time the estimated annual number of these tragedies has steadily risen, presumably reflecting improved data acquisition methods rather than a true increase in such events.

Still, incidence figures have varied widely. In their survey of reports from five countries, Link and Estes tallied incidence values of sudden deaths in athletes per 100,000 person-years between 0.4 and 3.6 (32). Such numbers were not dissimilar from those occurrences in the general population, causing the authors to provocatively speculate that "much of the data indicate a similar or lower incidence of sudden cardiac death in athletes compared to nonathletes, although the data are far from conclusive" (32). However, in the only study which has directly compared death rates in athletes and nonathletes in the general population, Corrado et al. found over a 20-year period in the Veneto region of Italy that deaths occurred at a rate of 2.3 per 100,000 per year in athletes <35 years old and 0.9 per 100,000 per year in nonathletes (14).

In their review of reports of sudden unexpected cardiac death in the literature, Asif and Harmon found that "studies of high quality and rigor" indicated an incidence of approximately 1:50,000 and between 1:50,000–1:80,000 deaths per athlete years in college and high school athletes in the United States, respectively (3). These authors noted that although previous reports have labeled certain forms of heart disease to be responsible for sudden death in young persons, "more comprehensive investigations in the United States and international populations [in] athletes, nonathletes, and military support that the most common finding on autopsy in young individuals with SCD [sudden cardiac death] is actually a structurally normal heart" (3).

In their survey of deaths in athletes ages 14–18 years in seven states over a period of six years, Harmon et al. described 69 cases annually of sudden cardiac death (23), a rate of 1:100,000 per athlete years. Of the 50 that had autopsies performed, the most common finding was left ventricular hypertrophy in 26%, while in 18% the post-mortem findings were normal.

In a subsequent study, Harmon et al. reported 79 cases yearly of what were labeled as sudden cardiac deaths in collegiate athletes, with a risk of 1:50,000 (22). However, 25% of the autopsies in 69 of these cases were completely normal (in fact, the most frequent finding). The deaths in such cases might be accounted for at least partially by electrical disorders of the heart (such as long QT syndrome) which would provide no evidence on autopsy (see below).

Such discrepancies in incidence figures presumably reflect variations in inclusion criteria (are deaths from chest trauma and sickle cell disease included?), definitions (what is an "athlete"?), geographical/genetic population differences, and means of ascertaining occurrences. Considering the available information, it might be reasonable to suggest that no more than 50–75 cases of sudden unexpected death from documented heart disease occur annually in the United States in athletes at or below college age, with an incidence of 1:80,000–1:200,000 athlete years (34).

In dealing with the fears of one's teenage son or daughter dying suddenly on the court or playing field, the extent of such a risk needs to be placed in proper perspective. According to the National Center for Health Statistics, between the years 1999 and 2006, an average of 16,375 teenagers died in the United States annually (40). Of these, 5,735 died in motor vehicle accidents, 550 from accidental poisonings, 393 from accidental drowning, and 163 as a result of "unintentional discharge of a firearm." In effect, the statistical chance of an adolescent succumbing in an automobile accident is almost 100 times that of the risk of death during athletic play.

Certain features of athletes and sports play at the interscholastic level have been linked to a greater risk for episodes of sudden death. The great majority of fatal events have occurred in two sports—football and basketball—which is at least partially explained by the greater numbers of athletes in these sports. Sudden death is more common in males than females and in African Americans compared to white athletes. (More on these discrepancies will be addressed in the sections that follow.)

Harbingers of Sudden Cardiac Death in Young Athletes

A number of cardiac conditions have been linked to sudden death in young athletes. These are characterized as being a) *rare* (with low frequencies in the general population, b) *predisposing to fatal arrhythmias* (which is generally highly unusual among the heart conditions in the pediatric age group), particularly during exercise, and c) *occult* (typically silent in respect to symptoms and findings on physical examination). It has generally been assumed that sudden death during sports participation does not occur in athletes whose heart is structurally and functionally normal; that is, a heart abnormality—electrical or physical—is expected to serve as a substrate for all of these tragedies. (Exceptions are cases of deaths from recreational use of cardio-toxic drugs [e.g., cocaine] and *commotio cordis*, in which death occurs due to a blow to the chest [usually a thrown ball], which triggers a fatal cardiac rhythm when it disturbs a vulnerable moment in the heart's electrical activity [39].)

If this is so, one is left with the difficulty of explaining the frequency of cases of athletes' sudden collapse and death in which autopsy findings are unrevealing of an underlying cardiac abnormality. As described above, in fact, in some series such is the most common post-mortem result. Were those all deaths from disorders of the heart's electrical conduction system? Were occult abnormalities, such as discrete coronary artery obstructions, missed on the autopsy? Are there factors predisposing athletes to sudden death of which we are unaware? Unfortunately, there are no easy answers here.

It should be recognized that all of these various forms of rare heart disease which pose a risk for sudden death do so via the common pathway of creating instability of the heart's electrical activity, most commonly *ventricular fibrillation*. Normally the electrical signal generated at the top of the heart travels through the atria and then the ventricles in specialized conduction fibers, which trigger atrial and then ventricular contraction. Ventricular fibrillation is characterized by a total chaotic disruption of normal electrical activity in the ventricle with critical and unacceptable loss of the heart's pumping capacity. In those rare cardiac abnormalities predisposing to sudden death, this arrhythmia is typically triggered by myocardial ischemia (inadequate blood perfusion of the ventricular muscle) occurring with the augmented cardiac metabolic demands of exercise.

The extent and means that risk of cardiac death with sport play can be detected via the routine pre-participation medical evaluation—clearly a needle-in-the-haystack situation—are currently topics of vigorous debate, even on an international scale (50). The idea here is one of *prevention*, detecting the would-be athlete who is at risk and precluding sports participation. Considering the unsettled imbroglio and emotional, divisive stands surrounding this approach, particularly regarding the use of the electrocardiogram and echocardiogram as routine screening tools, this author admits to a sense of relief that such arguments do not bear on evaluation and decision-making in the collapsed athlete and will henceforth be ignored here.

The most critical focus in the evaluation of the athlete who has collapsed during training or competition is that of ruling out any underlying cardiac disease that would pose a risk of fatal arrhythmia during future sports play. In the sections that follow the features and diagnostic assessment of four of the most common forms of heart disease considered responsible for sudden death in young athletes will be reviewed. The purpose here is to recognize the selection and ambiguities of diagnostic tools utilized in the attempts to detect underlying cardiac disease in the evaluation of an athlete who has suffered collapse.

Hypertrophic Cardiomyopathy

Hypertrophic cardiomyopathy (HCM) is a genetic heart muscle disease of unknown cause which is characterized by dramatic thickening of the ventricular walls. This enlargement involves both ventricles but is most prominent in the septum which divides the right and left ventricular chambers. In a fully grown healthy adolescent this septum is, on the average, about 8 mm thick, with an upper limit of normal of 12 mm. In patients with HCM, it is not uncommon for the septum to measure 20–30 mm, creating a large myocardial mass which compromises the volume of the left ventricular chamber, thereby limiting stroke volume and cardiac output. In some cases, particularly in adults, this myocardial mass encroaches on the left ventricular outflow tract, creating a point of obstruction.

Patients with HCM are faced with an increased risk for sudden death, particularly during strenuous exercise. What creates this risk is uncertain, but it is suspected that the difficulty of the coronary arterial circulation in perfusing the depths of the thickened ventricular muscle with adequate blood supply results in myocardial damage, particularly at times of increased metabolic demand, and, catastrophically, fatal ventricular arrhythmias.

Suspecting HCM in a young person is often problematic, since this myopathy is usually "silent," causing no symptoms and providing a deceptively normal physical examination. For this reason, athletes who die suddenly of unsuspected HCM have typically undergone a normal pre-participation medical evaluation comprised of an unremarkable medical history-taking and findings on cardiac auscultation. However, a small minority of adolescents with HCM may report chest pain, dizziness, collapse, shortness of breath, or palpitations, particularly during physical activity. Too, in approximately 20% of cases a history can be obtained of another family member with this disease.

While the history and physical examination are typically of little diagnostic value, the electrocardiogram is frequently abnormal in patients with HCM (for those who understand these things, abnormal Q waves and ST-T wave changes). However, it is the two-dimensional echocardiogram—an ultrasound examination—which provides the definitive diagnosis, permitting measurement of the thickness of the ventricular walls and interventricular septum, the dimensions of the left ventricular chamber, and the existence of any left ventricular outflow obstruction.

When these echocardiographic findings are typical, there is no difficulty in making the diagnosis of HCM. If the ventricular septum measures over 18 mm and the ratio of the thickness of the septum to the left ventricular free wall is >1.3, in the absence of any other explanation (such as pathologic narrowing of the aortic valve, or severe systemic hypertension), the diagnosis of HCM is confirmed (37). However, difficulty may sometimes arise in distinguishing HCM from findings in a normal heart, especially that of a trained athlete who is expected to have some degree of training-induced ventricular hypertrophy.

In the case of highly trained athletes the upper limit of normal for ventricular septal thickness might be 13–14 mm, the normal range defined by 95th percentile confidence limits above the expected average value. That means that 5% of such trained athletes—one in 20—might be expected to have a thickness over 13 mm. So, let's suppose the measurement is 15–16 mm. Is this one of few unusual athletes with a normal heart whose ventricular septal thickness is in that 5% category? Or, is this an athlete who has HCM, albeit with limited phenotypic expression, but still at risk for sudden death? Do we pat this young athlete on the back and congratulate him on his exceptional training program? Or, instead, do we prohibit him from any further participation in sports, explaining that he has a serious, potentially fatal heart condition? It's a rather pivotal decision, to be sure.

Fortunately, there are some means by which the weight of this difficult decision-making in borderline cases can be eased. Highly trained endurance athletes are expected to have an enlarged left ventricular chamber, evidence of high aerobic fitness (elevated maximal oxygen uptake on exercise testing), and normal or enhanced myocardial diastolic function. Patients with HCM, on the other hand, usually exhibit a diminished left ventricular chamber size, low aerobic fitness, and evidence of myocardial diastolic dysfunction. In cases where doubt still exists, a period of detraining has been suggested to untangle the situation, during which the physiological hypertrophy from training (in contrast to that of HCM) should be expected to regress.

Aberrant Coronary Arteries

In adult populations, the most common cause of sudden death during exercise is atherosclerotic coronary artery disease, in which fatty-fibrous plaques obstruct myocardial blood supply, causing myocardial necrosis and provoking fatal arrhythmias. Fortunately, adolescents do not suffer from this scenario, but, instead, unrecognized congenital anomalies of the coronary arteries, "mistakes" in the normal development of these structures *in utero*, can account for sudden death in the same fashion in young athletes.

During fetal development, the right coronary artery arises from the right sinus of the aortic valve and feeds the right ventricular musculature, while the left coronary artery departs from the left sinus. Following a short course as the main left coronary artery, it divides into the circumflex and left anterior descending coronary arteries which provide blood flow to the back and front of the left ventricle, respectively. Things can go awry in this scenario in a number of developmental errors which result in an abnormal origin and course of the left and right coronary arteries. These anomalies, then, are forms of *congenital* rather than acquired heart disease. The most common associated with risk for sudden death is when the left main artery arises off the right valve sinus and then courses in front of the aorta (between it and the pulmonary artery) to reach its branching point on the left side (59).

The incidence in the pediatric population of a left coronary artery arising from the right aortic valve sinus is probably between 1:1,000 and 1:4,000 (16,33). A study of sudden deaths occurring in military training indicated 21 cases among 6.3 million recruits, suggesting an incidence of 1:300,000 (17). Clearly, then, a large number of youths possess this anomalous coronary artery pattern without consequence.

Exactly how such aberrant coronary artery arrangements should provoke sudden death—and why such events should silently await the teen years—has not been clear. Some have felt that compression of the aberrant left coronary artery as it passes between the pulsating aorta and pulmonary artery—particularly with exercise—might be critical. Others have considered that the acute angle by which the aberrant left coronary artery departs the right aortic sinus could become functionally obstructive as blood flow increases with exercise. Intravascular ultrasound techniques have proven particularly instructive. In situations in which the aberrant left coronary artery passes *within* the aortic wall it becomes narrowed and easily compressed during heart muscle contraction (systole) (2). This variation on the anatomic themes appears to be that which poses the greatest risk for sudden death.

Almost invariably the first indication of the existence of an aberrant coronary artery is the sudden collapse and death of the athlete on the practice or playing field. These abnormalities are notoriously occult, preceding such tragic events by no symptoms whatsoever—although previous chest pain and syncopal collapse during exercise are rarely reported. Findings on physical examination and electrocardiogram are normal. Using modern high-resolution equipment, experienced cardiac ultrasonographers are usually able to visualize the origins of the coronary arteries from the base of the aorta as well as the initial trajectory of their course. In situations of doubt, as when such images cannot be obtained, MRI or computed tomography angiography are usually capable of visualizing coronary artery anatomy at the base of the aorta. Coronary angiography remains the definitive diagnostic technique.

Right Ventricular Cardiomyopathy

Right ventricular cardiomyopathy (also termed "arrhythmogenic right ventricle") is a peculiar disorder in which loss of myocardial fibers and replacement with fat is confined to the thin-walled, low pressure right ventricle. Such changes serve to trigger ventricular arrhythmias, particularly under the sympathetic stimulation of exercise, causing sudden death. This is a genetic disease, and a positive family history can be obtained in half of cases.

In keeping with the common theme of occult heart disease, patients with this disorder rarely describe any symptoms, although collapse with syncope and palpitations may rarely be reported. Physical examination and chest x-ray are typically normal. The electrocardiogram can reveal certain characteristic changes—wide QRS complexes in the right precordial leads with undulation of the ST segments (so-called epsilon waves). Echocardiogram in full-blown cases reveals right ventricular enlargement, focal right ventricular wall motion abnormalities, and echo density of the ventricular anterior wall.

One of the most intriguing aspects of this disease is the striking discrepancy of its frequency as a cause of sudden death in athletes in different geographical regions, particularly comparing reports from Italy and the United States. In the Veneto region of Italy, right ventricular cardiomyopathy is described as the most common cause of these events, accounting for over one-half among 47 deaths in one report (14). In the United States, on the other hand, this disorder barely appears on the lists of etiologies. In a report of 134 sudden deaths in athletes under 35 years, Maron et al. found only three cases of right ventricular cardiomyopathy. The explanation for such geographical differences remains to be forthcoming.

Long QT Syndrome

The electrical depolarization of the myocardial cell which triggers muscular contraction is mediated by ion transport across the cell membrane. While outward sodium ion current accounts for depolarization, inward potassium current is responsible for electrical recovery, or repolarization. Errors in gene actions which govern these electrochemical functions are reflected in a family of disorders known collectively as the "channelopathies." The most common of these, long QT syndrome, is itself composed of at least 13 different genetic-based variants with different clinical phenotypes. All are characterized by delayed ventricular repolarization (electrical recovery) after each heart beat, which is reflected on the electrocardiogram as a prolongation of the interval between the onset of the Q wave and the end of the T wave (QT interval). This effect augments the action of cytosolic calcium, which makes these patients susceptible to dangerous ventricular arrhythmias and sudden death (20). In most of the genetic subtypes such risk is exacerbated by exercise and emotional stress.

The diagnosis of long QT syndrome is established on a routine electrocardiogram tracing, which reveals a prolongation of the QT interval, corrected for heart rate. The accurate measurement of this interval is, however, sometimes problematic, since the slope of the termination of the T wave approaches the baseline in a gradual, asymptotic manner. The average corrected QT interval among healthy individuals is 0.40 seconds, with an upper limit of normal of 0.44–0.46 seconds, while persons with long QT syndrome often exhibit a QT interval of over 0.50 seconds. Exercise testing may be useful in interpreting borderline values. During a graded cycle or treadmill test, the value of the corrected QT interval in healthy subjects does not change. With long QT syndrome it may lengthen, particularly during the recovery phase, but such responses vary according to the genetic type (51).

Genetic testing is available to diagnose long QT syndrome and define the genetic variant involved. However, such testing is negative in about 25% of cases of long QT syndrome. As an electrical disorder, there are no physical clues that provide an identification of long QT syndrome on an autopsy examination. Genetic testing has been advocated in the post-mortem assessment of athletes who have died suddenly but in whom the standard autopsy has failed to reveal an anatomic cardiac cause (a so-called "molecular autopsy") (6). This approach has proven illuminating in establishing the frequency with which such electrical disorders can be responsible for these tragedies.

Several studies have consistently indicated that up to one-third of cases of unexplained sudden death in young people (not athletes) can be attributed to genetic defects responsible for cardiac channelopathies (58). For example, Bagnall et al. prospectively obtained clinical and post-mortem data on children and young adults ages 1–35 years in New Zealand and Australia who had suffered sudden death (4). Of 490 cases identified, 40% were of undetermined etiology. With genetic testing of blood obtained at autopsy, 27% of those were found to have a "clinically relevant cardiac gene mutation." The extent that the remainder of unexplained sudden deaths might be accounted for by an electrical abnormality such as one of the channelopathies (i.e., with normal genetic testing) or reflects some as yet unrecognized cause remains speculative.

Physiological Ventricular Hypertrophy

Can the physiologic training-induced ventricular hypertrophy of the athlete pose a risk for life-threatening arrhythmias? It's a provocative question with a long history. When Henschen first reported that cross-country skiers had enlarged hearts by chest percussion in 1898, he concluded that this finding reflected normal, healthy responses to athletic training (47). Still, it was not lost on physicians that cardiac enlargement, ventricular hypertrophy, and electrocardiographic changes observed in such athletes were not dissimilar to those observed in patients with heart disease. Despite such concerns, in what could be termed a mass natural experiment, the well-being of millions of athletes has supported the conclusion that, after all, Henschen was right, and such characteristics of the "athlete's heart" are physiologic and portend no risk.

In recent years, however, this controversy has surfaced once again. Evidence indicates that the myocardial thickening which is a normal response to sports training may, like the hypertrophy observed with heart disease, pose a risk for serious ventricular rhythm disorders and could potentially, in extremely rare cases, serve as a substrate for sudden unexpected death (49). Opinions on the matter, however, are sharply divided. Maron and Pellicia contend that "There is no evidence at present showing that athlete's heart remodeling leads to long-term disease progression, cardiovascular disability, or sudden cardiac death" (36). On the other hand, Hart has argued that "intensive athletic training is associated with a small but finite risk of sudden death, which may be a consequence of the cellular electrical changes of mild-to-moderate cardiac hypertrophy" (24).

There is no question that the cardiac electrical system is modified in response to athletic training. But the electrocardiographic findings—sinus bradycardia, first-degree heart block, left ventricular hypertrophy—reflect the normal physiological autonomic and structural changes with training. However, there is increasing evidence that disturbances in heart rhythm—sometimes significant ones—are more common in trained athletes than nonathletes. For example, Biffi et al. reported that on 24-hour continuous electrocardiographic tracings, 77% of 175 highly trained Italian athletes had some form of ventricular ectopy (premature ventricular beats), including 5% who exhibited periods of ventricular tachycardia (a recognized antecedent of ventricular fibrillation) (9). Following a period of detraining, the frequency of ventricular arrhythmias in these athletes declined.

Herm et al. reported findings on portable electrocardiographic recorders worn by 108 participants without known cardiac disease (ages 45–53 years) in a marathon race (26). All had run at least two marathon races in the previous five years and reported an average training mileage of 40 km per week. Mean finish time was 249 minutes. At least one episode of non-sustained ventricular tachycardia was recorded in 10 (9.3%) of the runners, while 7.5% showed transient ischemic ST-T wave changes. Whether such electrical events might have been triggered by occult coronary artery disease is not clear. However, others have described no ventricular arrhythmias in runners during marathon races (1,19).

It has been suggested that certain of the autopsy findings of ventricular hypertrophy in cases of sudden death in athletes may have been misinterpreted as examples of HCM. This conclusion is based on the observation that many of the demographic features of supposed HCM in such cases are not consistent with those typically seen in clinical cases of HCM (48). For example, almost all of the cases of sudden death from presumed HCM during sports play have occurred in males (55 of 56 sudden deaths in one review [42]), while there is no sex predilection in the general population of patients with HCM. Also, African-American athletes suffer from a disproportionately higher risk of sudden death from reported HCM. In one description of 158 sudden deaths in American athletes, the frequency of sudden death from HCM was actually greater in African Americans than in Caucasians (35). Among those patients with HCM in the general population, no racial bias is observed.

Males (compared to females) and African Americans (compared to Caucasians) have a relative greater degree of ventricular hypertrophy with sports training (5,45,56). Altogether, then, these observations suggest that at least some of the deaths attributed to HCM in athletes could have instead reflected fatal arrhythmias occurring secondary to training-induced physiological hypertrophy.

Concern has been raised that risk of serious arrhythmias in trained athletes might be related to abnormal stresses placed on the right ventricle (which pumps into a relatively higher vascular resistance during exercise than does the left ventricle) (15). Heidbuchel et al. described a group of 40 elite cyclists who were found to have complex ventricular arrhythmias, including ventricular tachycardia (25). The majority of these athletes showed right ventricular dilatation, and 59% satisfied diagnostic criteria for right ventricular cardiomyopathy. The authors suggested that extensive training might adversely affect the right ventricle, simulating the anatomic and electrocardiographic changes seen with right ventricular cardiomyopathy.

The question of risk of serious, life-threatening arrhythmias posed by training-induced hypertrophy remains unresolved. If such characteristics of the "athlete's heart" can cause sudden death, such occurrences are extraordinarily rare and thereby do not, unfortunately, lend themselves to conventional research approaches. A better understanding may come from greater insights regarding the unique electrophysiological responses to acute and chronic exercise in the hearts of trained athletes.

Not (Usually) Harbingers of Sudden Death

As noted previously, the great majority of recognized causes of collapse during sports competition in young athletes are more benign and typically bear little import to serious underlying disease. These are typically suspected from a description of the circumstances surrounding the event, and usually no additional clues can be obtained from the physical examination nor documentation obtained from laboratory tests. The good news is that most can be prevented in the future by easily accomplished measures. And even recurrences are associated with favorable outcomes when exercise-induced syncope is not related to heart disease (13). The unfortunate news is such historical information relies on subjective reports which may be unreliable or inaccurate and are usually impossible to confirm.

This creates difficulty in interpreting the level of importance of certain factors (weather, hydration status, etc.) as causative in the collapse of the athlete.

Here are a few possibilities:

Hyperthermia

The internal body heat generated by muscular effort is normally controlled by thermoregulatory responses of increased sweating and cutaneous vascular dilation for convective skin loss. In conditions in which the effectiveness of such response is limited by high levels of environmental temperature and humidity, vigorous exercise can cause an abnormal rise in body core temperature. Increased blood flow to the skin diminishes central blood volume, with a fall in cardiac filling, right atrial pressure, and stroke volume. Meanwhile, augmented sweating rate serves to accentuate all of these adverse effects. The end result is diminished cardiac output and cerebral blood flow, both of which contribute to the clinical spectrum of hyperthermia, ranging from fatigue and light-headedness (heat exhaustion) to overt cardiovascular collapse (heat stroke) (31).

The ambient temperature reported at the time of an athlete's collapse is obviously the best means of suspecting this etiology. Still, other factors should be considered, including

- Duration and intensity of the exercise. (Did collapse occur during the "warm-up" or at the end of a highly competitive race?)
- Was fluid intake sufficient (see below)? (In a dehydrated state the athlete is more susceptible to collapse from hyperthermia.)
- Where did the event occur? (In a cross-desert race or in a shaded forest trail?)
- Was the athlete accustomed (i.e., acclimated) to exercise in the heat? Was he or she highly fit? (Both factors provide resistance to heat injury.)

Dehydration

Maintenance of adequate body fluid content—and consequently of circulating blood volume—is critical for both optimizing exercise performance and preventing heat injury during sports play. Euhydration is essential for sustaining high levels of cardiac output, while thermoregulatory responses rely on a sufficient vascular volume to prevent exaggerated increase in body temperature. Therefore, the athlete who becomes dehydrated during training or competition suffers from a reduced exercise capacity while increasing the risk of symptoms of heat strain noted above, which include syncope and collapse.

It is often difficult to get a true sense of the hydration status of an athlete at the time of his or her collapse. Self-report of fluid intake can be unreliable (i.e., the athlete knows he "should have" consumed fluids before a distant race). Still, such an event occurring after three hours of highly competitive basketball in a 95-degree gymnasium without supplementary fluid intake, or when an unknowledgeable coach has restricted fluids from her athletes, are red flags to suggest dehydration as a central contributor to fatigue with syncope during sports play.

Neurocardiogenic Syncope

Dehydration may also trigger syncope by initiating vagal reflexes associated with low blood volume. In what is termed the Bezold-Jarisch reflex, diminished left ventricular volume stimulates sympathetic stretch receptors in the ventricular walls. This initiates a vagal reflex which causes heart slowing with vasodilatation, provoking syncope. The same process can be initiated by the high sympatho-adrenal effects of intense exercise, with reflex "vasovagal" responses and syncopal collapse (11).

Supportive evidence for this diagnosis can be obtained by performing a tilt-table test, which mimics the condition of increased sympathetic drive in combination with reduced left ventricular filling that can occur with competitive exercise (21). In this test, the subject is tilted on a table to a semi-upright position, with monitoring of heart rate and blood pressure as well as recording subjective feelings of dizziness or occurrence of overt syncope. While the specificity and sensitivity of this procedure have not been firmly established, a fall in blood pressure and pulse, in combination with dizziness or syncope, suggests an athlete who is particularly prone to neurocardiogenic syncope. Such susceptibility can often be suspected, too, by a history of dizziness on arising from bed in the morning or during standing in a hot shower.

The management of such an athlete usually consists initially of promoting fluid intake (to maintain left ventricular volume). Pharmacologic treatment is available as well, with options such as beta-blocker medication (to prevent sympathetic efferent triggers) and fludrocortisone (a corticosteroid which promotes fluid retention) (8).

Post-Exertional Venous Pooling

Much has been made of the expectation that syncope and collapse of an athlete immediately following a competition (e.g., after crossing the finish line) is less likely to reflect underlying cardiac disease than such events which occur during a competition. This distinction reflects the frequent occurrence of venous blood pooling in the lower extremities upon cessation of vigorous leg exercise. During running, the pumping action of the leg musculature maintains central blood volume, even in the presence of arterial vasodilation. This function ceases abruptly at the end of a race, causing pooling of blood in the dependent limb, a reduction in central blood volume, and a fall in cerebral blood flow, all leading to post-exertional syncope and collapse. This all supports the traditional coach's admonition to "keep moving after you finish!"

Psychogenic Hyperventilation

During the initial stages of a progressive exercise test, minute ventilation rises linearly in parallel with oxygen uptake, reflecting the increasing metabolic demands of exercising muscle. At higher work intensities, the buffering of a rise in blood lactate level by bicarbonate produces excessive carbon dioxide beyond that released as an end product of aerobic metabolism. This causes a disproportionate rise in minute ventilation in respect to oxygen uptake, which reflects, in effect, a *physiological hyperventilation*. The emotional stimulation of intense competition in a highly driven athlete can result in even greater levels of ventilation. This *psychogenic hyperventilation* causes the arterial partial pressure of carbon dioxide ($PaCO_2$) in the blood to fall and arterial pH to rise, changes which trigger vasoconstriction (closing off of arteries serving the brain) in the cerebral vascular circulation. It has been assumed that the consequent fall in cerebral blood flow might be responsible for mental derangements (confusion, dizziness) and overt syncope with collapse in athletes in highly competitive situations.

There is now increasing experimental evidence to support the validity of this scenario. Use of transcranial Doppler measurement of middle cerebral artery velocity and positron emission tomography (PET) confirm that hypocapnia (reduced $PaCO_2$) reduces cerebral blood flow as a consequence of cerebral vasoconstriction (28,57). For example, Bednarzcyk et al. measured cerebral blood flow and arterial blood gases in ten volunteers before and after five minutes of hyperventilation (at rest) (7). Baseline cerebral blood flow averaged 61 ml/min/100 gm tissue but fell to 31 ml/min/100 gm tissue with hyperventilation. At the same times, $PaCO_2$ declined from a mean value of 38 mm Hg to 20 mm Hg.

Normally, vigorous exercise triggers a 10–30% rise in cerebral blood flow (10). Any reduction consequent to the hypocapnia of hyperventilation would be expected to interfere with normal cerebral function, with mental confusion and alterations in consciousness. Such responses may reflect the influence of marked anxiety and determination during sports competition that override normal respiratory mechanisms designed to defend against such outcomes (52).

Collapse as a Manifestation of Exercise Fatigue

Could syncope or near-syncope with collapse along with mental confusion during athletic competition be simply a manifestation of high levels of exercise fatigue? According to the *central governor hypothesis*, the answer is "yes." This highly controversial concept, popularized by exercise physiologist Tim Noakes, proposes the existence of brain control centers which serve to limit exercise performance with the goal of preventing damaging bodily stress (44).

By the traditional concept, "fatigue" or "exhaustion" during sports competition is defined by the functional limits of the constellation of physiological and biochemical factors that contribute to exercise performance. The central governor hypothesis argues, instead, that it is the brain's perception of effort that establishes maximal effort. That is, according to this idea, the symptoms of fatigue which limit exercise are subjective "feelings" rather than a physiological state, and such unpleasant feelings (hyperpnea, dizziness, mental confusion—even collapse and collapse) are designed by the brain to protect against serious consequences of extremes of physical effort. As Noakes has put it, during exercise, "fatigue is not a physical event but rather an emotion" (34).

This is not, in fact, a new idea. In 1915 the Italian physiologist A. Mosso suggested that such a protective central controller acts such that "the fatigue increasing more rapidly than the amount of work done saves us from the injury which lesser sensibility would involve for the organism" (41). Ten years later, A.V. Hill agreed: At high exercise intensities, "[a governor] causes slowing of the circulation as soon as a serious degree of [oxygen] unsaturation occurs, since it would obviously be very dangerous for [the heart] to be able to exhaust itself very completely" (27).

This is no lack of evidence that human beings a) do possess exercise capacities beyond normal expectations and b) such transgressions into supra-maximal efforts can be accompanied by harmful and potentially fatal outcomes. Anecdotal reports of temporary extraordinary strength in life-and-death situations are common (e.g., lifting a car off a pinned accident victim), and such Herculean acts are recognized to cause torn muscles. In fact, human muscles have the capacity to generate sufficient force to break bones. Before the routine use of appropriate anesthesia, patients undergoing electro-convulsive shock therapy for mental disorders faced the risk of suffering fractures of the spine, humerus, femoral neck, and scapula. In a review of patients at Lancaster Moor Hospital in England between 1942 and 1952, Kelly found that muscle contractions from convulsions with shock therapy produced fractures or dislocations in 2.4% of 2,200 patients (30).

Other critical outcomes from excessive exercise might be prevented by such a protective central governor. *Rhabdomyolysis* is the process of muscle tissue destruction that can occur with unaccustomed severe exercise (46). This cell breakdown can trigger life-threatening complications of renal failure, electrolyte disturbances, cardiac arrhythmias, and death. Rhabdomyolysis and its complications not uncommonly occur in groups of athletes, such as in August of 2010 when over half of the high school football players in an Oregon training camp in the August heat were sent to the hospital with this condition (18).

Over-exertion in the heat can stress the limits of the body's thermoregulatory mechanisms and effect an unacceptable rise in core temperature. When that increase reaches over 40° C, potentially fatal heat stroke can occur, initiated by mental confusion, collapse, and seizures, eventuating in coma and death (12). It is not unlikely, too, that extreme levels of sympatho-adrenergic drive could trigger fatal cardiac arrhythmias or impair cardiac muscle function in the same manner as eventuates in the process of rhabdomyolysis in skeletal muscle. Evidence indicates that participation in ultra-endurance athletic events is accompanied by a transient depression of myocardial function (54).

That the human organism would possess a means of protecting itself from such catastrophic outcomes with extremes of exercise makes Darwinian sense. A central theme of mammalian physiology is the evolutionary-based preservation of homeostasis and protection against extreme perturbations of extrinsic (i.e., environmental) stresses. According to the central governor model, it is just the purpose and function of a controlling factor in the brain that accomplishes this, and it does so via two mechanisms: First, it creates the unpleasant sensations of fatigue (including dizziness, mental confusion, and syncope) that make the athlete terminate exercise. And, second, it reduces *central command*, the signals arising in the motor cortex of the brain which descend down the spinal cord to control the strength of skeletal muscular contractions (causing so-called "central fatigue").

This is a controversial topic, to be sure. Indeed, some have found this concept totally unacceptable, voicing their opinion in articles with titles such as "Is it time to retire the 'central governor'?" (55) and "The central governor model of exercise regulation teaches us precious little about the nature of mental fatigue and self-control failure" (29). Inzlicht and Marcora wrote that "the central governor model is biologically implausible and, worse, unfalsifiable, appearing more and more like some sort of all-knowing homunculus" (29). Noakes, in the true combative spirit of scientific debate, countered that "my conclusion is that the dominance of an authoritarian Kuhnian philosophy, which refuses to admit genuine error or the need to alter one's course of belief or action explains why there is little appetite in the exercise sciences for the acceptance of genuinely novel ideas such as the CGM" (43).

One specific criticism of the central governor model is that "it is difficult to see evidence of this ultimate function at work given just how easily this ultimate function is overturned by motivational incentives" (29). There are, in fact, examples of situations in which extremely highly levels of motivation and determination on the part of the athlete apparently overrides the "wisdom" of such a proposed central governor—heat injury when competing in hot ambient conditions, triathletes crawling to reach the finish line after near syncopal collapse, drill sergeants commanding recruits to excessive workloads leading to rhabdomyolysis. But such conditions, although highly publicized and visible, constitute a very tiny proportion of the millions of annual participants in athletic events. Whether the ability to override a central governor is "easily" accomplished is arguable.

> "So, I've reviewed all your laboratory tests, Scott, and they all turned out to be normal. The electrocardiogram revealed no evidence of any stress or enlargement of the heart, and the heart rhythm was normal. On your echocardiogram there were no abnormalities of heart structure or function. When you performed the exercise stress test, we found, as expected, high levels of fitness. Your heart responded with a normal rate and rhythm, and the electrocardiogram showed no signs of any decrease in blood flow to the heart muscle. On the tilt test you showed no exaggerations of changes

in blood pressure or heart rate. All your blood test were also normal—unremarkable blood count, sugar and electrolyte levels. So, putting this together, there is nothing here to suggest that your collapse was a signal that you have some underlying heart disease."

"So, then, what do think caused me to collapse?"

"I think it's most likely that in the heat of the moment near the finish line you started breathing too fast—that's called hyperventilation—which caused some chemical changes in your blood that made you faint. Or, as a second possibility, that same excitement led to such forceful contractions of your heart that your brain made a response—that's termed a 'vasovagal reaction'—which made your heart slow down, leading you to lose—or almost lose—consciousness. Neither of these two possible causes is really serious. I mean they don't pose any risk for something terrible happening to you if they should occur again.

"Based on what we know, then, I'm going to clear you to play basketball. My advice would be to make sure you've drunk plenty of fluids before, during, and after practices and competitions. And think about controlling your breathing. If you have additional episodes of collapse we should take a close look at you again with some follow-up tests.

"We must acknowledge here that we can never be 100% sure that this is a wise decision. Could we have missed some dangerous problem that went undiscovered? There is always a very small possibility. We could restrict you from sports, a conservative approach that one might argue would reduce some undisclosed risk of future bad outcome. But in my opinion, there would be a price to pay by doing this. We would be depriving you of your psychological and social and physical well-being, something that would seriously diminish your enjoyment and quality of life. Nothing we do in life, not a single decision, is without some element or degree of risk. If we are all in agreement, this is the course we'll take for now."

References

1 Aagaard P, Sahlen A, Bergfeldt L, et al. Heart rate and its variability in responses to running-associations with troponin. *Med Sci Sports Exerc.* 2014;46:1624–1630.
2. Angelini P. Coronary artery anomalies: an entity in search of an identity. *Circulation.* 2007;115:1296–1305.
3. Asif IM, Harmon KG. Incidence and etiology of sudden cardiac death: new updates for athletic departments. *Sports Health.* 2017;9:268–279.
4. Bagnall RD, Weintraub RG, Ingles J, et al. A prospective study of sudden cardiac death among children and young adults. *N Engl J Med.* 2016;374:2441–2452.
5. Basavarajaiah S, Boraita A, Whyte G, et al. Ethnic differences in left ventricular remodeling in highly-trained athletes. *J Am Coll Cardiol.* 2008;51:2256–2262.
6. Basso C, Carturan E, Pilichou K, Rizzo S, Corrado D, Thiene G. Sudden cardiac death with normal heart: molecular autopsy. *Cardiovasc Pathol.* 2010;19:321–325.

7. Bednarczyk EM, Rutherford WF, Leisure GP, et al. Hyperventilation-induced reduction in cerebral blood flow: assessment by positron emission tomography. *DICP*. 1990;24:456–460.
8. Benditt DG. Neurally mediated syncopal syndromes: pathophysiological concepts and clinical evaluation. *Pacing Clin Electrophysiol*. 1997;20:572–584.
9. Biffi A, Maron BJ, DiGiacinto, et al. Relation between training induced left ventricular hypertrophy and risk for ventricular tachyarrhythmias in elite athletes. *Am J Cardiol*. 2008;101:1792–1795.
10. Braz ID, Fisher JP. The impact of age on cerebral perfusion, oxygenation and metabolism during exercise in humans. *J Physiol*. 2016;16:4471–4483.
11. Calkins H, Seifert M, Morady F. Clinical presentation and long-term follow-up of athletes with exercise-induced vasodepressor syncope. *Am Heart J*. 1995;129:1159–1164.
12. Cheshire WP. Thermoregulatory disorders and illness related to heat and cold stress. *Auton Neurosci*. 2016;196:91–104.
13. Colivicchi F, Ammirati F, Biffi A, Verdile L, Pelliccia A, Santini M. Exercise-related syncope in young competitive athletes without evidence of structural heart disease. *Eur Heart J*. 2002;23:1125–1130.
14. Corrado D, Basso C, Rizzoli G, Schiavon M, Thiene G. Does sports activity enhance the risk of sudden death in adolescents and young adults? *J Am Coll Cardiol*. 2003;42:1959–1963.
15. D'Andrea A, Morello A, Iacono AM, et al. Right ventricular changes in highly trained athletes: between physiology and pathophysiology. *J Cardiovasc Echogr*. 2015;25:97–102.
16. Davis JA, Cecchin F, Jones TK. Major coronary anomalies in a pediatric population: incidence and clinical importance. *J Am Coll Cardiol*. 2001;37:593–597.
17. Eckart RE, Scoville SI, Campbell CI, et al. Sudden death in young adults: a 25-year review of autopsies in military recruits. *Ann Intern Med*. 2004;141:829–834.
18. Eichner ER. An outbreak of muscle breakdown: a morality play in four acts. *Curr Sports Med Rep*. 2010;9:325–326.
19. Franco V, Callaway C, Salcido D, et al. Characterization of electrocardiogram changes throughout a marathon. *Eur J Appl Physiol*. 2014;114:1725–135.
20. Gomez AT, Prutkin JM, Rao AL. Evaluation and management of athletes with long QT syndrome: an evolved paradigm. *Sports Health*. 2016;8:527–535.
21. Grubb BP, Temesy-Armos PN, Samoil D, Wolfe DA, Hahn H, Elliott L. Title table testing in the evaluation and management of athletes with recurrent exercise-induced syncope. *Med Sci Sports Exerc*. 1993;25:24–28.
22. Harmon KG, Asif IM, Maleszewski JJ, et al. Incidence, etiology, and comparative frequency of sudden cardiac death in NCAA athletes: a decade in review. *Circulation*. 2015;132:10–19.
23. Harmon KG, Asif IM, Maleszewski JJ, et al. Incidence and etiology of sudden cardiac arrest and death in high school athletes in the United States. *Mayo Clin Proc*. 2016;91:1493–1502.
24. Hart G. Exercise-induced cardiac hypertrophy: a substrate for sudden cardiac death in athletes? *Exp Physiol*. 2003;88:639–644.
25. Heidbuchel H, Hoogsten J, Fagard R, et al. High prevalence of right ventricular involvement in endurance athletes with ventricular arrhythmias. *Eur Heart J*. 2003;24:1473–1480.
26. Herm J, Topper A, Wutzler A, et al. Frequency of exercise-induced ST-T segment deviations and cardiac arrhythmias in recreational endurance athletes during a marathon race: results of the prospective observational Berlin Beat of Running study. *BMJ Open*. 2017;7:e015798.

27. Hill AV. Muscular exercise, lactic acid, and the supply and utilization of oxygen. *Proc Royal Soc Brit.* 1924:97:438–475.
28. Immink RV, Pott FC, Secher NH, van Lieshout JJ. Hyperventilation, cerebral perfusion, and syncope. *J Appl Physiol.* 2014;116:844–851.
29. Inzlicht M, Marcora SM. The central governor model of exercise regulation teaches us precious little about the nature of mental fatigue and self-control failure. *Front Psychol.* 2016;7:656.
30. Kelly JP. Fractures complicating electro-convulsive therapy and chronic epilepsy. *J Bone Joint Surg.* 1954;36:70–79.
31. Kenefick RW, Sawka MN. Heat exhaustion and dehydration as causes of marathon collapse. *Sports Med.* 2007;37:378–381.
32. Link MS, Estes NAM. Sudden cardiac death in the athlete. *Circulation.* 2012;1 25:2511–2516.
33. Lytrivi ID, Wong AH, Ko HH. Echocardiographic diagnosis of clinically silent congenital coronary artery anomalies. *Int J Cardiol.* 2008;126:386–393.
34. Maron BJ. Historical perspectives on sudden death in young athletes with evolution over 35 years. *Am J Cardiol.* 2015;116:1461–1468.
35. Maron BJ, Carney KP, Lever HM. Relation of race to sudden cardiac death in competitive athletes with hypertrophic cardiomyopathy. *J Am Coll Cardiol.* 2003:41:974–980.
36. Maron BJ, Pellicia A. The heart of trained athletes: cardiac remodeling and risks of sports, including sudden death. *Circulation.* 2006;114:1633–1644.
37. Maron BJ, Pellicia A, Sprito P. Cardiac disorders in young trained athletes. *Circulation.* 1995;91:1596–1601.
38. Maron BJ, Shirani J, Poliac LC, Mathenge R, Roberts WO, Mueller F. Sudden death in young competitive athletes: clinical, demographic, and pathological profiles. *JAMA.* 1996;276:199–204.
39. Menezes RG, Fatima H, Hussain SA, et al. Commotio cordis: a review. *Med Sci Law.* 2017;57:146–151.
40. Minino AM. *Mortality Among Teenagers Aged 12–19 Years: United States, 1999–2006. NCHS Data Brief No. 37.* Hyattsville, MD: National Center for Health Statistics; 2010.
41. Mosso A. *Fatigue.* London: Allen & Unwin; 1915.
42. Mueller FO, Cantu RC, Van Camp SP. *Catastrophic Injuries in High School and College Sports.* Champaign, IL: Human Kinetics; 1996. pp. 23–29.
43. Noakes TD. Is it time to retire the A.V. Hill model? A rebuttal to the article by Professor Roy Shepard. *Sports Med.* 2011;41:263–277.
44. Noakes TD. Fatigue is a brain-derived emotion that regulates the exercise behavior to ensure the protection of whole body homeostasis. *Front Physiol.* 2012;3:82.
45. Pellicia A, Maron BJ, Culasso F, et al. The athlete's heart in women: echocardiographic characteristics of highly-trained elite female athletes. *JAMA.* 1996;276:211–215.
46. Rawson E, Clarkson PM, Tarnopolsky MA. Perspectives on exertional rhabdomyolysis. *Sports Med.* 2017;47 Suppl 1:S33–S49.
47. Rost R. The athlete's heart: what did we learn from Henschen, what Henschen could have learned from us. *J Sports Med Phys Fitness.* 1990;30:339–346.
48. Rowland T. Sudden unexpected death in young athletes: reconsidering "hypertrophic cardiomyopathy." *Pediatrics.* 2009;123:1217–1222.
49. Rowland T. Is the "athlete's heart" arrhythmogenic? Implications for sudden cardiac death. *Sports Med.* 2011;41:401–411.

50. Rowland T. Prevention of sudden cardiac death in young athletes: controversies and conundrums. *Med Sports Sci*. 2011;56:171–186.
51. Rowland T. Exercise electrocardiography. In: Rowland T, editor. *Cardiopulmonary Exercise Testing in Children and Adolescents*. Champaign, IL: Human Kinetics; 2018. pp. 51–64.
52. Saltzman HA, Heyman A, Sieker HO. Correlation of clinical and physiologic manifestations of sustained hyperventilation. *N Engl J Med*. 1963;268:1431–1436.
53. Saposnick G, Redelmeier D, Ruff CC, Tobler PN. Cognitive biases associated with medical decisions: a systematic review. *BMC Med Inform Decision Making*. 2016;16:138.
54. Shave R, George K, Whyte G, Hart E, Middleton N. Postexercise changes in left ventricular function: the evidence so far. *Med Sci Sports Exerc*. 2008;40:1393–1399.
55. Shephard RJ. Is it time to retire the 'central governor'? *Sports Med*. 2009;39:709–721.
56. Smith D, DeBlois J, Wharton M, Rowland T. Influence of sex on ventricular remodeling in collegiate athletes. *J Sports Med Phys Fitness*. 2012;52:11–10.
57. Smith KJ, Ainslie PN. Regulation of cerebral blood flow and metabolism during exercise. *Exp Physiol*. 2017;102:1356–1371.
58. Tester DJ, Ackerman MJ. The role of molecular autopsy in unexplained sudden cardiac death. *Curr Opin Cardiol*. 2006;21:166–172.
59. Villa ADM, Sammut E, Nair A, Rajani R, Bonami R, Chiribiri A. Coronary artery anomalies overview: the normal and abnormal. *World J Radiol*. 2016;8:537–555.

6

IS THERE BIOLOGICAL REGULATION OF PHYSICAL ACTIVITY?

The evidence—at least in adults—is beyond compelling: engaging in regular physical activity engenders health and emotional well-being. On this point there is little argument. The accumulated research information over the past several decades clearly indicates that habitual activity reduces the risk of major diseases which constitute the majority of mortality and morbidity in the population (i.e., myocardial infarction, stroke, diabetes, obesity, osteoporosis, and so forth) (7). Current public health efforts to improve the level of physical activity in the population consequently are based on a strong scientific foundation.

(In children, establishing evidence for the health-activity link is more problematic, since the disease outcomes influenced by physical activity do not typically surface until the adult years. Still, efforts to increase the activity habits of youth for salutary outcomes are founded on two reasonable assumptions: a) the subclinical genesis of the adult illnesses ameliorated by physical activity often occurs during the pediatric years, and dampening the pathologic progression of these diseases early in life will be expected to pay dividends in reducing the frequency of their clinical outcomes in later years, and b) habits of regular activity may be instilled in youth that then persist through a lifetime [55].)

Strategies to improve habits of physical activity hinge to a large extent on recognizing the factors which determine one's level of physical activity. Consequently, an entire research industry has been built on identifying just what motivates (or fails to motivate) an individual to get off the couch and engage in regular exercise. Often such determinants—perhaps better stated as "correlates"—are environmental in nature (access to recreational facilities, climate, neighborhood design); others are social (family and peer support) or psychological (self-concept, self-image) (22,58).

Implicit in designing strategies for promotion of exercise is the assumption that an individual's decision to exercise or not is just that—a conscious decision. It is a cognitive *choice* whether to take the elevator or the stairs. One *decides* to read a book or shoot some hoops in the driveway. In short, such strategies assume that the extent of involvement in physical activity is a matter of individual *free will*. The strategy, then, is to manipulate the factors which influence that active, conscious decision to exercise or not.

But now comes a different idea, one suggesting the presence of an involuntary control over physical activity which operates outside of consciousness or human will. Put precisely, the concept is that *there exists within the brain an inherent, biological center which controls an individual's level of daily motor activity*. The proposed evolutionary explanation for such an activity controller within the central nervous system rests in its contribution to maintaining the body's energy balance. Its existence would therefore be consistent with the function of other feedback systems in the body which serve to precisely maintain the *milieu intérieur* (temperature, pH, body fluid content, blood oxygenation, etc.) (56). Too, the concept of the brain serving in a pro-active manner, directing body functions rather than acting simply as a passive reflex afferent-efferent relay station, is consistent with current neurophysiological concepts (26). "The idea that an involuntary biologic controller of physical activity should exist, then, has gained conceptual credibility, having shifted from being deemed bizarre to being integrated into the current of mainstream thinking" (56).

This chapter will review arguments for the reality of such a biological control of physical activity and will address its proposed evolutionary basis. It is difficult to argue that the evidence supporting its existence is not convincing and its proposed rationale unreasonable. However, at the same time, the implications of the function of such involuntary control remain clouded in uncertainty. Specifically, one cannot review this material without raising a number of critical unanswered questions: How important is this biological control in influencing activity compared with environmental and psychosocial factors? Is its importance a function of age? (One thinks here of determinants of motor activity in a six-month old infant compared to those influencing a 30-year-old executive.) How easy is it to "override" central control of activity? Are there forces that can alter a biological activity "set point"? Can disturbance in the normal function of the biological control of physical activity be held responsible for chronic energy imbalance (i.e., obesity)? Until such questions can be answered, the "meaning" of a biologic control of physical activity will remain an unresolved but potentially significant issue.

It is not difficult to be skeptical that an occult governor, without our conscious direction, dictates how much we move around all day. Indeed, it seems counterintuitive that an individual does not make his or her own decisions regarding participation in physical activities. One weighs pros and cons, looks at alternatives, and makes decisions—what career to pursue, whom to marry, where to live, how much to exercise—based on purposeful contemplation. *Homo sapiens*, as opposed other animals, possess the capacity to *deliberate*.

But, on this matter we may be fooled. Abundant evidence has accumulated, based largely on new neuroimaging techniques, that decisions we once felt were our own actually originate in the depths of the subconscious (44). As the neurologist Robert Burton has written, "common sense is merely the strong sense of what is familiar and right, not a truth or guarantee of fact ... Feelings about our involuntarily generated subconscious thoughts often feel like deliberate actions of the conscious minds. . . . Our brains possess involuntary mechanisms that make unbiased thought impossible yet create the illusion that we are rational creatures capable of fully understanding the mind created by the same mechanisms. . . . Hiring the mind as a consultant for understanding the mind feels like the metaphoric equivalent of asking a known con man for his self-appraisal and letter reference" (12).

What all of this is saying is that the reality of a biological control of physical activity—versus one's free choice to exercise or not—is just another example of the ages-old philosophical conundrum: Do human beings possess free will, whereby one dictates his own decisions in life, or are we at the mercy of determinism, in which such actions are established by subconscious factors, ones out of conscious control, be they cultural, biological, or experiential. (A deterministic outlook holds that every action we take in our lives, every event, is established by the event that preceded it. And that event is determined by the one before it, and so on, backwards in time. A strict determinist would argue, then, that your decision of what movie to see tonight is, in fact, a reflection of—is pre-determined by—events surrounding the "Big Bang" 14 billion years ago.)

We've encountered this free will versus determinism conundrum before in this book—in Chapter 1 when arguing whether one's physical abilities in response to training are limited by a genetic ceiling or by one's will to train intensely. And in Chapter 11 we will struggle with the question of whether one's pace in a distance race is controlled by a subconscious central governor or consciously elected by one's own personal strategizing. Now, in a similar vein, can involvement in physical activity reflect the actions of a subconscious, involuntary central controller and/or a matter of personal choice? (For those beginning to suspect that a good number of other controversies in the realm of exercise science might also involve issues of free will versus determinism, Mark Balaguer's excellent book *Free Will* [MIT Press, 2014] is recommended.)

The issue of free will versus determinism is not simply an academic one. Indeed, within this debate lie serious ethical and legal questions (e.g., is a criminal truly responsible for his own heinous actions?). One might be tempted to contend that the question of whether one consciously decides to take a walk before dinner or not does not share in this import. But this may not be true. If an involuntary controller of physical activity acts to maintain body energy balance, this governor serves a critical biological function, and derangement of such a regulator of energy expenditure could eventuate in adverse health outcomes (i.e., obesity).

To summarize the basic point: "Is the amount that we move around during the course of a day a matter of free will, of conscious decision-making, susceptible to modification through education, interventional programs, and manipulation of the environment? Or, is activity energy expenditure deterministic, hard-wired by eons of evolutionary pressures into the brain as an intrinsic, involuntary controller of activity that is largely resistant to extrinsic forces? Or is it a matter, somehow, of both" (56)?

Lines of Evidence

Taken collectively, a number of observations provide substantial support for the existence of an involuntary, biologic control of daily energy expenditure via motor activity. Particularly striking is the diversity of the sources of this information, which includes evidence from human and animal activity levels over the life span, genetic studies of twins, biochemical effects, outcomes from surgical interventions in animals, and even intrauterine sex differences in physical activity.

Progressive Decline of Physical Activity Energy Expenditure Throughout Life

Perhaps the most convincing argument supporting the influence of biologic regulation of physical activity comes from the observation that levels of physical activity (when adjusted appropriately for body size), whether assessed as energy expenditure or by measures of motion, decline progressively over the course of a lifetime. Some have contended, alternatively, that psychological and social factors might be responsible for this pattern (34). Indeed, the downward trend in physical activity with age, particularly in young persons, has been interpreted from a public health standpoint as a cause for concern, a disturbing manifestation of increasingly sedentary lifestyles (17). However, while psychosocial factors are clearly important in dictating activity levels (54), an influential role of biologic control is evidenced by similar downward trends over the life span consistently observed throughout the animal kingdom.

In Human Beings

Virtually from the time that a toddler becomes fully ambulatory, the level of daily energy expenditure in physical activity, expressed in respect to body size, steadily declines throughout the human lifetime. The fall-off is most sharp during the pediatric years, levels off to some extent in mid-adulthood, and then declines again more sharply in the elderly.

In cross-sectional data accumulated by Turin in 22 international studies, average total daily energy expenditure between the ages of 2 and 18 years (measured by the doubly labeled water technique) fell from 83 to 48 kcal/kg (a 44% decrease) (67). In a similar study, Black et al. subtracted values for the basal metabolic rate from total energy expenditure to identify specifically daily activity energy expenditure (4). Between the ages of 1 and 17 years, the average daily activity energy expenditure fell from 0.105 to 0.065 MJ/kg in males (−38%) and from 0.110 to 0.83 MJ/kg in females (−25%).

A number of studies which have measured physical activity in the same individuals over time have confirmed the magnitude of fall in physical activity during childhood as indicated in these cross-sectional reports. Using oxygen uptake-calibrated heart rate measures, the reports of Saris et al. (59) and Verschuur and Kemper (69) indicated a fall in mass-specific caloric expenditure through physical activity approaching 50% between the ages of 6 and 18 years. An equivalent magnitude of decline in reported physical activity in boys and girls over a similar time period was described in the longitudinal investigation by McMurray and his colleagues (49). In a compilation of 26 such studies, Dumuth et al. calculated an average decline in activity in youth between the ages of 10 and 19 years (most assessed by questionnaire) of 7.0% per year (23).

Similar trends, though not quite so dramatic, have been recorded during the mid-adult years. In a cross-sectional study, Caspersen et al. found a decline (by questionnaire) in "regular sustained exercise" of 7% and 9% in males and females between the ages of 18–29 and 75 years (16). The Amsterdam Longitudinal Growth and Health Study involved a series of six assessments of physical activity (by questionnaire) between the ages of 13 and 27 years (68). During this 14-year period, estimated exercise energy expenditure declined from 4,990 to 2,910 METs (metabolic equivalents) in males (−42%) and from 3,810 to 3,180 METs in females (−17%). The greatest rate of decrease was observed in the early adolescent period. Similar magnitudes of decline were recorded in the Cardiovascular Risk in Young Finns project (63).

In the elderly years this pattern of progressive decline in physical activity persists. In a longitudinal study over 10 years of 33 Dutch men ages 65–84, Bijnen and colleagues found that total time spent in physical activities declined by 33% (3). The authors contended that this decrease was not caused by a deterioration in functional status. Starling et al. described an inverse relationship between physical activity energy expenditure and chronological age in women 52–85 years ($r = -0.44$) (62).

No single study has examined exercise energy expenditure or quantified daily physical activity across the entire human life span. Still, a mosaic which could be constructed from the above information would clearly indicate a substantial continuous decrement of these measures over time. The size-related daily motor activity of an elderly individual is a small fraction of that displayed by a 4-year-old child.

And in Animals

As noted above, the conclusion that the steady decline in physical activity over the life span in humans is not simply psychosocial in origin but reflects a biological-based progression is evidenced by similar trends observed among animals. In fact, virtually every animal species that has been studied demonstrates a progressive fall in motor activity with age.

Ingram has published an extensive review of the research literature addressing patterns of animal motor activity over a life span (32). Among rodents, the most common animal studied, 23 reports revealed a typical decline pf over 50% in exploratory and wheel-running activity (measured by infrared sensor and motion detectors) between the ages of 6 and 30 months. Ingram concluded that "age-related decline in laboratory rodent species is a well-established phenomenon."

Other animals display similar patterns. At one end of the size scale, Bolanowski et al. reported a decline in physical activity with age of the nematode *Caenorhabditis elegans*, a microscopic worm that lives for less than a month's time (5). Their findings were based on counting the frequency of waves of the organism's body over one minute visualized under a microscope (which declined from 80 to 20 between the ages of 4 and 14 days). Similar declines in spontaneous activity over a life span have been reported in fruit flies (43), house flies (72), and monkeys (33). The only animal which may not display such an age-related decline in activity is the giant squid (oceanographer Grant Cumming, personal communication). That's because, contrary to other animals, the squid may continue to grow throughout its life cycle, creating a continuously increasing need for volume of food intake, and, by necessity, searching behavior.

Influence of Sex

In virtually every study which has been conducted on the sex influences on physical activity, males have been found to be more active than females. In the meta-analysis of Eaton and Enns of 127 studies in subjects ages 2 months to 30 years, males predominated throughout, and the statistical significance between sex groups widened with increasing age (24). Sallis et al. reviewed nine studies in youths 6–18 years old and found that boys averaged 14% greater activity than girls by self-report and 23% higher levels of activity when assessed by heart rate (57).

Traditionally, it has been assumed that such differences in habitual physical activity by sex are explained by psycho-social factors, reflecting cultural stereotypes of masculinity and femininity. Two observations, however, have suggested that sex differences in activity levels may have a biological as well as a psychosocial basis: a) sex differences in motor activity have been observed in early infancy, even *in utero*, well before social influences on activity would be expected, and b) evidence exists that sex differences in physical activity might be at least partially explained by discrepancies between males and females in level of biological maturation.

A meta-analysis performed in 1986 of 14 studies revealed that males were significantly more physically active than females between birth and the age of 11 months (25). A follow-up analysis of the literature performed a decade later included 46 studies and again revealed male infants to be more active than females, although with a broad overlap (14). The authors concluded that

> Given such convergent data, we favour the interpretation that these early sex differences are largely innate and biological in origin. . . . This early sex difference presumably influences, and interacts with, gender-specific socialization processes to amplify sex differences as the child ages.

The initial review disclosed that even prenatally male fetuses were more active than females, a difference that did not reach statistical significance. However, only six studies were involved, which was considered to be an inadequate number to answer the question. Using ultrasound to measure fetal leg movements, Almli et al. found that males were more active than females on serial measurements at 30, 34, and 37 weeks gestation (1). However, such findings could not be confirmed by others (52). It is difficult to explain these sex differences at such an early age if determination of spontaneous motor activity was not, at least to some extent, under a genetic-based, biologic control.

We tend to think of the serial changes in physical and physiological function that turn a child into an adult during the course of the pediatric years as a predictable, deterministic process. True, but the *tempo*, the rate of such height and bone formation and development of secondary sexual characteristics, is highly variable from one child to the next. Some experience biological development faster than others, and, as a consequence, a child's chronological age does not always fit his or her biological age—as any fifth grade class photo makes obvious.

At any given chronological age, girls, on the average, demonstrate advanced biological development by 1–2 years compared to boys. Eaton and Yu initially suggested that the lower levels of physical activity in girls compared to boys might be explained by their advanced biological developmental age (25). By this proposal, then, the decline in motor activity over time during childhood was linked to biological rather than chronological age.

Lauren Sherar and her Canadian colleagues sought to find out (61). In a cross-sectional study they measured physical activity levels by questionnaire in 70 boys and 68 girls between the ages of 9 and 18 years. As expected, when activity levels were plotted against chronological age, boys were more active than girls. Bu when aligned in respect to biological age (established by estimated peak height velocity), the sex differences in activity level disappeared. Similar findings were reported by Thompson et al. (65) and Cairney et al. (13).

The concept advanced by Eaton and Yu seems to bear credibility. These results do in fact support the conclusion that "sex differences in physical activity during childhood and adolescence [in respect to chronological age] are explained by the differential tempo of sexual maturation in males and females, pointing to a biological rather than a sociocultural influence" (56).

Neurochemical Mechanisms

A biological model for motor activity regulation demands a neurochemical mechanism by which such a controller would operate. In fact, this issue has been the focus of a considerable volume of research attention, predominantly, by necessity, in animals. These investigations have provided a convincing argument that the activity of dopamine-dependent neural pathways in the brain are central to altering motor activity. In its action as a neurotransmitter, dopamine is produced by neurons in different locations throughout the brain, each with a specific function. In respect to its effect on physical activity, two loci are of particular interest—the pars compacta in the substantia nigra, located in the basal ganglia, and the ventral tegmental area in the midbrain.

Data provided in studies of rodents appears to indicate that the former locus regulates the amount of daily spontaneous physical activity, while the latter affects motivation to exercise through reward-seeking (i.e., pleasure) behavior. The examples would be, for the first, the amount that a mouse moves about in its cage all day, and, for the second, the reason such an animal is compelled to run on a wheel at all hours of the night. (As will be noted later, the same dichotomy of dopamine-stimulated exercise behavior might be manifest in humans as the extent of energy expenditure via physical activity in the former and compulsive desire for a daily 5-mile run in the latter.)

Here is a quick summary of some of the experimental data supporting these constructs. In mice selected for particular high levels of wheel running, Bronikowski et al. described a 20% increase in dopamine receptors compared to control mice (10). Active and inactive animals have been shown to exhibit different expression of dopamine receptors (38). Electrical stimulation of the substantia nigra and ventral tegmental area of rats causes an increase in spontaneous motor activity (41). When dopamine antagonists are administered to rats (either systemically or directly into the nucleus accumbens) open-field and spontaneous activity decreases (27). Motor activity and dopamine function decrease in parallel as animals age (53).

It should be noted for completeness that dopamine is not the only chemical agent in the brain that has been suspected to control spontaneous motor activity in animals (most prominently among the other candidates: ghrelin, melanocortin receptors, orexin-A, and nitric oxide). In fact, in 2008 Teske et al. provided a list of 26 such agents (64), in response to which Garland et al. commented that "various correlates of generalized locomotor activity have long been the subject of considerable research, but central themes are difficult to extract" (27). That is, any true cause-and-effect mechanisms derived from observed associations of chemical agent with activity levels are not easily deciphered.

So much for animals. What about humans? Could the "decision" to engage in physical activities reflect variations in dopamine function within the central nervous system? In the title of their 2010 article, Knab and Lightfoot asked this very question: "Does the difference between physically active and couch potato lie in the dopamine system?" (39). What these authors were asking, in effect, is can the neurochemical basis of physical activity which seems well-founded in rodents be transferred to human beings? Predictably, the answer to both questions is unknown.

There does exist some indirect evidence for such a function of dopamine and other neurotransmitters in humans. As in animals, the aging human demonstrates parallel declines in habitual physical activity and dopamine function (53). Motor disorders such as in Parkinson's disease, anorexia nervosa, and attention deficit hyperactivity disorder have all been associated with disorders of dopamine function (56). However, in a study of over 8,000 Dutch individuals Huppertz et al. could demonstrate no relationship between gene alleles affecting dopamine receptors and leisure-time exercise behavior (31). Still, this investigation concerned questionnaire responses to time spent in self-initiated physical activities rather than measured levels of general physical activity.

Effects of Brain Dysfunction on Motor Activity

Perturbations of brain function—either experimentally induced or naturally occurring—have been documented to alter motor activity levels. In his review of published studies in animals, Viggiano listed those which revealed augmented motor activity following experimentally generated lesions in 12 different regions of the brain (70). Activity levels in animals can be affected by concussions. In a study of male mice, Budinich et al. found that animals became hyperactive after a traumatic brain injury (11). These studies indicate that functional or physical disruption of brain centers may trigger alterations of motor activity.

Not surprisingly, no information is available regarding the effects of surgically induced brain lesions on activity in humans. Moreover, changes in behaviors in those with central nervous system pathology (cerebral vascular accidents, tumors) may reflect associated influences such as medications, emotional instability, associated pain symptoms and sleep disturbances. However, the story surrounding one particular brain tumor in humans may be instructive. Craniopharyngioma is a tumor located at the base of the brain in the area of the hypothalamus, the structure important in control of energy balance. Following surgical removal of this tumor, patients often become obese, which has traditionally been considered due to excessive food intake (hyperphagia). However, Harz and colleagues estimated volume of food intake in these post-operative patients as well as their daily physical activity (by accelerometer) (30). Contrary to expectations, they found that a fall in physical activity rather than an excessive caloric intake was the principal cause of their obesity. The authors postulated that this reduction in activity might reflect hypothalamic damage, hypothyroidism, or changes in autonomic nervous system activity.

Other forms of central nervous system dysfunction in humans are linked to altered motor behavior. For example, attention deficit hyperactivity disorder (ADHD) is a common disorder in youth characterized by excessive motor behavior. Its etiology is unknown, but considerable evidence points to a disturbance of dopamine and catecholamine function in the central nervous system (50). For example, a number of genes have been identified which are both associated with ADHD and control of dopamine receptor function and transport (48).

Hyperactivity has been described in up to 80% of cases of anorexia nervosa (42), a finding that has been attributed to the purposeful strategy of these patients to lose weight. However, evidence exists that this hyperactivity has a pathogenic basis as a manifestation of disturbed dopamine function (15,20). That conclusion has been supported by findings of hyperactivity in animal models of anorexia nervosa (2).

A Genetic Basis

It should follow that the existence of a biological controller of physical activity necessitates an underlying genetic basis. The phenotypic expression of genetic information is recognized to be regulated not only by gene structure but also by extra-genetic influences (epigenetic, environmental, etc.), but in the final analysis it should be expected that the actions of certain gene alleles should be identifiable that direct a central governor in the brain to establish energy expenditure through physical activity. In fact, current research continues to provide—at a remarkably increasing pace—clear-cut evidence for such genetic control in both animals (40) and human beings (71). (Indeed, by the time this book is published the sum of such data will presumably have already risen by some exponential rate.) Not only does this information provide support for biological regulation of physical activity but it offers to provide insights into a genetic basis for disturbances of energy balance such as that underlying obesity (29).

The influence of genetic information on physical activity levels is derived from a number of sources:

- Early epidemiological twin studies provided evidence for a strong genetic control over levels of habitual physical activity. Based on calculations from differences in activity in identical (monozygotic) versus fraternal (dizygotic) twins, the hereditary influence on activity was considered to be at least 50% (compared to environment and gene-environment interaction) (8).
- Animals can be successfully bred for level of daily motor activity. In the study by Garland and Kelly, each successive generation of mice exhibited progressively increasing wheel-running time, reaching a peak of a 250% rise at 6–8 weeks of age (27). Of interest, in that study both daily motor movement and wheel-running time increased with breeding, suggesting a genetic control of both forms of dopamine-driven activity.

- Gene loci linked to the phenotypic expression of physical activity have been identified thanks to dramatic advances in the analytical tools available to molecular geneticists. In animals, several such linkage studies have identified areas of chromosomes responsible for the augmented motor activity observed in selectively bred hyperactive mice (47). Still, these have accounted for only 7–17% of the variability in activity levels, causing Kelly and Pomp to conclude that "the presence of a complex architecture for voluntary activity likely involves many genes with relatively small effects" (36). As of 2014, nine linkage studies in humans had identified an association between specific gene regions and physical activity (40), and 15 candidate genes had been located that are connected with daily energy expenditure (21).

It should be recognized that "evidence for genetic control of physical activity strongly supports, but does not necessarily imply, the existence of a central nervous system controller of physical activity in humans. Gene action plays a role in personality (energetic or laconic), psychological traits (such as level of self-image), somatotype (endomorphic or ectomorphic), and abilities in motor performance (the skilled will prefer to exercise). All of these biologically influenced factors might be expected to contribute to habits of physical activity, independent of a central control mechanism" (56).

The "Meaning" of Biologic Control of Physical Activity

It is difficult to argue that the information provided in the previous section does not provide a compelling argument for the existence of a biological controller of physical activity in humans. To emphasize again, the remarkable diversity of the lines of this evidence is particularly striking. But now we move on to the next question: *why* should such a regulatory mechanism exist? What is its physiological "*raison d'être*"?

Such questions seeking to "explain" biological phenomena are typically addressed through the lens of Darwinian evolutionary pressures. That is, what survival advantage, what benefit to reproductive capacity, might this process offer—if not at present at least in the deep historical past? In this case, it is reasonable to propose that the "purpose" of biological control of physical activity lies in its contribution to the maintenance of body energy balance. Such balance—avoiding extremes of weight gain or loss—is critical for survival. And the means available for human beings to match energy "in" to energy "out" are, in fact, limited.

Maintenance of Energy Balance

The ability of the human body to preserve a constant body weight within very narrow limits is not often appreciated (35). Despite often-times wide swings in caloric intake and exercise energy expenditure, the weight of a typical adult quite remarkably varies by only about 0.5% over a 6–10 week period (37). Such constancy demands a close matching over time of energy intake by food consumption with energy losses, principally via the basal metabolic rate, physical activity, and thermic effect of food. The relative contribution of each of these mechanisms of energy loss varies widely between different individuals. In a study of adults living for 24 hours in a respiratory chamber with no vigorous activity, the participants demonstrated a total daily energy expenditure of 2,292 kcal/day. Of this total, average basal metabolic rate, spontaneous physical activity, and thermal effect of food contributed 79%, 17%, and 7%, respectively (51). At the other extreme, cyclists competing in the Tour de France were found to expend an average of over 6,000 kcal per day, which represented 70% of total energy expenditure (60).

That biological factors should control physical activity as a major component of the energy balance equation is immediately suggested by the observation that the other major determinants of energy balance (dietary intake, basal metabolic rate, thermal effect of food) are clearly of biological origin, dictated by involuntary regulatory processes. It is important to recognize, too, that the size-relative values of the principal factors influencing energy balance—caloric intake, basal metabolic rate, and physical activity—all decrease in parallel with age, particularly during the childhood years. Between the ages of 6 and 18 years the basal metabolic rate in boys declines from 53 to 44 kcal/m^2 BSA, a fall of 17%. During that same age span caloric energy intake and activity energy expenditure decrease by about one-half (9) (Figure 6.1). This provides an intriguing observation: not only

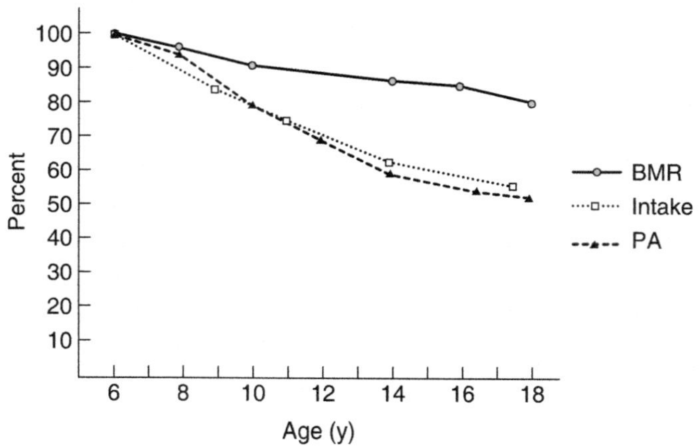

FIGURE 6.1 As children grow, parallel declines are observed in mass-specific metabolic rate (BMR), daily caloric intake (Intake), and daily energy expenditure by physical activity (PA).

Reprinted by permission from T.W. Rowland, "The Childhood Obesity Epidemic: Putting the Dynamics Into Thermodynamics," *Pediatric Exercise Science* 16 (2004):87–93.

must the magnitude of these determinants of energy balance be matched with near-zero tolerance, but any supreme energy balance controller in the human brain must also recognize and balance their *rate of change* over time. How this magic is accomplished remains mysterious. (A full discussion of the interplay between these determinants of energy balance can be found in reference 56.)

So far, no one knows precisely how a biologic control of physical activity would work. The complexity of such a system has been emphasized by Garland et al.:

> Very little is known about the neurobiology of voluntary exercise, spontaneous physical activity or sedentary behavior in healthy animals. Various neural correlates of generalized locomotor activity have long been the subject of considerable research, but central themes are difficult to extract. In general, locomotor activity in both humans and rodents is controlled by a complex cascade of neurochemical interactions that coordinate central neural inputs with motor outputs. . . . [In addition] a litany of other neural systems beyond those required for basic motor control become relevant, including those involved in aversion, conditioning, learning and the desire for and perception of both exogenous and endogenous rewards.
>
> *(28)*

Still, reasonable assumptions concerning the operation of such central control can be made using the well-documented mechanisms surrounding the biological regulation of caloric intake as a model. In this complex feedback loop, information regarding nutritional status is transmitted from several peripheral sites to a regulatory center in the hypothalamus. Based on "insights" into the energy balance status, this center regulates, via dopamine-related processes, eating behavior (i.e., augmenting or diminishing food intake by appetite).

A biological control of exercise energy expenditure might be expected to operate in a similar fashion (56). Afferent input regarding activity energy expenditure status could originate from several peripheral sources, including metabolic, pressure, and thermal receptors within muscle tissue. This information would then be transmitted to the hypothalamus, where efferent commands to increase or decrease activity could be initiated as necessary to maintain total energy balance (Figure 6.2).

These concepts presuppose an overall executive controller of all the elements in the energy balance equation which operates to maintain that balance within very narrow limits, as dictated by Darwinian evolutionary pressures. To achieve this, such a master controller, then, has at its disposal the capacity to adjust caloric intake (by appetite) and involvement in physical activity as variables which can be adjusted to sustain this balance.

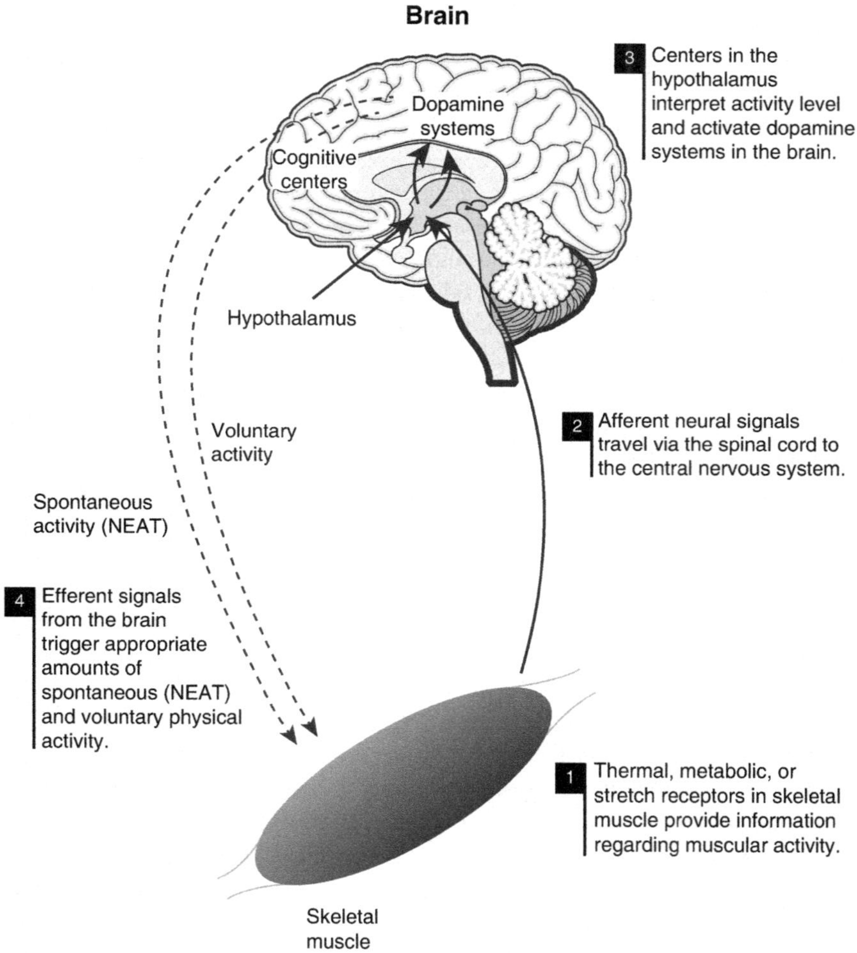

FIGURE 6.2 Hypothetical construct of the means by which a controller of activity energy expenditure in the brain might operate through afferent and efferent feedback mechanisms.

Reprinted by permission from T.W. Rowland, *Biological Regulation of Physical Activity (Champaign, IL:* Human Kinetics, 2017), 120.

Expressions of Biological Control of Activity

So far in this chapter we have skirted the issue of just what is meant by "physical activity" or "energy expenditure via motor activity." In fact, just what forms of motor activity would a purported central biological mechanism control? As we now address this issue in human beings we can harken back to an earlier discussion that identified two separate forms of physical activities in rodents driven by discrete dopamine systems in the brain—one manifest by how much an animal moves around during the course of a day (a general level of physical activity) while the other a motivationally directed reward type of activity which generates "pleasure" (the example being obsessive wheel running by rodents in a cage).

The same dichotomy might be operant in humans as well. Some have considered a biological regulator of energy expenditure as working mainly by influencing activities collectively known as *non-exercise activity thermogenesis (NEAT)*. These are all the non-planned spontaneous motions made during everyday living, such as energy expenditure from posture, fidgeting, holding a book, moving about the house, and climbing stairs. The estimates of the amount of energy expended via NEAT have varied widely (from 15% to 50% of total daily energy expenditure) and are clearly individual- and time-of-day-dependent (45). Clearly, the accumulated contribution of such "minor" forms of activity over the course of a day is far from non-trivial. That a biological controller might act primarily by influencing NEAT, and that such regulation would serve in the interests of body energy balance, is evidenced by studies indicating increases in NEAT in response to overfeeding (46) and fall in NEAT in cases of negative energy balance (45).

The second form of physical activity, which has been termed "hedonistic," includes those purposeful physical activities we choose to do for pleasure—skiing, playing basketball, distance running, and so forth. If the analogy with rodents holds, these activities—just like compulsive wheel running in cages—would also have a biological basis, driven by dopamine systems in the brain. Some have contended, however, that engagement in these hedonistic forms of physical activity are instead under the control of purposeful cognitive decision-making. As such, one's desires to participate in a couple of sets of tennis or take a hike in the country should override any biologic controller. As Borer has argued, "our understanding of the regulation of energy balance is impeded by preoccupation with a homeostatic view of this mechanism and comparative inattention to non-homeostatic motivational and physiological processes controlling feeding, spontaneous physical activity, and metabolism" (6).

The advocate of a biologic regulation of physical activity would counter, though, with the argument that, yes, you did actively *decide* to dance until dawn in a nightclub, but over time a central involuntary control would counter with a decrease in spontaneous activity (NEAT?) that would maintain overall exercise energy expenditure at a certain level important for energy balance and a stable body weight. The parallel situation occurs when one binges on a Thanksgiving Day dinner, when afterwards physiological regulation of appetite "averages out" caloric intake over time so that body weight remains essentially unchanged. That is, voluntary increases in physical activity and dietary intake can eoverride central physiological regulatory mechanisms, but only temporarily.

Experimental evidence supporting or refuting the ideas of either of these camps of opinion is not currently at hand. Perhaps a compromise proposal is in order: a control center situated in the hypothalamus of the brain considers afferent input on level of voluntary food intake and engagement in physical activities—the day-to-day flux in both as we conduct our lives—then adjusts each via appetite and motor activity to achieve a required energy balance in the body.

Implications

Perhaps the most to-the-point question that comes out of all this information is this: What is the degree of impact on levels of physical activity dictated by a central biological controller in respect to that of the traditionally considered environmental and psychological factors? Which leads to the more particular question of how does the concept of an involuntary control of physical activity fit into schemes for promoting physical fitness in the population? At present, there is no answer available to respond to either of these critical queries. It can be hoped that future research efforts will provide improved insights.

Biological regulatory mechanisms (e.g., for acid-base status, temperature, fluid content, etc.) are generally considered deterministic and immutable in their role of maintaining, in a strict manner, the constancy of the body's physiological processes. Still, such set points can change (witness the rise in target temperature response to pyrogenic stimuli when one develops a fever). Animal hibernation is, in fact, a classic example of biological set points not only being modified but essentially eliminated altogether. Too, examples in which cognitive will can override biologic control can be cited (starvation during hunger strikes, heat stroke with sports competition). Thus, the plasticity of a regulator of physical activity in response to cognitively determined behaviors remains to be determined.

Could a Biological Controller of Physical Activity be Altered by Pharmacological Intervention?

There exists a long list of chemical agents that when administered to animals and/or human beings will alter physical activity behavior (66,70). Based on this finding, Thorburn and Proietto have suggested that pharmacological therapy might prove useful in increasing physical activity and thereby favorably affecting energy balance in individuals with obesity (66). Drugs which operate by decreasing appetite have been utilized in overweight persons, with variable success, but at present, none are available with the intention of augmenting motor activity.

The potential for this pharmacological approach has not gone unnoticed. Castaneda et al. have suggested that future pharmacological means of improving levels of spontaneous physical activity could be highly successful in managing those with obesity, since physical activity possesses the greatest variability among the contributors to energy expenditure (18). Ceccarini and colleagues concluded that:

> In light of the recent difficulties in finding drugs with a safe and durable impact on body weight, an alternative approach to be employed in the future may be represented by stimulating physical activity and leptin sensitivity or

reproducing its beneficial effect on weight control. Identification of gene variants positively associated with beneficial effects of increasing locomotor activity in obese individuals may further help in the selection of subsets of patients potentially responding to such therapeutic approach.

(19)

A Final Thought

To finish this chapter, a final speculation: Resolution of this controversy surrounding whether one's participation in daily physical activity is controlled by personal choice, influenced by alterable environmental factors and/or the dictates of a subconscious governor of motor activity working to maintain energy balance might be expected to be of high interest to philosophical thinkers. Particularly this might serve to enlighten those stuck in the quagmire of classic arguments of free will versus determinism. Here, quite astoundingly, would be a philosophical "nut" cracked by scientific investigation. Neat.

References

1. Almli CR, Ball RH, Wheeler ME. Human fetal and neonatal movement patterns: gender differences and fetal-to-neonatal continuity. *Dev Psychobiol.* 2001;38:252–273.
2. Barry VC, Klawans HL. On the role of dopamine in the pathophysiology of anorexia nervosa. *J Neurol Trans.* 1976;38:107–122.
3. Bijnen FCH, Feskens EJM, Caspersen CJ, Mosterd WL, Kromhout D. Age, period, and cohort effects on physical activity among elderly men during 10 years of follow-up: the Zutphen Elderly Study. *J Gerontol.* 1998;53A:M235–M241.
4. Black AE, Coward WA, Cole TJ, Prentice AM. Human energy expenditure in affluent societies. *Eur J Clin Nutr.* 1996;50:72–92.
5. Bolanowski MA, Russell RL, Jacobson LA. Quantitative measures of aging in the nematode *Caenorhabditis elegans. Mech Ageing Dev.* 1981;15:279–295.
6. Borer KT. Nonhomeostatic control of human appetite and physical activity in regulation of energy balance. *Exerc Sport Sci Rev.* 2010;38:114–121.
7. Bouchard C, Blair SN, Haskell WL. *Physical Activity and Health. Second Edition.* Champaign, IL: Human Kinetics; 2012.
8. Bouchard C, Malina RM, Pérusse L. *Genetics of Fitness and Physical Performance.* Champaign, IL: Human Kinetics; 1997. p. 66.
9. Briefel RR, McDowell MA, Alaimo K. Total energy intake of the US population: the third National Health and Nutrition Examination Survey, 1988–1991. *Am J Clin Nutr.* 1995;62 Suppl:1072S–1080S.
10. Bronikowski AM, Rhodes JS, Garland TJ, Prolla TA, Awad TA, Gammie SC. The evolution of gene expression in mouse hippocampus in response to selective breeding for increased locomotor activity. *Evol Int J Org Evol.* 2004;58:2079–2086.
11. Budinich CS, Tucker LB, Lowe D, Rosenberger JG, McCabe JT. Short and long-term motor and behavioral effects of diazoxide and dimethyl sulfoxide administration in the mouse after traumatic brain injury. *Pharm Biochem Behav.* 2013;108 Suppl C:66–73.
12. Burton RA. *A Skeptics Guide to the Mind.* New York: St. Marin's Griffin; 2013.

13. Cairney J, Veldhuisen S, Kwan M, Hay J, Faught BE. Biological age and sex-related declines in physical activity during adolescence. *Med Sci Sports Exerc.* 2013;46:730–735.
14. Campbell DW, Eaton WO. Sex differences in the activity level of infants. *Inf Child Develop.* 1999;8:1–17.
15. Casper RC. The "drive for activity" and "restlessness" in anorexia nervosa: potential pathways. *J Affec Disord.* 2006;92:99–107.
16. Caspersen CJ, Pereira MA, Curran KM. Changes in physical activity patterns in the United States, by sex and cross-sectional age. *Med Sci Sports Exerc.* 2000;32:1601–1609.
17. Caspersen CJ, Powell KE, Christenson GM. Physical activity, exercise, and physical fitness: definitions and distinctions for health-related research. *Public Health Rep.* 1985;100:126–131.
18. Castenada TR, Jurgens H, Weidmer P. Obesity and the neuroendocrine control of energy homeostasis: the role of spontaneous locomotor activity. *J Nutr.* 2005;135:1314–1319.
19. Ceccarini G, Maffei M, Vitti P, Santini F. Fuel homeostasis and locomotor behavior: role of leptin and melanocortin pathways. *J Endocrin Invest.* 2015;38:125–131.
20. Davis C. Eating disorders and hyperactivity: a psychobiological perspective. *Can J Psychiatry.* 1997;42:168–175.
21. DeMoor MHM, Liu Y-J, Boomsma DI, et al. Genome-wide association study of exercise behavior in Dutch and American adults. *Med Sci Sports Exerc.* 2009;41:1887–1895.
22. Dishman RK, Sallis JF, Orenstein D. The determinants of physical activity and exercise. *Public Health Rep.* 1981;4:421–438.
23. Dumuth D, Gigante D, Domingues M, Kohl HW. Physical activity change during adolescence: a systematic review and pooled analysis. *Int J Epidemiol.* 2011;40:685–698.
24. Eaton WO, Enns LR. Sex differences in human motor activity level. *Psychol Bull.* 1986;100:19–28.
25. Eaton WO, Yu AP. Are sex differences in child moor activity a function of sex differences in maturational status? *Child Dev.* 1989;60:1005–1011.
26. Engel AK. Dynamic predictions: oscillations and synchrony in top-down processing. *Nature Rev.* 2001;2:704–716.
27. Garland T, Kelly SA. Phenotype plasticity and experimental evolution. *J Exp Biol.* 2006;209:2344–2361.
28. Garland T, Schutz H, Chappell MA, et al. The biological control of voluntary exercise, spontaneous activity and daily energy expenditure in relation to obesity: human and rodent perspectives. *J Exp Biol.* 2011;214:206–229.
29. Graff M, Scott RA, Justice AE, et al. Genome-wide physical activity interactions in adiposity—a meta-analysis of 200,452 adults. *PLoS Genet.* 2017;13:e1006528.
30. Harz KJ, Muller HL, Waldek E, Pudel V, Roth C. Obesity in patents with craniopharyngioma: assessment of food intake and movement counts indicating physical activity. *J Clin Endocrinol Metab.* 2003;88:5227–5231.
31. Huppertz C, Meike B, Broen-Blokhuis MM, et al. The dopamine reward system and leisure time exercise behavior: a candidate allele study. *Biomed Res Int.* 2014;2014:591717.
32. Ingram DK. Age-related decline in physical activity: generalizations to nonhumans. *Med Sci Sports Exerc.* 2000;32:1623–1629.
33. Janicke B, Coper D, Janicke UA. Motor behavior of different-aged Cercopithecidae: silver-leafed monkey (*Presbytis cristatus* esch.), lion-tailed monkey (*Macaca Silenus L.*), moor macaque (*Macaca maura Cuv.*) as observed in the zoological garden. *Gerontology.* 1986;32:133–140.

34. Katzmarzyk PT. Physical activity and fitness with age, sex, and ethnic differences. In: Bouchard C, Blair SN, Haskell WL, editors. *Physical Activity and Health. Second Edition.* Champaign, IL: Human Kinetics; 2012. pp. 39–51.
35. Keesey RE, Hirvonen MD. Body weight set points: determination and adjustment. *J Nutr.* 1997;127:1875S–1883S.
36. Kelly SA, Pomp D. Genetic determinants of voluntary exercise. *Trends Gen.* 2013; 29:348–357.
37. Khosa T. Billewicz WZ. Measurement of changes in body weight. *Br J Nutr.* 1964;18:227–239.
38. Knab AM, Bowen RS, Hamilton AT, Gulledge AA, Lightfoot JT. Altered dopaminergic profiles: implications for the regulation of voluntary physical activity. *Behav Brain Res.* 2009;204:147–152.
39. Knab AM, Lightfoot JT. Does the difference between physically active and couch potato lie in the dopamine system? *Int J Biol Sci.* 2010;6:133–150.
40. Kostrzewa E, Kas MJ. The use of mouse models to unravel genetic architecture of physical activity: a review. *Genes Brain Behav.* 2014;13:87–103.
41. Kotz CM, Wang C, Teske JA, et al. Orexin A mediation of time spent moving in rats: neural mechanisms. *Neuroscience.* 2006;142:29–36.
42. Kron L, Katz JL, Weiner H. Hyperactivity in anorexia nervosa: a fundamental feature. *Compr Psychiatry.* 1978;19:433–440.
43. LeBourg E, Lints FA. Hypergravity and aging in Drosophila melanogaster. 5. Patterns of movement. *Gerontology.* 1992;28:65–70.
44. Lehrer J. *How We Decide.* Boston: Mariner Books; 2009.
45. Levine JA. Non-exercise activity thermogenesis. *Proc Nutr Soc.* 2003;62:667–679.
46. Levine JA, Eberhardt NL, Jensen MD. Role of nonexercise activity thermogenesis in resistance to fat gain in humans. *Science.* 1999;283:212–214.
47. Lightfoot JT, Leamy J, Pomp D, et al. Strain screen and haplotype association mapping of wheel running in inbred mouse strains. *J Appl Physiol.* 2010;109:623–634.
48. Madras BK, Miller GM, Fischman AJ. The dopamine transporter and attention-deficit/hyperactivity disorder. *Biol Psychiatry.* 2005;57:1397–1409.
49. McMurray RG, Harrell JS, Bangdiwala SI, Hu J. Tracking of physical activity and aerobic power from childhood through adolescence. *Med Sci Sports Exerc.* 2003;35:1914–1922.
50. Prince J. Catecholamine dysfunction in attention-deficit/hyperactivity disorder: an update. *J Clin Psychopharmacol.* 2008;28 Suppl 2:S39–S45.
51. Ravussin E, Lillioja S, Anderson TE, Christin L, Bogardus C. Determinants of 24-hour energy expenditure in man. *J Clin Invest.* 1986;78:1568–1578.
52. Robles de Medina PG, Visser GH, Huizink AC, Buitelaar JK, Mulder EJ. Fetal behavior does not differ between boys and girls. *Early Hum Develop.* 2003;7:17–26.
53. Roth GS, Joseph JA. Cellular and molecular mechanisms of impaired dopamine function with aging. *Ann NY Acad Sci.* 1994;719:129–135.
54. Rowland T. Adolescence: a "risk factor" for physical inactivity. *Pres Council Phys Fitn Sports Res Dig.* 199;3:1–5.
55. Rowland T. Promoting physical activity for children's health: rationale and strategies. *Sports Med.* 2007;37:929–936.
56. Rowland T. *Biologic Regulation of Physical Activity.* Champaign, IL: Human Kinetics; 2017.
57. Sallis JF, Buono MJ, Roby JJ, Micale FG, Nelson JA. Seven-day recall and other physical activity self-reports in children and adolescents. *Med Sci Sports Exerc.* 1993;25:99–108.

58. Sallis JF. Prochaska JJ, Taylor WC. A review of correlates of physical activity of children and adolescents. *Med Sci Sports Exerc.* 2000;32:963–975.
59. Saris WHM, Elvers JWH, van't Hof MA, Binkhorst RA. Changes in physical activity of children aged 6 to 12 years. In: Rutenfranz J, Mocellin R, Klimt F, editors. *Children and Exercise XII.* Champaign, IL: Human Kinetics; 1986. pp. 121–130.
60. Saris WHM, van Erp-Baart MA, Westerterp KR, ten Hoor F. Study on food intake and energy expenditure during extreme sustained exercise: the Tour de France. *Int J Sports Med.* 1989;10 Suppl 1:S26–S31.
61. Sherar LB, Esliger DW, Baxter-Jones ADG, Tremblay MS. Age and gender differences in youth physical activity: does physical maturity matter? *Med Sci Sports Exerc.* 2007;39:830–835.
62. Starling RD, Toth MJ, Matthews DE, Poehlman ET. Energy requirements and physical activity of older free-living African Americans: a doubly-labeled water study. *J Clin Endocrinol Metab.* 1998;83:1529–1534.
63. Telama R, Yang X. Decline of physical activity from youth to young adulthood in Finland. *Med Sci Sports Exerc.* 2000;21:1617–1622.
64. Teske JA, Billington CJ, Kotz CM. Neuropeptidergic mediators of spontaneous physical activity and non-exercise thermogenesis. *Neuroendocrinology.* 2008;87:71–90.
65. Thompson AM, Baxter-Jones ADG, Mirwald RL, Bailey DA. Comparison of physical activity in male and female children: does maturation matter? *Med Sci Sports Exerc.* 2003;35:1684–1690.
66. Thorburn AW, Proietto J. Biological determinants of spontaneous physical activity. *Obes Rev.* 2000;1:87–94.
67. Turin E. Energy requirements of children and adolescents. *Pub Health Nutr.* 2005; 8:968–993.
68. Van Mechelen W, Twisk JWR, Post GB, Snel J, Kemper HCG. Physical activity of young people: the Amsterdam longitudinal growth and health study. *Med Sci Sports Exerc.* 2000;32:1610–1616.
69. Verschuur R, Kemper HCG. Habitual physical activity in Dutch teenagers measured by heart rate. In: Binkhorst RA, Kemper HCG, Saris WHM, editors. *Children and Exercise XI.* Champaign, IL: Human Kinetics; 1985. pp. 194–202.
70. Viggiano D. The hyperactive syndrome: metanalysis of genetic alterations, pharmacological treatments and brain lesions which increase locomotor activity. *Brain Behav Res.* 2008;194:1–14.
71. de Vilhena e Santos DM, Katzmarzyk PT, Seabra AF, Maia JA. Genetics of physical activity and physical inactivity in humans. *Behav Genet.* 2012;42:559–578.
72. Zou S, Liedo P, Altamirano-Robles L, et al. Recording life-time behavior and movement in an invertebrate model. *PLoS ONE.* 2011;6:e18151.

7

HOW CAN A BASEBALL PLAYER HIT A 95-MPH FASTBALL?

This controversy pits the scientists against the athletes (a relationship that has, admittedly, not always been the warmest). The question: Can a major league batter successfully hit a 95-mph fastball?

According to the scientists, the answer is "no." And here's why. The pitch, delivered 60.5 feet away, crosses home plate in about 0.5 seconds. In that space of time the batter must decide if, when, and where to swing a bat which measures 2.75 inches across to strike a ball of 2.85 inches in diameter. The time required between deciding to attempt to hit the pitch and the initiation of muscular activity is around .200 seconds, and then it takes .180 seconds to swing the bat. That means that the decision to swing or not at the pitch must be made when the ball is not yet half way to the plate, and the swing must be started at a point when the ball has reached about 60% of its flight path. (To put this into perspective, the blink of an eye takes about .300-.400 seconds.) Just to start with, then, any success in striking the ball with the bat would seem to be an insurmountable challenge bordering on the miraculous.

Even more importantly, though, the angular velocity in the batter's field of vision as the ball crosses home plate is over 500 degrees per second. The fastest angular velocity that a human being's visual apparatus is capable of following is expected to be about 70 degrees per second. This means that the batter must lose sight of the ball well before it reaches the plate. The location and timing of the swing, then, is only a matter of a good guess. That a batter could actually connect ball and bat in such a situation, assuredly, must be no more than a matter of chance (that is to say, like, almost never).

Meanwhile a first baseman for the Boston Red Sox who is currently sporting a .250 batting average can only read this with much amusement. Out on the diamond, hitting a 95-mph fastball is, contrary to all theoretical expectations, a reality often achieved. Obviously, in this controversy the athletes are correct. But why? How do these extraordinary masters of applied physics manage to perform—not consistently but nonetheless with astounding frequency—an "impossible" task that makes the game of baseball so enjoyable to play and watch?

The issue is of more than academic interest. If hitters could appreciate the factors that explain just how they can accomplish this remarkable feat, and if such determinants were capable of being improved through training, a world of possibilities might be uncovered that could lead to batting champion success. While much has been learned about the vagaries of physics underpinning the game of baseball, though, much remains mysterious (53).

Hitting a pitched baseball presents two specific challenges: successful judgments of timing—*when* to swing—and space—*where* to swing. The former is termed *coincident timing*, while the latter requires the independent facility of *visual tracking* of the ball. The trick for the batter, then, is to somehow defy the proscribed limits expected by physical principles in accomplishing these tasks and deliver a shot through the gap just outside the diving shortstop's glove.

Tracking the Ball

"Watching the ball" is the oft-repeated mantra critical for success in playing all ball sports. If you want to hit a baseball, so it goes, you have to know where to swing. Do major league players possess super-human physical and physiological qualities that enable them to do this better than the rest of us? Do they utilize "tricks" that permit them to bypass the expected limits of human performance? Or have the normal limits of visual tracking of a baseball simply been underestimated? The answers to these questions are not altogether clear.

When the eye is following a moving object, it must keep the image of that object on the *fovea*, the small region in the central portion of the retina of the eye that provides for accurate vision. Once the image wanders from the fovea, which only occupies 1–2° of the visual field, one's vision becomes impaired. An image only five degrees away from the fovea results in a loss of visual perception of 70%. It is possible for the eye to track (i.e., maintain a moving object on the fovea) by "smooth pursuit movements" as long as the angular velocity of the object across the field of vision is normally less than 60–70° per second. At a higher velocity, the eye cannot "keep up," and begins to use jumps of visual focus, called *saccades*, to define the path of the object.

Saccades therefore play an important role in serving as a "default" mechanism when angular velocities exceed those that can be satisfied by continuous tracking with the eyes. They also serve to provide a full picture of one's surroundings, as the eye must move in a continuous series of saccades to enable the brain to compose a visual collage which appears to the consciousness as a three-dimensional picture of reality. Saccadic motions of the eye normally are no greater than about 15°, and are extremely rapid (up to 900° per second); during the movement itself vision is temporarily suppressed to prevent blurring that would otherwise occur. Use of saccades in following a moving object like a pitched baseball can be either voluntary or reflex (i.e., automatic). Saccades and continuous pursuit motions of the eye are independent neuro-visual functions. Both mature during childhood and are expected to reach adult mature levels by adolescence (23).

Visual tracking patterns in non-athletic individuals have been described by Schalen (45). Eye motions were measured as subjects followed on a screen a spot of light moving at speeds varying from 10° to 60° per second. Continuous tracking ability was observed to decline once angular velocities reached 40–50° per second. Superimposed saccades were observed in most of the participants and their frequency and amplitude were directly related to the speed of the light target. Interestingly, although this was the general pattern among the study participants, three followed the light totally free of saccades, indicating that a "smooth pursuit system can function above optimal velocity limits." The author suggested that "this type of tracking may be explained by a high degree of attention and motivation."

Do differences in visual tracking and use of saccades explain the talent of major league baseball players to hit a fastball? Electrical engineers Terry Bahill and Tom LaRitz, in a study they conducted "for the fun of it," set out to try to find some answers (6). They instrumented graduate students, members of the Carnegie Mellon University baseball team, and a single professional player for the Pittsburgh Pirates, to determine their eye and head motions in response to a simulated baseball pitch (a white plastic ball pulled by a motor down a string at speeds between 60–100 mph). In assessing their results, the definition of two measures must be appreciated. The first, which might be termed the horizontal *visual angle*, is that created between the batter's direction of vision (where his eyes are pointed) and the line connecting the pitching mound to home plate (essentially, the flight path of the pitched ball). As the pitch is delivered, this angle is almost zero, then increases very slowly (to about 5 degrees during most of the ball's path to the plate). It quickly increases just as it approaches the batter, reaching 90 degrees when the ball actually crosses the plate. In considerations of tracking the ball, then, the image of the ball is traveling almost directly toward the batter for the great majority of the pitch but suddenly deviates to a right angle, perpendicular to the line of vision, as it traverses home plate.

The other measure, alluded to earlier, is the *angular velocity*, the speed in degrees of arc per second that the ball passes through in the batter's field of vision. The limits of the ability of the eyes to continuously track the ball by smooth pursuit movements are defined by this measure. As noted previously, it is not expected that the human eye can track a baseball which is moving at an angular velocity of over 60–80° per second.

Bahill and LaRitz found in their study that the students could track the ball as it approached until the point when the visual angle reached 16°, which occurred when the ball was 9 feet in front of the plate. When the angle reached 50°, at two feet in front of the plate, the image of the ball was displaced a full 34° off the foveal region of retina (the focus point of visual acuity). The fastest smooth pursuit velocity for the eyes was 50° per second with an additional 20° per second provided for the head, well beneath the average angular velocity of the ball (507° per second) between the visual angle of 16° and 50°.

The single professional player managed to keep his eye on the ball longer in its path than the students, with an acceptable position error until the ball was 5.5 feet from the plate with a visual angle of 24°. But at the 50° visual angle point, the image, which was moving at a remarkable angular velocity of 1,100° per second, was 16° off the fovea.

Interestingly, the investigators found in this small group of subjects that the use of a saccade when the eye lost the capacity for continuous pursuit tracking as the ball neared home plate was uncommon. In fact, this was observed in only one subject, who watched the ball in the first half of its trajectory before performing a saccadic movement ahead of the ball, which allowed him to actually observe the ball striking the bat.

From the findings in this study it could be concluded that a batter can visually track an oncoming pitch by smooth pursuit eye movements for most of the path of the ball, but at a distance of 5–7 feet in front of the plate he will "lose it." The eye has the capacity for performing a saccadic motion ahead of the ball at this point and then letting the ball "catch up," but the remaining distance/time to the plate is sufficiently short that this may not be a common strategy. Consequently, one cannot normally watch the ball to the point of contact with the bat. However, as Bahill and LaRitz commented, "Why would a batter want to see the ball hit his bat? He could not, because of his slow reaction time, use the information gained in the last portion of the ball's flight to alter the course of the bat." They felt, instead, that information gained earlier in the ball's flight obtained by continuous visual tracking is utilized to predict the ball's location when it crosses the plate. And, not surprisingly, professional baseball players are more adept at such tracking and prediction than nonplayers.

It is intuitively obvious that the slower the speed of the pitch, the closer to the plate the batter can track it. Which raises an interesting question—how slow does the pitch have to be before a batter can visualize it all the way to the bat? Watts and Bahill performed a computer simulation to answer just that nagging question (53). Using a very conservative upper limit of trackable angular velocity of 300° per second, they found the expected direct correlation between the pitch speed and the distance that the tracking eye would lose sight of the ball in front of the plate. The remarkable finding was that with the slowest pitch that would still reach the plate (20 mph in slow pitch softball) the batter would still lose the ball in his or her vision 3–4 feet in front of the plate. Conclusion: It is impossible to throw a pitch slow enough that the batter can actually track it all the way to bat.

Several studies have indicated that baseball players are superior to nonathletes in *dynamic visual acuity (DVA)*, defined as the capacity to discriminate the characteristics of an object moving in the field of vision (18,39,51,52). These investigations measured the ability of subjects to recognize the direction of the gap in a C-shaped target as it is projected on a screen with increasing velocities. Rouse et. al, for example, found an average DVA of 82° and 70° per second in baseball players and nonathletes, respectively (39). Superior DVA in athletes compared to nonathletes has, in fact, been demonstrated in a number of sports, including volleyball, basketball, tennis, and motor sports.

In the study of Uchida et al., in which baseball players had a 33% greater DVA than nonplayers, the authors concluded that "the better DVA of athletes is primarily due to an improved ability to track moving targets with their eyes" (50). A number of authors have contended that, in turn, this superior tracking ability is a consequence of an enhanced use of saccadic movements.

Again, the idea here is that saccadic eye movements serve as a "default" means of recognizing the trajectory of the ball when its angular velocity in the batter's field of vision exceeds that which can be achieved by smooth pursuit movements of the eyes. The saccade (or series of saccades) then jumps ahead of the path of the ball, allowing it to "catch up" in one's vision.

There is, however, very little research information which would document the use of saccades in accounting for the superior tracking abilities of baseball hitters. In the sport of cricket, the batsman faces a similar visual task as in baseball—the ball is delivered at a speed of up to 80 mph by the bowler before it strikes the ground and then must be struck on the rebound by the batsman. Land and McLeod reported that from the time of its release the batsman's eyes follow the ball but then make a predictive saccade to the point where the ball is expected to strike the ground. The ball is then followed by the eyes for the 100–200 ms after it bounces (20). Importantly, the saccade was found to be quicker in good compared to poor batsmen.

Bahill and LaRitz have pointed out that in baseball "the anticipatory saccade must be made before the end of the trajectory, because saccadic suppression prevents us from seeing during saccades. This suppression of vision extends about 20 ms after the saccade. So if you want to see the ball hit the bat, you must make your anticipatory saccade early in the trajectory" (6).

A number of investigations have been performed, in fact, which have addressed the question of which portion of a pitched baseball's path to the plate can be best utilized by the batter in predicting the location of the ball when it crosses the plate (9,14). To reiterate the task: It takes 500 ms for the pitched ball to reach the plate, so a swing/no-swing decision must be made by the batter in that time span. The batter's visual reaction time amounts to 200 ms, and the duration for the swing itself 180 ms. Theoretically, then, without some kind of super-power, the batter must make the decision to swing or not 120 ms into the pitch; that is, when the spinning baseball has only traveled a distance of about 18 feet, or 26% of its trajectory. Presumably, then, the successful batter possesses the means of adjusting the swing based on later visual information, either via superior visual tracking or use of saccades.

Early studies suggested that baseball hitters do not, in fact, focus on the ball during its entire flight and emphasized the importance particularly of prediction based on early portions of its trajectory. Two recent studies have shed some light on this matter.

Based on those earlier reports, Patricia De Lucia and Edward Cochran from Adelphi University theorized that hiding the first portion of the pitch from the batter would be most detrimental to hitting performance (9). To test this, they examined the ability of nine college ball players to successfully strike a 60-mph pitch from a ball machine when vision was obscured by a screen during the first, middle, and third portions of the pitched, compared with a control non-obscured pitch. Somewhat surprisingly, the batters demonstrated good success in all the obscured conditions, making contact with the ball on 64% of pitches compared to 78% in the control condition. The lowest success rate (57%) was observed when the middle portion of the pitch was obscured; no significant differences from the control condition were seen when vision was blocked in the first and third portions of the ball trajectory. The authors concluded that the most significant take-away message from this investigation was that "batters can extract sufficient perceptual information for batting regardless of which segment of the trajectory is blocked."

Takatoshi Higuchi and his colleagues took a different approach with a similar testing protocol, examining the effect of pitch trajectory occlusion on the accuracy of the batter in striking the ball on the ideal "sweet spot" of the bat (14). In this study, ten college baseball players attempted to strike a delivered ball at speeds of 72 and 91 mph in three conditions: no occlusion, and while wearing a visual occlusion device that blocked the flight of the pitched ball beginning 150 ms after the ball release and 150 ms before arrival at the batter (total pitch times for the two speeds were 548 and 453 ms). Again, little difference was seen in the three conditions. The only significant difference from the control non-obstructed condition was a greater variability of the ball-bat contact location in the short-axis direction during the first third of the pitch. This study supported the idea that "visual information about the final one-third of the ball trajectory did not contribute significantly toward improving baseball hitting accuracy." As R.K. Adair contended in his book *The Physics of Baseball*, "If it weren't psychologically upsetting, the batter could just as well close his eyes after the ball is halfway to the plate, or if it were a night game, management could turn out the lights—the hitter would hit the ball just as well" (3).

Conclusions from these two studies should be tempered by certain limitations of the experimental procedure, as pointed out by the authors themselves. In the former study the pitch speed was slow and the testing apparatus was considered to be a "distraction." The same might be said of the visual occlusive device worn in the second study, in which ball delivery was limited to the strike zone above the outer half of home plate from the batter "for participant's safety." Both studies, then, describe an "artificial batting situation," and relevance of the findings to the real world of a night game at Fenway Park is problematic.

Other authors have emphasized the importance of batter recognition of events in the early phase of the delivered pitch. In a study of junior college baseball players, Gray found that swing/no-swing decisions were correlated with the launch angle of the pitcher's delivery (13). It was pointed out, however, that in that study other potential influences, such as observed ball rotation, gravitational drop rate, and so forth were not accounted for in this analysis. Gray contended that "it is more likely that the batter uses visual information about the ball's crossing height to *adjust* [italics mine] the movement parameters for the first phase of the swing" (13). (Whether a hitter can functionally adjust the direction of the bat in mid-swing has been argued [10,32], but the recognized ability of a batter to abort a swing would seem to clearly indicate this is possible.)

Hitting A Curveball

The foregoing discussion is based on the erroneous premise that the batter stepping up to the plate can anticipate a fastball approaching in a predictable straight trajectory. Of course, this isn't true. In fact, the wily pitcher can act to make the ball move in a number of directions—curveball, slider, knuckle ball, and so forth, which compounds the challenge of the batter to accurately predict the path of the ball to contact with his swinging bat. A full discussion of the flight paths of these pitches in the pitcher's arsenal and how they might be recognized by a batter is beyond the scope of this chapter. However, a brief look at the challenges provided by a curveball is in order.

According to Newton's First Law of Motion, an object moving forward in space can be deviated from its forward path by an external force, and in the case of a pitched baseball this is provided by *Bernoulli's principle*. The latter holds that the faster the velocity of a fluid—be it liquid or gaseous, like air—the lower its pressure. And that, in a nutshell, is what makes a curveball curve.

When throwing a curve, the pitcher puts a twist on the ball with his fingers that imparts topspin, meaning that, if the ball is moving right to left, it is turning counter-clockwise. A small layer of air which adheres to the stitches of the ball on the top, which is spinning forward in the direction of the pitch, encounters the oncoming air at 70 mph. Meanwhile, the air flowing over the bottom of the ball is spinning away from the direction of the pitch and the oncoming air. Consequently, air flows slower over the top than the bottom, causing a downward pressure differential, and the ball drops during its path to the plate. The same dynamics can be used to apply side spin to a pitch, particularly with a sidearm delivery, causing the ball to curve laterally. Most curveballs delivered at the big-league level arrive at the plate with a combination of the two motions (53).

A talented pitcher can deliver a curveball that drops by as much as 17 inches, with the extent of the curve being influenced by factors such as the radius of the ball, the amount of spin, the speed of the pitch, and the density of the surrounding air. Since the latter effect declines with altitude, it is said that it is more difficult to throw a good curveball at Coors Field in Denver than in Yankee Stadium and virtually impossible, theoretically, at the top of Mount Everest (29).

A thrown curveball describes a continuous arc from its delivery to its arrival at the plate. In fact, as Allman has pointed out, "if [a ball] travels sideways and there were no gravity . . . a curveball would form a circle with a more than 2,000-foot diameter, circumnavigating Baltimore's stadium and parking lot" and, finally, returning to the pitcher (4). It has always been intriguing, though, that as seen from the batter's perception, the curveball suddenly "breaks" down or laterally about 5–10 feet in front of the plate. That is, the batter cannot discern any curve of the pitch until just before it reaches home plate. This peculiarity, which, of course, is what makes a curveball so difficult to hit, has been ascribed to a visual illusion caused by the changing visual angle of the ball in the batter's vision or to a transition between central and peripheral vision (46).

Even the best batters will acknowledge the difficulty in connecting with a well-thrown curveball, particularly one which breaks toward the lower outside border of the plate. One not thrown so well, such as a curve ending up high in the strike zone (a "hanging curve"), on the other hand, is highly susceptible to being driven out of the park. If a curve breaks early, there may be sufficient time of visual tracking to permit the pitch recognition and location. Hitters employ other clues in dealing with curveballs. The pattern of pitches by the pitcher (i.e., some are curveball specialists and others rarely will deliver one), the pitch count, the pitches thrown to previous batters, etc., can help a batter better guess if a curveball is likely coming. Sometimes give-away quirks in a pitcher's windup or delivery are predictive, and some players feel they can detect on oncoming curve by observing the rotation of the seams on the ball (17).

Pitching-Hitting Handedness Discordance

Traditional baseball wisdom contends that batters hit more successfully (and, consequently, pitchers fare worse) when facing a player of opposite handedness. That's why a coach will often bring in a right-handed pitcher to relieve a lefty when facing a right-handed batter in the final innings of a tight game. But just what accounts for these handedness advantages is not altogether clear. "This difference in most batters' ability is perplexing," wrote Bahill and LaRitz (6), "since our computer analysis shows that for an overhand fastball the only difference is a 2° offset in the beginning; there is no difference in either angular position or angular velocity over the last fourth of the pitch. . . . We suspect, with little evidence, that for a right-handed batter the right-handed pitcher is harder to hit than the left-handed pitcher only for the curve ball."

A curveball thrown by a right-handed pitcher will deviate down and out, away from a right-handed batter, but down and in, toward the left-handed batter (and vice versa for a left-handed pitcher). It has been suggested that the differences in batting success related to handedness might reflect a moment's hesitation from fear. Bahill and LaRitz quote the comments of Karl Schurr of Bowling Green University: "When a right-handed batter sees a ball thrown by a right-handed pitcher coming straight at his head he doesn't know if it is a curve ball that will cross the plate for a strike, or a wild fastball that will hit his head. On the other hand, the left-handed pitcher would have to be wild as a March hare to raise as much adrenaline in the batter."

Getting Real

The astute reader may have by now voiced a criticism that has been commonly made concerning the above studies: none have examined visual features of baseball players at bat in the setting of actual baseball play. The technological challenges of performing such a study with instrumented subjects are understandably formidable, particularly the difficulty of pupillary constriction in response to sunlight. Unfortunately, then, that findings in these reports can be confidently transposed to actual baseball competition remains problematic. As Abernethy et al. have emphasized, such artificial testing situations might provide spurious outcomes in respect to those in actual field settings by a) eliminating an advantage that an expert might possess by experience, b) creating unrecognized floor or ceiling effects, and c) making experts behave differently by depriving them of information they would have used in a more realistic setting (1).

Robert Singer and his co-workers at the University of Florida sought to remedy this problem in their study of tennis players returning serve (47). Here the challenge is not dissimilar to the hitting of a pitched baseball. The ball is delivered approximately 80 feet away at a velocity that can approach 150 mph, demanding a decision as to when and where to swing the racket early in the flight of the ball. Too, the angular velocity when it reaches the receiver far exceeds that humanly possible to track, necessitating accurate prediction and use of saccades (40).

Singer et al. studied serve returns in five instrumented, highly ranked collegiate tennis players on lit courts at night (thereby obviating pupillary constriction in the sun) (47). Mean serve velocity from delivery to point of ball-racket contact was approximately 35 m per second (80 mph). A variety of visual strategies were observed in the five players. Two used a continuous visual pursuit to track the ball throughout its course, while two did not track the ball at all but instead made exclusive use of anticipatory saccades. The other player used both techniques. These findings, although in a small number of subjects, would suggest that considerable inter-individual variation might be observed in visual tracking strategies in highly trained talented athletes.

Similarly, David Mann and colleagues sought to examine visual-motor performance in two elite cricket batters in a "natural setting" (24). They found that two features of the response of these batters to a delivered ball in a simulated realistic setting separated them from two club players: first, the more skilled batmen directed their gaze by larger and earlier saccadic motions ahead of the ball, a "strategy that ensured they could 'park' their gaze ahead of the ball so that gaze could 'lie-in-wait' for the ball to arrive." By this means, in fact, these players could visualize the point of contact of the ball with the bat. This ability was enhanced by a second distinctive characteristic, the ability to couple movements of the head to the trajectory of the ball.

In their discussion of this study, the authors questioned the veracity of traditional dogma that holds that saccades are performed by athletes watching a ball as a default mechanism when velocity exceeds that by continuous visual tracking. They found that saccades were utilized even when gaze was accurately following the flight of the ball, consistent with the findings of Croft et al. that in junior cricket players predictive saccades are employed regardless of the velocity of the ball (8).

Neurophysiological Studies

The descriptive studies outlined above provide some indications that major league batters possess high visual skills that permit their rather extraordinary capacity to strike a high velocity pitch. The neurological mechanisms in the central nervous system that might provide for this exceptional expertise are just beginning to be addressed (28).

The past several decades have witnessed the development of a number of noninvasive diagnostic measures that provide insights into brain anatomical features and neurophysiological function that distinguish athletes from nonathletes. These include functional magnetic resonance imaging (fMRI, which defines regional blood flow as an indicator of metabolic activity), transcranial magnetic stimulation (whereby magnetic impulses activate corticospinal activity), and electroencephalography (EEG, recording neuronal electrical activity). *Event-related potentials (ERP)* are recorded as voltage fluctuations from EEG recordings. One such ERP peak, designated as "P300" (since it occurs about 300 ms after a stimulus), has been particularly utilized as a marker of cognitive processing.

Studies utilizing these techniques indicate that visual pursuit is a function of a widely divergent set of brain areas, including the cerebellum, dorsal vermis, caudal fastigial nucleus, medial superior cortical area, and so on. Saccades are triggered by a totally independent set of neurological determinants which, again, involve a variety of circuits in the cerebellum, brain stem, and frontal and parietal cerebral regions (see ref. 23).

How these two neurological functions might operate in a unique fashion in baseball hitters has not yet been examined. In fact, although noninvasive studies have substantiated neurophysiological and anatomic differences in trained animals and expert musicians, the issues surrounding athletic expertise are just beginning to be explored (28). Initial investigations appear to indicate that neurophysiological adaptations are skill-specific and that athletes tend to demonstrate superior neurological efficiency (as an expression of a greater reliance on automaticity of motor responses compared to the cognitive attention necessary in less trained individuals).

Two studies have been performed examining P300 responses in baseball players (27,33). Radio et al. examined ERP as a marker of perceptual decision-making in advanced versus intermediate skilled baseball hitters as they sat watching an oncoming pitch projected on a screen (33). The participants were told to quickly press one of two buttons in response to whether the pitch was a fastball or curveball. The unique feature of this study was that the hitters were told in advance of each pitch which kind of pitch would "arrive," but in a certain percentage of times the cue provided was false (the players were warned this would be the case). As expected the reaction times for the accurate pre-cued pitches were faster than the false ones, but in each case the reaction times were faster in the more skilled players. Overall, responses were similar to fastballs, but the advanced hitters demonstrated faster accuracy in recognizing curveballs.

P300 latency (delay time) and amplitude were measured in respect to the stimulus onset defined as the point of the pitcher windup and the ball in the ear region in the pitcher's hand. Compared with the advanced players, the intermediate skilled hitters produced higher P300 amplitudes in responding to curveballs and shorter latencies for both types of pitches. The authors concluded that these ERP differences reflected greater automaticity by more talented players and "a more limited attentional capacity" in the intermediate batters.

Nakamoto and Mori compared Go/No-go decisions in college baseball players compared to nonplayers (27). Average P300 latency and amplitude were not different between the groups for Go decisions, but in the No-go trials P300 amplitude was greater in the baseball players. These authors suggested that this finding reflected the players' stronger inhibitory capacities when making batting decisions.

Training or Inheritance?

Despite all theoretical expectations, major league baseball players are capable of—sometimes—hitting a 95-mph fastball. Such facility appears to be explained at least in part by their superior abilities in visual tracking, use of saccades, and dynamic acuity, superimposed on experience and pitch prediction. All this enables these hitters to predict accurately on a certain percentage of attempts the location of the ball as it arrives over the plate, even when its path may deviate at the last moment.

The visual superiority of baseball hitters versus the rest of us might be attributed at least partially to a high degree of motivation and focus. Indeed, professional players might well be suspected of a high degree of motivation in focusing on arriving pitches, given their considerable remuneration in successfully doing so. On the other hand, it is well documented that sports performers who are anxious and under emotional stress experience a deterioration in the efficiency of visual search strategies (21). Too, one's peripheral vision is typically impaired and reaction time diminished in the intensity of strenuous exercise (5).

Most likely, however, such attributes contributing to batting skills arise from real neurophysiological advantages. Which raises the next question: are such abilities inherent, a matter of genetic endowment? Or, on the contrary, are they acquired, learned through training and experience? That is, does one become a formidable major league hitter *because* he is endowed with certain neuro-visual gifts or, rather, do hours of training and experience *engender* such skills?

The simple straightforward answer here is that no one knows for certain. The issue bears considerable importance for baseball players, since, if effective, employment of specific training techniques to improve visual skills might be a valuable means of improving batting skills. That visual training techniques can actually improve such visual functions, and whether any such improvement might translate into improved physical performance, has long been debated (26). As Abernethy and Wood noted, there exists convincing evidence that visual drills can improve measures of visual function, but "some caution needs to be exercised when extrapolating this evidence to the use of visual training in athletes. One reason for this caution is that many of the reported improvements with visual training have been in patients with visual defects. Because of possible ceiling for general visual improvement, it does not necessarily follow that comparable improvements can or will occur for people entering a visual training program with normal or above-normal visual function" (2).

Some authors have suggested that visual training techniques can improve batting performance (36). For example, Joseph Clark and co-authors (which included Baseball Hall of Fame catcher Johnny Bench) claimed that a visual training program was responsible for a rise in the average batting average of the University of Cincinnati baseball team from .251 to .285 between 2011 and 2012 (7).

Abernethy and Wood examined the effect of two visual training programs on visual and motor performance in a group of 40 non-athletic college students (2). The training procedures involved four weeks of exercises previously contended to improve visual skills and motor abilities (36). Measures of static visual acuity, dynamic visual acuity, phoria, vergence, stereopsis, depth perception, reaction time, eye tracking, and coincident timing failed to improve with training compared to those of a control, non-training group of students. Moreover, no effects of training were observed in a tennis forehand task. The authors concluded that generalized visual training programs "do not appear to provide the improvements in either basic visual function or motor performance relevant to sport that they claim to produce."

In 1993 Hitzeman and Beckerman reviewed the extant literature at the time and concluded that "There is little evidence demonstrating that a regimen of visual training will achieve an improvement in the visual skills of athletes. Although there have been some reports of enhanced visual ability following periods of training, so few studies have been performed and so many questions have been raised about experimental design that no conclusive favorable opinion can be offered" (15). In addition, they concluded that "There is even less agreement concerning whether enhancement of visual skills will lead to improved athletic performance." It would not seem that convincing evidence has been offered since that time to alter that opinion.

Coincident Timing

So much for the visual skills of baseball hitters in locating the *where* of successful batting. We move on now to the challenge of *when* to swing—the fine timing of ball arrival and swing of the bat to launch a hit. This skill set involves A) recognizing the speed of the oncoming ball, and B) perfectly timed performance of a cascade of decision to swing → visual motor delay → the coordination of muscular activation that swings the bat. The challenge then is matching A to B. And, to the essence of the challenge, A is arriving in half a second at 95 mph, and B must be enacted in a time of about 300 ms. Not unexpectedly, the margin of error in this "successful interception" is extraordinarily small. It has been suggested that coincidental timing of bat-meets-ball must be as precise as ± 9 ms—a little less than one-hundredth of a second—to strike a 90-mph fastball (12,34). And yet, begging credulity, it happens.

Judging Pitch Speed

How does one judge the velocity of an object moving in the field of vision? The quick answer might be that the observer estimates such speed by an awareness of the rate of displacement of the object in respect to its surroundings or background. Clearly, though, there are other factors involved. For instance, one would have great difficulty comparing the velocity of a jet airplane flying overhead at 30,000 feet with one flying at an altitude of just 2,000 feet. Similarly, it would be virtually impossible to recognize that the speed of a locomotive headed directly toward an observer was actually traveling at the same speed as one that is crossing directly across the field of vision of someone sitting in an automobile at a railroad crossing.

For a batter viewing an oncoming pitch, the major part of the trajectory of a fastball is directly toward the batter, with only a tiny visual angle (the same situation as the oncoming locomotive). Consequently, from the batter's perspective the ball, traveling at a speed of 95 mph, is barely moving against the background field of vision. Only when the ball approaches the front of the plate does the visual angle begin to suddenly increase. How then to judge its speed?

It is generally believed that recognizing velocity of a pitch to estimate time to contact with the swing of the bat is achieved predominantly by observing the rate of increase in the size of the ball in the batter's vision as it approaches the plate (34,35). That is, the faster it arrives, the more rapid is the increase in angular displacement on the retina of the ball's image. One can describe here mathematically what the brain achieves reflexively:

$$V = \left(D^2/s\right)\left(d\theta/dt\right)$$

where D is distance, s is the radius of the ball, and $\left(d\theta/dt\right)$ the angular rate of expansion of the ball's image on the retina.

(D. Regan has pointed out that such calculations were used by the author and astronomer Fred Hoyle in his science fiction novel *The Black Cloud* to estimate the time that it would take a black cloud out in space to hit the Earth [34]. Regan notes, however, that such estimation of time to disastrous earthly contact would be spurious if the cloud was simply growing in size without movement.)

Binocular vision can provide information of velocity of moving objects in the field of vision which are close to the observer. The ball creates images in right and left retinae that are moving in opposite directions, creating *binocular disparity*, offering estimation of ball velocity. Traditional wisdom has held that this binocular depth perception is only operant for short-distance viewing (i.e., under 10 m). Regan has pointed out, however, that a great deal of inter-individual variation exists in the "relative sensitivity" to monocular and binocular information (34), and it is possible that information provided by binocular vision may be important for certain baseball hitters.

Swinging the Bat

The other side of time-to-contact challenge—the physical swing of the bat—involves a cascade of finely orchestrated neuromuscular functions, an act of almost unconceivable complexity. It starts with the cognitive or reflexive decision to initiate the swing with the firing of millions of neurons in motor centers of the brain, each a matter of transcellular membrane ion movement, networking with an order more of connecting synapses and serving to initiate a "generalized motor program." This in turn generates an efferent electrical signal down the spinal cord to the motor neurons which are responsible for triggering skeletal muscular contraction. All this occurs in about 200 milliseconds. Then, in a smoothly coordinated sequence, the muscles of not only the shoulder and arm but also the upper and lower body segments must be activated in a precise pattern to effect the swing of the bat, this requiring an additional 180 ms.

Clearly professional baseball players possess superior skills in such coincident timing of bat and ball, but by just what mechanism this link of perceptual and motor systems is achieved is not altogether clear. Most have considered that visual information indicating the critical time-to-contact serves as the triggering event (43). There exist two schools of thought regarding the means by which the batter then adjusts the muscular event of the swing to coincide with this temporal point of ball arrival. By the concept of *predictive control*, batters utilize a pre-determined motor response which is learned and organized in anticipation of the pitch. The batter has at his disposal a repertoire of such established actions and selects a programmed pattern in response to a particular pitch. The alternative model, *prospective control*, holds that adaptations of a batter's swing are necessary during the process of the pitch and that modifications of the motor pattern as the ball arrives at the plate are critical for successful coincident timing.

While the latter concept has been met with some skepticism (i.e., arguing that tight temporal constraints are too prohibitive for such adjustments) (49), there are certain "anecdotal observations" that seem to clearly indicate the baseball hitters are capable of such last-millisecond modification of their swings: hitters are capable of performing a "check" swing on recognizing a bad pitch, can strike a ball which deviates in direction just before the plate, and are capable by wrist action at the last moment to direct the ball to a certain part of the field (44). Sarpeshkar et al. noted that "when intercepting targets that follow a curvilinear flight path, there is reason to believe that movement control is less likely to be *predictive* and more likely to be *prospective*" (44). The findings of Le Runigo et al. in tennis players suggested that such expertise in late interceptive skill might be at least partially explained by a shorter visual-motor delay time in elite players (22). There is currently no clear argument for one of these models over the other (50); it remains possible that both concepts could hold true.

Given the tight temporal constraints of coincident timing, a number of studies have focused on the role of anticipation—gaining information before the release of the ball—in hitting expertise (25,43). For example, batters not uncommonly take a preparatory step forward and transfer body weight as the pitch is delivered, thereby shortening the total time for muscular activation in the swing of the bat (16). Compared to nonathletes, baseball hitters have been found to focus on particular pre-pitch cues, such as the pitching elbow and arm or ball release point (19). As noted previously, the character of the pitch to be delivered may be anticipated by experienced batters by factors such as the pitch count (31), the number of runners on base, or the pitcher's personal pattern.

As Muller and Abernethy have underscored, "it is important to note that experts are not only better able to acquire information from the same time periods as nonexperts, but they are also able to acquire advance cues from probability information from movement patterns that less-skilled performers cannot acquire. . . . [This] early information specifies the appropriate ballpark for the response . . ." (25). The ability of batters to utilize such anticipatory cues appears to be a developmental/experiential matter, as these skills ae not typically demonstrated before the age of 15 years (54).

Slowing Down Time

Questions of the meaning and nature of time have troubled thinkers since ancient times. Modern-day physicists have regarded time as a block, in which past, present, and future are not distinguished, or as a part of a space-time continuum that constitutes a fourth dimension of reality. In the daily lives of average human beings, however, time is normally observed as a constant flow of the present, turning an unpredictable future into memories of the past, flowing continuously and objectively, like the current of a river. Still, sometimes the experience of the passage of time is altered in a subjective manner, as at a boring meeting, where time "drags," while when having fun, time "flies."

Within the context of this uncertainty of just what time "is," one must consider those fascinating anecdotal events—typically stressful ones—when individuals claim that time was suspended. In the processes of an automobile accident, for example, victims will often describe their sensation that "everything slowed down, like in slow motion." Psychiatric researchers Russell Noyes and Roy Kletti compiled accounts of 61 such events, concluding that such episodes of retarded time and motion, usually surrounding life-threatening circumstances, are "a disputed phenomenon for which there is, nevertheless, a wealth of anecdotal evidence" (30). These events have been ascribed to heightened arousal and fear (38), or as a manifestation of "narrowing and sharpening of the focus of attention."

(If, based on its apparent inconsistency with daily experience, the concept of time "slowing" seems to be rather unreal, the reader may consult the works of Albert Einstein, who revealed that time does not, in fact, proceed in an objective, deterministic manner. Rather, the passage of time is relative in respect to the velocity of the person measuring it. And *time dilation*, or slowing, can be observed when extreme velocities of such persons are involved. Of course, to the average human, whose daily experiences do not approach any speed approaching that of light, this might be argued to have no practical bearing. However, the fact remains that the rate of passage of time should not be uncritically expected to be fixed and immutable.)

This phenomenon has been reported during play by champion athletes as well. Players with names like Michael Jordan, Jimmy Connors, and Apolo Ohno have all described critical moments in intensive competition when the action suddenly slows down and becomes quiet. Tim Gallwey, in his classic book *The Inner Game of Tennis*, describes how the ball can become larger and drift slower in the field of vision when one focuses intensively to return a shot (11). In baseball, too, quoting the late neurologist Oliver Sacks, "A baseball may be approaching at close to a hundred miles per hour, and yet, as many people have described, the ball may seem to be almost immobile in the air, its very seams strikingly visible, and the batter finds himself in a suddenly enlarged and spacious timescape, where he has all the time he needs to hit the ball" (42). He attributed such slowing of time by athletes, which proffers a hitting advantage, to the effect of training experience. "Their neural representation becomes so ingrained in the nervous system as to be almost second nature, no longer in need of conscious effort or decision. One level of brain activity may be working automatically, while another, the conscious level, fashioning a perception of time, a perception that is elastic and can be compressed or expanded" (41).

Psychologists Matthew Rhodes and David McCabe from Colorado State University contended that this ability to "slow the world down" by athletes is linked to level of sports expertise (37). However, the direction of the causative arrow here would be unclear: Does the expertise of an elite athlete *enable* him to slow time? Or, conversely, does one become more likely to reach elite status *because* he or she is endowed with such ability?

It should be noted here that some have questioned the veracity of such time-slowing events. As Marc Wittmann wrote in his book *Felt Time. The Science of How We Experience Time*, "It remains unclear whether people in such situations really experience slow motion, or whether—after the event, and on the basis of the emotional charge of what they have gone through—they simply believe that they felt everything happening more slowly" (55). Such phenomena are, not surprisingly, difficult to study experimentally. In one investigation that attempted to do so, the capacity for temporal resolution of subjects was initially established as the shortest time they could distinguish between two successive flashing lights (48). They then performed the same task while being dropped in a free fall from a 31-m tower in an amusement park. As they plummeted in this terrifying experience, their temporal resolution—that is, their objective ability to sense time—did not change.

Some Final Remarks

So, in summary, yes, a baseball batter at the plate is capable of hitting a delivered high velocity pitch. And, yes, by the expected constraints of time, the unpredictability of the path of the ball, and the near impossibility of coincidental timing of hundredths of a second for successful ball-bat contact, this should be nigh on impossible. In this chapter a number of avenues of explanation have been explored that might account for the hitters' extraordinary skill. We have seen that certain visual skills—particularly abilities in tracking and use of saccades—may distinguish batters from nonplayers. Too, neurophysiological differences between the two may account for the players' greater facility at coincident timing. And hitters may more intelligently make use of anticipatory cues to pitch type and location. However, none of these specific advantages seems to provide the type of "aha!" explanation that would be hoped for.

Perhaps a more "holistic" explanation may be in order—that professional batters are better able to synthesize all the bits of information necessary to connect ball with bat. By experience they have learned to produce this skill as an outcome of recognizing global patterns that provides an overall perceptual advantage for the professional batter at the plate. That is, "the expert's advantage appears to be perceptual. . . . how domain-specific visual information is interpreted and used to guide action" (2). The ultimate answer, then, may be the athlete's brain is better wired to recognize *patterns*, constructed to confront the physical elements of the challenge facing them at the plate. Awaiting insights from future research, one can best be advised to simply sit back with a favorite libation and enjoy the beauty of the game.

References

1. Abernethy B, Thomas KT, Thomas JT. Strategies for improving understanding of motor expertise (mistakes we have made and things we have learned!!). In: Starkes JL, Allard F, editors. *Cognitive Issues in Motor Expertise.* Amsterdam: Elsevier Science Publishers; 1993. pp. 317–356.
2. Abernethy B, Wood JM. Do generalized visual training programmes for sport really work? An experimental investigation. *J Sport Sci.* 2001;19:203–222.
3. Adair RK. *The Physics of Baseball.* New York: Harper Collins; 1985.
4. Allman WF. Pitching rainbows: the untold physics of the curve ball. In: Schrier EW, Allman WF, editors. *Newton at the Bat. The Science in Sports.* New York: Charles Scribner's Sons; 1984. pp. 3–14.
5. Ando S. Peripheral visual perception during exercise: why we cannot see. *Exerc Sport Sci Rev.* 2013;41:87–92.
6. Bahill AT, LaRitz T. Why can't batters keep their eyes on the ball? *American Scientist.* 1984:72:249–253.
7. Clark JF, Ellis JK, Bench J, Khoury J, Graman P. High-performance vision training improves batting statistics for University of Cincinnati baseball players. *PLoS ONE.* 2012;7:e29109.
8. Croft JL, Button C, Dicks M. Visual strategies of sub-elite cricket batsmen in response to different ball velocities. *Hum Movement Sci.* 2010;29:751–763.
9. De Lucia PR, Cochran EL. Perceptual information for batting can be extracted throughout a ball's trajectory. *Percept Mot Skills.* 1985;61:143–150.
10. Fitch HL, Turvey MT. On the control of activity: some remarks from an ecological point of view. In: Landers D, Christina R, editors. *Psychology of Motor Behavior and Sport.* Champaign, IL: Human Kinetics; 1978, pp. 3–35.
11. Gallwey WT. *The Inner Game of Tennis.* New York: Random House; 1974.
12. Gray R. Behavior of college baseball players in a virtual batting task. *J Exper Psychol: Human Percept Perf.* 2002;28:1131–1148.
13. Gray R. Expert baseball batters have greater sensitivity in making swing decisions. *Res Q Exerc Sport.* 2010;81:373–378.
14. Higuchi T, et al. Contribution of visual information about ball trajectory to baseball hitting accuracy. *PLoS ONE.* 2016;11:e0148498.
15. Hitzeman SA, Beckerman SA. What the literature says about sports vision. *Optom Clin.* 1993;3:145–169.
16. Hubbard AW, Send CN. Visual movements of batters. *Res Q.* 1954;25:42–57.
17. Hyllegard R. The role of baseball seam pattern in pitch recognition. *J Sport Exerc Psychol.* 1991;13:80–84.1
18. Ishigaki H, Miyao M. Differences in dynamic visual acuity between athletes and non-athletes. *Percept Mot Skills.* 1993;77:835–839.
19. Kato T, Fukuda T. Visual search strategies of baseball batters: eye movements during the preparatory phase of batting. *Percept Mot Skills.* 2002;94:380–386.

20. Land MF, McLeod P. From eye movements to actions: how batsmen hit the ball. *Nat Neurosci*. 2000;3:1340–1345.
21. Janelle CM. Anxiety, arousal and visual attention: a mechanistic account of performance variability. *J Sports Sci*. 2002;20:237–251.
22. Le Runigo C, Benguigui N, Bardy BG. Visuo-motor delay, information-movement coupling, and expertise in ball sports. *J Sports Sci*. 2010;28:327–337.
23. Luna B, Velanova K, Geier CF. Development of eye-moment control. *Brain Cogn*. 2008;68:293–308.
24. Mann DL, Spratford W, Abernethy B. The head tracks and gaze predicts: how the world's best batters hit a ball. *PLoS ONE*. 2013;8:e58289.
25. Muller S, Abernethy B. Expert anticipatory skill in striking sports: a review and a model. *Res Q Exerc Sport*. 2012;83:175–187.
26. Muller S, Fadde PJ, Harbaugh AG. Adaptability of expert visual anticipation in baseball batting. *J Sport Sci*. 2017;35:1682–1690.
27. Nakamoto H, Mori S. Effects of stimulus-response compatibility in mediating expert performance in baseball players. *Brain Res*. 2008;1189:179–188.
28. Nakata H, Yoshie M, Miura A, Kudo K. Characteristics of the athletes' brain: evidence from neurophysiology and neuroimaging. *Brain Res Rev*. 2010;62:197–211.
29. National Aeronautics and Space Administration. https://www,grc,nasa.gov/www/k-12/airplace/btraj.html.
30. Noyes R, Kletti R. Depersonalization in response to life threatening danger. *Comp Psychiatr*. 1977;18:375–384,
31. Paull G, Glencross D. Expert perception and decision making in baseball. *Int J Sport Psychol*. 1997;28:35–56.
32. Peper L, Bootsma RJ, Mestre DR, Bakker FC. Catching balls: how to get the hand to the right place at the right time. *J Exper Psychol*. 1994;20:591–612.
33. Radio SJ, Janelle CM, Barba DA, Frehlich SG. Perceptual decision making for baseball pitch recognition: using P300 latency and amplitude to index attentional processing. *Res Q Exerc Sport*. 2001;72:22–31.
34. Regan D. Visual factors in hitting and catching. *J Sport Sci*. 1997;15:533–558.
35. Regan D, Gray R. Hitting what one wants to hit and missing what one wants to miss. *Vision Res*. 2001;41:3321–3329.
36. Revien L, Gabor M. *Sports Vision: Dr. Revien's Eye Exercises for Athletes*. New York: Workman Publishing; 1981.
37. Rhodes MG, McCabe DP. Expertise makes the world slow down: judgements of duration are influenced by domain knowledge. *Q J Exp Psychol*. 2009;62:2313–2319.
38. Roth M, Harper M. Temporal lobe epilepsy and the phobic anxiety-depersonalization syndrome. II: practical and theoretical considerations. *Comp Psychiat*. 1962;3:215–226.
39. Rouse MW, DeLand P, Christian R, Hawley J. A comparison of dynamic visual acuity between athletes and nonathletes. *J Am Optom Assoc*. 1988;59:946–950.
40. Rowland TW. *Tennisology: Inside the Science of Serves, Nerves, and On-Court Dominance*. Champaign, IL: Human Kinetics; 2014.
41. Sacks O. Speed. *The New Yorker*. 2004; August 23:60–69.
42. Sacks O. *The River of Consciousness*. New York: Alfred A. Knopf; 2017.
43. Sarpheshkar V, Mann DL. Biomechanics and visual-motor control: how it has, is, and will be used for reveal the secrets of hitting a cricket ball. *Sports Biomech*. 2011;10:306–323.
44. Sarpeshkar V, Mann DL, Spratford W, Abernethy B. The influence of ball-swing on the timing and coordination of a natural interceptive task. *Hum Movement Sci*. 2017;54:82–100.

45. Schalen L. Quantification of tracking eye movements in normal subjects. *Acta Otolaryngol.* 1980;90:404–413.
46. Shapiro A, Lu Z-L, Huang C-B, Knight E, Ennis R. Transitions between central and peripheral vision create spatial/temporal distortions: a hypothesis concerning the perceived break of a curveball. *PLoS.* 2010;5:e13296.
47. Singer RN, Williams AM, Frehlich SG, et al. New frontiers in visual search: an exploratory study in live tennis situations. *Res Q Exerc Sport.* 1998;69:290–296.
48. Stetson C, Fiesta MP, Eagleman DM. Does time really slow down during a frightening event? *PLoS ONE.* 2007;2:e1295.
49. Tresilian JR. Perceptual information for the timing of interceptive action. *Perception.* 1990;19:223–239.
50. Tresilian JR. The accuracy of interceptive action in time and space. *Exerc Sport Sci Rev.* 2004;32:167–173,
51. Uchida Y, Kudoh D, Higuchi T, Honda M, Kanosue K. Dynamic visual acuity in baseball players is due to superior tracking abilities. *Med Sci Sports Exerc.* 2013;45:319–325.
52. Uchida Y, Kudoh D, Murakami A, Honda M, Kitazawa S. Origins of superior dynamic visual acuity in baseball players: superior eye movements or superior image processing. *PLoS ONE.* 2007;7:e31530.
53. Watts RG, Bahill AT. *Keep Your Eye on the Ball. Curve Balls, Knuckle Balls, and Fallacies of Baseball.* New York: W.H. Freeman and Company; 2000.
54. Weissenstenier J, Abernethy B, Farrow D, Muller S. The development of anticipation: a cross-sectional examination of the practice experiences contributing to skill in cricket batting. *J Sports Exerc Physiol.* 2008;30:663–684.
55. Wittmann M. *Felt Time. The Science of How We Experience Time.* Cambridge, MA: MIT Press; 2017. p. 35.

8

WHAT IS THE "PURPOSE" OF THE CARDIOVASCULAR SYSTEM?

"Sea water."

A stunned silence. Sea water? That's right. In the opening of television's 1957 Bell Science Series program *Hemo the Magnificent*, Dr. Frank Baxter (the scientist) is asked by the god-like Hemo, as proof of his (Dr. Baxter's) understanding, to reveal the secret of the circulation of blood in the human body. To the god's astonishment, Dr. Baxter smiles, and with a knowing twinkle in his eye, comes up with the correct, but seemingly odd, answer: "Sea water."

He goes on to explain: Living beings have inhabited the Earth for about 3.8 billion years, and for at least the first half of this period of time the ancient seas were populated entirely by primitive single-celled organisms. To sustain life, these *prokaryocytes* required direct contact with the surrounding water, by which they obtained food and oxygen and released waste products. When cells joined together to gain the advantages offered by multi-cellular organisms, special channels and spaces developed so that individual cells still maintained direct contact with their life-sustaining aqueous medium.

About 400 million years ago, though, new challenges arose when living beings began to abandon the security of the seas to emerge onto the land. How to keep from simply drying up? How were oxygen and water to be supplied to interior cells? What was to keep toxic waste materials from building up? And how was an energy source (i.e., food) to be made available? Only those animals which could solve these challenges would persist.

The answer for these new emigrants to the land was to take the sea with them. By a bewildering variety of means they devised vessels and pumps that would circulate self-contained sea water to bathe each and every cell of the body. All these closed circulatory systems have been developed to serve an identical purpose—feed each of those cells with life-sustaining sea water.

Today each of the trillions of individual cells in the human body goes about its specialized business in the same milieu as they would have billions of years ago—surrounded by sea water—that salty brine—by which it maintains its form, obtains oxygen and nourishment, and eliminates metabolic wastes and heat. And it's all thanks to the circulation of blood—a self-contained sea. We human beings, as well as the rest of modern-day terrestrial life, would seem to be not much different than an astronaut setting out from a space station for an extra-vehicular excursion. Far removed from the life-sustaining environment from which we all came, we carry that milieu with us, self-contained mini-replicas of an historical past. And so, "sea water" it is.

An enlightening and entertaining program of popularized science, this. Particularly nicely described is the mystique of how Nature accommodates environmental stresses and organizes itself to confront extrinsic challenges in order to sustain life via evolutionary adaptation. But beneath this pleasant veneer of scientific insight lies a subtext of more profound and, indeed contentious, issues that illustrate, equally well, the limits of our comprehension of just "how things really work."

To start with, what is one talking about when assuming that the cardiovascular system has a "purpose"? The *Oxford English Dictionary* defines the word as "The reason for which something is done or made or exists; an intention, an aim." Can one accurately or appropriately consider a biological function to have an intention, an aim? But of course, one quickly responds. The description of the evolutionary basis for the development of the cardiovascular system so nicely described above by the good Dr. Baxter clearly demonstrates this. Its purpose? Obviously to preserve an appropriate aqueous environment needed by all cells for survival. And if we project ahead in this discussion a bit and think about the purpose of the circulation of blood during exercise we can construct a long list—increased oxygen delivery to support augmented aerobic metabolic demands, shunting of blood flow to the skin for dispersal of heat, elimination of carbon dioxide and buffering of lactic acid, transport of critical hormonal influences, and so forth. There wouldn't seem to be much of an issue here.

In reaching such a conclusion, however—that a physiological system has an objective, or a goal—one finds oneself stepping out on some rather thin philosophical ice. Indeed, "purpose" signifies *teleology*, or goal directedness. Biologists have long sought to avoid teleological explanations, which for many has implied a belief in a divine creator, or god, which has designed such purposefulness of nature. How else, such believers claim, can one explain biological "purpose"? The multifarious functions of the cardiovascular system, would go the argument, can only be explained by some underlying design, one devised by a master designer.

The scientific world, of course, is generally in disagreement. Biologists would see "objectives" in living systems as reflecting a different form of definition of goal-directedness, one that can be defined and tested by scientific methods. One which does not depend on the existence of any such theological architect. Indeed, to avoid this contentious quicksand, scientists have adopted the term *teleonomy* to indicate purposeful behavior exhibited by biological processes which reflect scientifically plausible explanations divorced from any assumption of divine intervention (11,15).

Let's back up a bit and examine the origins of this thinking. At that inevitable moment of one's death the chemical composition of the body—all those atoms of carbon, and hydrogen, and oxygen—is identical to that of an hour previous, when enjoying the living state. Yet, life has been extinguished. Departed. What, in fact, exactly has vanished? Observations and queries like these once supported in the 18th century the concept of "vitalism," which argued for the existence of a unique "life force" that distinguishes living from non-living matter. Such a force, so went the reasoning, makes unique the existence of biological beings. In this era of molecular genetics, complex adaptive systems, and biological relativity, this idea has long been discredited. Still, the debate over what constitutes the essential nature of living beings remains on the table, with no ultimate resolution in sight. What, in fact, is it that has vanished at the point of death?

As the chemist Addy Pross has nicely put it, "Yes, it is true in this modern era we know unequivocally that there is no *élan vital*, that living things are made up of the same 'dead' molecules as non-living ones, but somehow the manner in which those molecules interact in a holistic ensemble results in something very special—us, and every living thing on this planet. So, paradoxically, despite the profound advances in molecular biology over the past half-century, we still do not understand what life is, how it relates to the inanimate world, and how it emerged" (15).

As was noted in the Preface of this book, a particularly intriguing observation arises in the midst of such conversations—the uncontestable recognition that "all living things behave as if they have an agenda" and that biological processes demonstrate a "purposeful character" (15). The question at hand—the purpose of the cardiovascular system—can thus be considered in the global context of similar questions of goal-directedness observed throughout the biological world. That biological matter is typified by such purposeful behavior—teleonomy—can be examined in the light of two corollary observations. First, to underscore the point, such goal-directed behaviors in living beings are performed with the same chemical constituents—and under the same constraints imposed by physical laws—as non-living matter. Thus, the answer as to how all this purposeful behavior can be explained must be revealed not in the constituent elements of living matter but rather in how those elements are organized.

Secondly, in contrast to living beings, non-organic inanimate matter cannot be considered to serve any recognized "purpose." It follows, then, that it can be expected that within any proposed explanation, matters of "organization" and "purpose" comprise, at least in part, the essential differences which distinguish living from non-living matter. Addressing questions of organization and purposefulness in life forms is thus likely to offer important insights into this age-old conundrum.

The last corollary—goal-directed processes in living matter versus the non-purposeful nature of inanimate objects—perhaps demands some argument. Non-living objects possess, intrinsically, no purpose. It seems like a rather stark statement. With his laws of physical motion, Isaac Newton in 1687 provided rules of behavior of physical objects and their motion, be it at scales of heavenly bodies in space or everyday objects in human daily lives. Here, for the first time, were described the rules governing an objective, rational, predictable universe. It was one that proved most satisfying to the human mind, for it assured the beauty of an ordered universe, and, as a corollary, some "meaning" (and, as an extension, some reason, beyond that of simple chance, for human existence).

But Newton failed to answer the question of *why* these laws might exist. As for *cause*, Newton found no problem in ascribing these laws of motion in an orderly, clockwork universe to the work of God. "The Newtonian model of the universe . . . was paralleled by the image of a monarchical God who ruled the world from above by imposing his divine law on it. The fundamental laws of nature searched for by scientists were thus seen as the laws of God, invariable and eternal, to which the world was subjected" (6). So whatever purpose that might be attributed to these laws lay somewhere in the inscrutable wisdom of such a divine power at the controls of the universe.

About a century later, the French mathematician Pierre-Simon Laplace refined Newton's Laws, concluding that based on these physical principles all future trajectories of both celestial and earth-bound bodies could be predicted with certainty. He did, however, provide a different take on any causal agent or goal-directedness that underlay these principles. Upon being asked why a Divine Being was not indicated in his synthesis, Laplace famously replied "I had no need for that hypothesis." As an alternative explanation he espoused the idea of *causal determinism*, whereby all future occurrences are caused by prior events—antecedent conditions—in compliance with the physical laws of nature. (This, of course, leaves one with the conundrum of what caused [and for what purpose] the whole inexorable chain of events to get started in the first place?)

Now, over 200 years later, despite enormous leaps in our understanding of the nature of the universe at all scales from astronomical to subatomic, the exasperating question remains, unanswered. For what purpose is there "something rather than nothing"?

(Libraries are filled with the works of thinkers since antiquity struggling with this question. For those wishing a contemporary "good read" on this issue, the reader may wish to consult Jim Holt's *Why Does the World Exist? An Existential*

Detective Story [W.W. Norton Company, 2012], in which a number of savants are quoted with perhaps due pessimism on the dilemma:

William James:	the question is "the darkest in all philosophy"
Bernard Lovell:	pondering on the issue can "tear the individual's mind asunder"
Arthur Schopenhauer:	"The lower a man is in an intellectual respect, the less puzzling and mysterious existence itself is to him")

Some might claim that we cannot dismiss the idea that a certain physical object has a "purpose." Take the standard vacuum cleaner, for instance. It's composed of a carefully crafted combination of metals, rollers, wires, bags, and so forth. But none of those physical parts by themselves, or even in combination, have any purpose. They just sit there, inert. It is only through the creative intervention of a human being that a switch is turned on and this device serves the purpose of cleaning up a rug. The purpose, the goal, the objectives of an inanimate object can only be described in terms of human intention. When we speak teleologically of inanimate objects, then, we must have some explanatory supreme being—mortal or otherwise—in mind. Perhaps there does exist an ultimate intrinsic purpose to objects in the physical universe (would it not be disturbing to us if there were not?), but, if so, up to now it's been a well-kept secret.

Biological Purposefulness

An examination of the purpose of biological processes must begin with a retrospective look back—way back—some 3.8 billion years at that propitious event labeled the "origin of life." If only one could recognize at that point in time the nature of the *something* that transpired—the magic of *abiogenesis* that turned chemistry into biology—the "secret of life" would be revealed. Disappointingly, the details are murky at best, and the truth of the origin of living matter on this planet has been, and will continue to be, open to a good deal of speculation and controversy.

Many hold to the "primordial soup" story that, as the initial step, carbon-containing molecules like methane and carbon dioxide which were floating in the early seas became organized by lightning strikes or solar radiation, forming organic molecules of greater complexity. The credibility of such a scenario was supported in the 1950s when Harold Urey and Stanley Miller, working at the University of Chicago, demonstrated in their laboratory that amino acids, the building blocks of proteins, could be produced by passing an electric current though such a mixture of molecules that approximated the supposed chemical composition of such primitive seas. (As critics have noted, however, this did nothing to actually verify the truth of such a hypothesis.)

As an alternative to this story of abiogenesis, some have weighed in on the possible importance of super-hot underwater volcanic vents in this process, proposing that life originated on the ocean floor. Others have contended that early organic compounds may have been seeded on Earth by meteorites and comets arriving from outer space.

While the details of abiogenesis are uncertain, it seems clear that this was a singular historical event. One and done. Life came from non-life at some point very long ago, but to the best of anyone's knowledge, this feat has never been repeated, at last not on this planet. There has never been any contemporary evidence of living matter having been generated from inorganic material. All this points to the conclusion that the chemical/environmental/electrical conditions that somehow initiated life existed only at a unique time in the history of the Earth. In our time, only life begets life.

Reflecting the beliefs of many scientists, the chemist Addy Pross has contended that organic matter, following the fortuitous events that eventuated in the initiation of life, was perpetuated in biological forms by two central characteristics: first, the capacity for self-replication and, second, the ability to utilize energy, a necessary attribute required to avoid the inevitable entropic decay dictated by the Second Law of Thermodynamics (15). That energy is ultimately derived from the nuclear reactions within the Sun, captured by plants through photosynthesis, and available to animals either by consuming plants or each other. These, in fact, continue to represent the defining features of all living beings. "The Second Law [of Thermodynamics] is the statement that organized systems spontaneously trend toward disorganization, toward disorder. Nature prefers chaos to order, so disorganization is the natural order. . . . Within living systems, however, the highly organized state that is absolutely essential for viable biological function is somehow maintained with remarkable precision" (15). As an extension of this idea, says Pross, "Death is just the reversion of a system from the kinetic replicative world back to the thermodynamic world, the world of 'regular' chemistry."

A compelling explanation remains elusive for just how carbon-containing organic compounds came to be created from simple inorganic molecules to "make" life. That's a sufficient mystery. But then how these compounds "learned" to replicate themselves is another conundrum altogether. A number of possible explanations have been offered, which are reviewed by Pross in his book *What is Life? How Chemistry Becomes Biology* (15).

The persistence of living matter, then, depended on a mechanism by which the faculty for self-replication would be sustained. In this part of the story biologists are now on more familiar ground, since evolutionary pressure to provide for reproductive capacity is the central theme provided by the paradigmatic concepts of Darwinian natural selection. This holds that characteristics of living beings are explained by millions of years of selective pressures, whereby phenotypic variations which are more advantageous to survival and reproductive success will persist.

Stripped down to its basic essentials, then, the story goes like this: A change in a phenotypic characteristic occurs from a previous A to a new B. If B is more advantageous than A in that it enhances survival and reproductive capacity, the organism will be better sustained in those with B than those stuck with A. That new and improved phenotype B, then, is exhibited as a seeming "purpose," one that is based entirely on self-preservation—and requiring no directive agent for its survival. The development of goal-directedness by the Darwinian model is one of self-actualization. One does not have to get tangled up in terms of "teleology" here but can speak instead of a biological or natural purpose.

For most biologists, the concepts inherent in the Darwinian model of evolution are central to the contemporary interpretation of physiological processes, but the details remain open to debate and discussion. Most argument has involved the source of the phenotypic variations upon which survival pressures act. At one end, proponents of Neo-Darwinism believe such variation arises from chance mutation of genetic material. From this viewpoint, alteration in genetic material is completely random, serving as "blind chance" with no room for purpose or function (11). This opinion reflects a traditional, but now questioned, gene-centered concept of biological function whereby a "program" is set by one's gene complement, which serves as a blueprint for all phenotypic expression and biological activity.

At the other end of opinion are those who see phenotypic variability as an expression of the interaction of non-genetic influences (system interactions, environmental, epigenetic) that can affect the expression of gene function. By this argument, genes do not actively dictate biological function; instead genetic material is passive, acted upon by the hierarchical nature of living beings and their environment. The analogy here is that the DNA coded information in one's genes is like a musical score. The printed notes on the page certainly do not constitute "music," instead awaiting an instrument or human voice to make it so. Similarly, the entire human organism, at all system levels and interactions, in conjunction with environmental influences, "plays" the gene. In this way phenotypic variation as a prelude to natural selection can serve as another avenue for defining biological "purpose." This argument holds that "all levels can contribute to generating biological function that characterizes life. . . [and] that organisms themselves are the source of the creative process in evolution, not random mutations of DNA" (11).

When one considers the "purpose" of the cardiovascular system, then, the teleological issue of Divine Intervention can be easily side-stepped by interpreting its critical functions as self-actualizing outcomes of natural selection or, as some would argue, determinants of the phenotypic variations themselves which are acted upon by this selection process. In either or both cases, a directive agent "is not necessary for this hypothesis." (Parenthetically, it is of interest to note that the essence of such goal-directedness has in many cases shifted from its original selective "intent." Cardiovascular responses enable locomotion today in the same manner that they did millions of years ago, but now, instead of selective survival advantages of gaining food, avoiding enemies and escaping adverse environmental extremes, enhancement of cardiovascular function provides certain health advantages and, not the least, one's capacity to participate in local 5-km road races.)

Biological Organization

In its function, the cardiovascular system is a classic example of a *complex system*, one of interacting multiple components. In such complex systems, as discussed previously in this book, the overall function of the system displays emergent qualities, one that is not explainable by the individual contributing actions of its component parts. It is, in effect, a classic example of "the whole is greater than its parts." Complex systems are self-organizing, meaning that they operate without a greater directing agent, and are typified by a hierarchical structure, with multiple strata of subsystems that support the system function. Feedback loops, nonlinearity, and variability combining both random (stochastic) and deterministic (predictably regular) features are all characteristics of complex systems. Importantly, the function of complex systems involves relationships and interactions within the components of the system, the subsystems, other body systems, and the environment. The nervous system and all the rest (pulmonary, hematological, gastrointestinal, immunological, thermoregulatory, endocrinological, and so forth) are each examples of complex systems.

Although it is now recognized that living beings operate through the activities of such systems, their extraordinary, "mind-numbing" complexity (by the classic definition) has proven daunting. Indeed, insights into the means by which complex systems achieve inter- and intra-system communication, the essential biological principles underlying these systems, their evolutionary development (what selective pressures did they serve?), and even the best means of measuring their operational activities remain at an embryonic level. Still, the "answers" to the fundamental nature of life appear to exist in this holistic model, rather than a reductionist approach which calls for deciphering the features of individual constituents of biological systems. Pross noted that "the enormous complexity of biological systems often makes the reductionist methodology difficult to implement, and it is that difficulty that has been responsible for the burgeoning anti-reductionist, holistic approach to biological systems of recent decades" (11).

It should be noted that the inter-relatedness of complex systems is not unique to biological matter but is observed in the physical world as well. While "the really important processes that define living systems are interactions between scales and levels" (11), "complexity is not the cause nor the essence of the life phenomenon; complexity is its *consequence*. Replication induced complexity, not the other way around" (15). Indeed, the literature of physics describes similar holistic concepts—a "universal connectedness of things and events": "The properties of a particle can only be understood in terms of its activity—of its interactions with the surrounding environment—and that particle, therefore, cannot be seen as an isolated entity, but has to be understood as an integrated part of the whole. . . . In modern physics, the image of the universe as a machine has been replaced by that of an interconnected dynamic whole whose parts are essentially interdependent and have to be understood as patterns of a cosmic process" (6).

One of the keys to understanding biological complex systems, particularly as it relates to system "purpose," lies in recognizing the features of the hierarchical set of subsystems that serve as the system infrastructure. The nature of such hierarchical structures observed in complex systems can be conveniently understood by an analogy with a symphony orchestra. Consider yourself seated in Symphony Hall enjoying a performance of Beethoven's Seventh Symphony. That music you're listening to is the emergent outcome of a complex system—the symphony orchestra. The individual musical instruments constitute the components of that system, but true to the nature of complexity, none of them are, in fact, producing Beethoven's Seventh. Only the components acting together, in the proper relationship as Ludwig demanded, establish that extraordinary functional emergent outcome.

But that's just the top stratum of the hierarchical structure. Below is a layer of the mechanics by which each instrument produces musical sound. In the clarinet the fluctuations of a wooden reed cause a sympathetic vibration in a column of air in the instrument's long cylinder, the frequency of which is governed by the geometry created by the opening and closing of holes in the column. The performer him- or herself occupies another stratum, an extraordinarily complex one in its own right, which includes the cerebral-visual recognition of musical notes, translated to a muscular cascade that "plays" the instrument, all of this governed by an extraordinarily precise inherent biological clock. In the next stratum lie the electrical currents which trigger muscular activation, and another layer below that is occupied by ions passing in and out of cell boundaries that create action potentials. And these proceedings must engage yet another subsystem which makes energy accessible for muscular contraction.

There are a few observations that should be noted here. First, this group of substrata which lie beneath the final emergent function is termed "hierarchical" because each level serves for the function in the stratum "above" it, effectively relinquishing its autonomy to a greater good. Note, too, that in each level, the form of physiological or biochemical activity is totally independent of the other levels. That is, an increase in transmembrane electrical gradient caused by transport of ions has nothing in common with the vibration of the air in a clarinet. That the brain can trigger a precisely timed arpeggio of notes via the fingers of the hand has nothing in common with the vibration qualities of the clarinet's reed. This is really quite a striking observation, since all of the subsystems must operate in cooperation and harmony to create Beethoven's masterpiece. There must exist, then, a means by which the different levels communicate with each other. They have to know what the other levels are "doing." Yet how the subsystems in the hierarchical structure of a complex system accomplish this remains a mystery.

Finally, and not least, it is obvious that the entire structure of co-dependent elements is a tenuous and vulnerable one—an error in any of its multitude of parts would seem to forecast system doom and failure. For this reason, and presumably thanks to Darwinian evolutionary pressures, complex systems are characterized by the presence of redundancies—backup processes in case of such malfunction.

In biological systems "[levels of organization] can be arranged in ascending order of size: atoms, molecules, networks, organelles, cells, tissues, organs, whole-body systems, and the whole organism. Each level can be viewed as assembling the components of the level below, and then itself forming a component for the level above" (11). With these concepts in mind, the hierarchical nature of the complex system at hand—the cardiovascular—can be readily appreciated. The emergent quality of this system is the flow of blood through the circulation, but one can begin with the most elementary of substrata, ionized atoms whose transport across cell membranes by protein molecules generates electrical currents, which releases calcium in the cell's sarcoplasmic reticulum, which facilitates sliding of actin-myosin filaments, which in unison with many others provides for contractile tissue, which generates force to expel blood from the ventricle, which is governed by the resistance created by arterioles downstream. The entire system must coordinate its function with other systems—particularly pulmonary, metabolic, and thermoregulatory, and so forth—to control adequacy of circulatory blood flow.

Matters of "purpose" of the cardiovascular system can be realized within the context of this hierarchical structure. Specifically, "functional significance, purpose and therefore teleological causation arise as inter-scale interactions in which components at the lower scale are constrained in a functional way by the properties at a higher scale. . . . [This] does not entail that there is some overall purpose, an intelligent designer or other theological assumption. It simply means 'purpose.' Those purposes arise from the inter-scale interactions. Processes at higher scales give purpose to processes at lower scales" (11).

Consider the sodium ion. It has no function—an atom, inert piece of matter. Yet moving up a level of hierarchy, the action of protein transporters that escort Na^{++} across cell membranes "creates" a recognizable function for the sodium ion—to produce an action potential which can serve to innervate the contractile process in heart muscle cells. The ability of a piece of cardiac muscle to contract has no purpose whatsoever. But place it into the orchestrated contractility of the heart and its purpose to eject stroke volume is clear.

As Noble has noted, "goal-directedness is therefore a relative property. Goals are always relative to some particular context, internal or external to the organism. . . . Purpose or function depends on the level we are considering. It has no meaning below the level at which the relevant function is integrated." Noble describes this as the principle of "biological relativity," which holds that "there is no privileged level of causation in biology: living organisms are multi-level open stochastic systems in which the behavior at any level depends on higher and lower levels and cannot be fully understood in isolation. Just as Special Relativity and General Relativity [in the physical realm] can be succinctly phrased by saying that there is no global (privileged) frame of reference, Biological Relativity can be phrased as saying there is no global frame of causality in organisms" (11).

Noble goes on to state that "the reason why we can identify goal-directed behavior in living organisms is that we can understand the processes by which the behavior emerges" (11). That is to say that all these individual processes within the hierarchical structure can be ascribed to Darwinian selective forces, isolated from any directional force other than its own ability for survival in order to assure replication. The idea of purposefulness progresses, then, in a level-dependent fashion in complex organisms. What is interesting in all of this goal-directedness is observed in organisms which are restricted to the level of a single cell (that is, without an overriding superior level to which to relinquish autonomy and authority).

In his book *Dance to the Tune of Life. Biological Relativity*, the British physiologist Denis Noble colorfully relates his experience in first observing a film of a living unicellular amoeba: "Nothing stood still. Everything was streaming this way and that as the organism moved around. When it found an object that was sensed (I assumed chemically) to be food the movements became beautifully coordinated as two extensions called pseudopodia (false feet) encircled the object, eventually allowing it to be taken in as a membrane coated vesicle to be digested. This tiny organism had a 'nose': the chemical receptors on its membrane surface. It had 'muscles': in fact, formed of protein molecules, some of them very similar to those of our cells, only not organized into separate muscular organs. It clearly had a 'nervous system' to connect the two together, although it had no nerves as we know them. It had a clear goal to feed itself. It knows when and how to reproduce itself in an intricately coordinated activity when it makes its genes dance as they and their predecessors have done for at least one billion years."

Purpose at the System Level

The previous sections of this chapter have presented the purpose of the cardiovascular system—as a model for all the others—in terms of Darwinian natural selection and within the context of the hierarchical structure of biological systems. We have seen how the relationships between the different levels of subsystems define that purpose, all within the self-organizing function of a complex system. The emergent quality of such a system—the "end product" of successive layers of subsystem function—contributes to an ultimate purpose: maintaining the replicative capacity and energy-utilization mechanisms required for sustaining living beings.

In this section we turn to the inter-relationships between individual components of the cardiovascular system itself. These might be listed as including a) a hollow muscular pump (the heart), b) an electrical network triggering the pump to contract (the cardiac conduction system), c) a timing mechanism which regulates the rate of that contraction (the sinoatrial node), d) a fractal network of blood-transporting vessels, and e) a series of peripheral resistors in that network to regulate blood flow (the arterioles). The goal here is to illustrate the principle of complex systems—that none of these individual components of the system explain its emergent quality, the circulation of blood. Instead, each interacts with the others to comprise an incredibly precisely orchestrated spectacle to accomplish this goal. The purpose of the cardiovascular system is thus defined and served by such interplay that exists between its constituent parts.

Such function will be examined in the context of the response of the cardiovascular system to physical exercise, during which its purposes become amplified and most clearly evident. The list of such critical contributions to exercise is impressively long. Indeed, without increased circulatory blood flow—which in itself obviously contributes nothing to actual locomotion itself—physical exercise would be impossible. Some examples:

A) Transport of oxygen to contracting muscle to provide for aerobic energy metabolism.
B) Removal of byproducts of cellular metabolism (carbon dioxide).
C) Buffering of lactic acid produced in cellular metabolism.
D) Increased blood flow to the cutaneous circulation for heat dissipation.
E) Transport of hormonal modifiers of exercise function (epinephrine, cortisol).

What causes the level of circulatory flow to rise in response to an acute bout of endurance exercise? A long-standing heart-centric model, still commonly found in biology and philosophy texts, holds that a) an increase in heart rate and b) an exaggerated contraction of ventricular myocardium to expel greater stroke volume combine to augment cardiac output and thereby increase circulatory flow. Current evidence, however, supports an alternative complex systems approach to answering this question, a model whereby control of the rate of circulatory blood flow resides in the vascular tone of the peripheral arterioles which define the resistance in the circuit.

This story begins in the 1840s in the laboratory of Jean Léonard Marie Poiseuille, the French physician and experimenter who studied the dynamics of fluid flow through fine bore glass tubes. From these he devised Poiseuille's Law, which holds that

$$V = (\pi p r^4)/(8\eta l)$$

Where V is the flow rate, p is the pressure gradient between the ends of the tube, r is the radius of the tube, l is the tube's length, and η is the viscosity of the fluid. Put more simply

Q (rate of blood flow) is related to P (blood pressure)/R (resistance)

(Those versed in electrical circuitry will recognize this as the analog to Ohm's Law, which indicates that the current in amperes is equal to the voltage divided by the resistance.) Poiseuille's Law states, then, that the rate of circulatory blood flow can be influenced directly by the cardiac pump, which is responsible for generating P, the pressure in the circulation, and/or inversely by R, the resistance in the vascular circuit created by the tone of the muscular walls surrounding the peripheral arterioles. As will be reviewed in more detail below, during exercise the primary driving factor for increasing circulatory flow is the latter—a fall in peripheral vascular resistance via arteriolar vasodilatation, while cardiac function maintains P. For this reason, circulatory control by the Poiseuille equation is sometimes termed the *peripheral model.*

An Historical Perspective

The first true insights into the physiological function of the heart were provided by Patterson and Starling in 1914 (13). In their description of the "law of the heart," the stretching of muscle fibers of the ventricles triggered an increase in the force of myocardial contraction, which in turn resulted in an augmentation of stroke volume and cardiac output. It was assumed at that time, then, that during exercise an exaggeration of this process would be responsible for increasing blood circulation—a *central* or *cardiocentric model* that accounted for cardiovascular responses to exercise.

Research in both dogs and humans in the 1950s, however, indicated this conclusion was erroneous. During increases in exercise intensity, measured stroke volume was found to be relatively stable, not increasing. And at the same time the diastolic dimension of the left ventricle did not enlarge, as would have been predicted by the central model. Moreover, studies in which heart rate was artificially increased by electrical pacing revealed a resultant *decline* in stroke volume, as well as no increase in cardiac output as would be expected with the cardiocentric model (17).

It was concluded, then, that the critical factor dictating control of the rate of the circulation of blood with exercise lies in the decline in peripheral vascular resistance resulting from arteriolar dilatation. As Guyton wrote in 1967, "The primary cause of augmented cardiac output is believed to be the local vasodilatation in the skeletal muscle. The heart has relatively little effect on the normal regulation of cardiac output" (8). Bevegard and Shepherd agreed: "The heart serves as a force-feed pump designed to discharge whatever volume it receives by increasing its rate or stroke volume. Unless there is dilatation of resistance vessels in some systemic vascular bed, mediated by local, humoral, or nervous mechanisms, an increased rate will not result in an increase in cardiac output" (3). A number of empiric findings in more recent studies have supported the validity of this peripheral model of circulatory control with exercise:

> During a treadmill or cycle exercise test of progressively increasing work to exhaustion, the calculated total body peripheral vascular resistance falls by approximately 60%.
>
> *(18)*

It makes "sense" (in a Darwinian context) that the rate of circulatory blood flow should be regulated by the activity level of the body functions that it serves. In this case the direct link appears to occur as a matching of such flow with the increasing metabolic requirements of contracting skeletal muscle fibers. In fact, the magnitude of circulatory blood flow is closely coupled with cellular oxygen uptake, causing Guyton to suggest that a fall in cellular oxygen level might be the factor that serves to augment, or autoregulate, blood flow to metabolic rate via arteriolar vasodilatation (8). More recently a number of agents have been identified which are produced locally at the cellular level and are capable of causing arteriolar vasodilatation in response to augmented cellular metabolic activity (acetylcholine, potassium ions, inorganic phosphate, carbon dioxide, adenosine). At present, however, no single chemical factor has been found entirely accountable.

That this fall in arteriolar vascular resistance—the denominator in the Poiseuille equation—serves as the controlling factor in rate of circulatory flow is the key premise of the peripheral model. As such, the dynamics of the circulatory system with exercise mimic that of a natural-occurring or surgically induced arteriovenous fistula, which bypasses the arteriolar bed and lowers systemic vascular resistance. As a consequence, the rate of circulatory flow is increased in those with such a fistula, without any direct effect on the heart (4).

> As exercise intensity rises to level of exhaustion, heart rate increases approximately three-fold over resting values.

Rate of spontaneous discharge of action potentials from the sinoatrial node is increased during exercise by superimposed sympathetic nervous stimulation as well as that from circulating catecholamines. Heart rate is tightly coupled with workload to levels approximating 75% maximal effort, when an unexplained tapering of the former is often observed. Values of maximal heart rate vary inversely with age and are influenced by exercise modality (treadmill, cycle), testing protocol, and form of exercise (walking, running). As a general statement, the heart must complete a cycle of systole and diastole in the approximate time frame of 0.3 seconds at peak exercise.

> Cardiac stroke volume rises by approximately 25% in the early stages of progressive upright exercise but then remains relatively stable to the point of exhaustion.
>
> *(22)*

This pattern has been consistently observed by numerous measurement techniques (indirect Fick, CO_2 rebreathing, Doppler echocardiography, thermodilution, thoracic bioimpedance) and in all subject populations (children, adults, males/females, athletes). The initial rise appears to reflect mobilization of blood sequestered in the lower extremities when assuming the upright position (2). When standing or sitting, gravity draws up to 500–1,000 ml of blood from the central circulation into the dependent extremity. As a consequence, stroke volume and cardiac output fall by 20% to 40%. At the onset of upright exercise this sequestered blood is mobilized by peripheral vasodilatation and the contractile action of skeletal muscle (24). Central blood volume, stroke volume, and cardiac output are thereby restored to levels in the supine position, this rise accounting for the initial increase in stroke volume during upright exercise (Figure 8.1). As expected, then, during progressive exercise performed in conditions independent of the effects of gravity (supine exercise, swimming, zero-gravity in space, arm exercise) stroke volume response is typically "flat," without any initial rise at onset of exercise (19).

The bottom line, then, is that except for the cardiac re-filling phenomenon at the onset of upright exercise, stroke volume does not effectively change as exercise intensity rises. This pattern, corroborated by contemporary findings, upholds earlier observations made in the 1950s and supports the validity of the peripheral rather than central model of circulatory control.

> End-diastolic size of the left ventricle remains stable or decreases slightly during the course of an acute bout of progressive exercise.
>
> *(14,20)*

Contrary to a popular misconception, the ventricles of the heart do not enlarge during exercise. Instead, the "volume load" of circulatory support imposed by

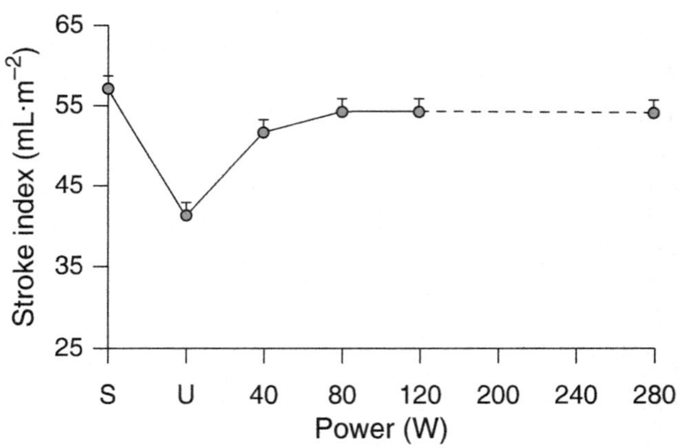

FIGURE 8.1 When assuming the upright position (U) after lying supine (S), stroke volume falls by about 25%, an effect of gravitational blood-pooling in the lower extremities, reducing central volume. With the onset of upright exercise, this dependent blood in the lower extremities is mobilized by muscular contraction, and central volume and stroke volume are restored. Stroke volume then remains stable with increasing exercise work to exhaustion.

Reprinted by permission from T. Rowland and V. Unnithan, "Stroke Volume Dynamics During Progressive Exercise in Healthy Adolescents," *Pediatric Exercise Science* 25 (2013): 173–185.

endurance exercise is satisfied by an increased heart rate with a stable (or even slightly decreasing) ventricular end diastolic dimension. This constancy of end-diastolic dimension can be assumed to reflect a similar stability of left ventricular end diastolic pressure. All this indicates that the constancy of stroke volume (except for the initial re-filling rise) during progressive exercise is accompanied by a stable volume of ventricular preload.

> Myocardial contractility (the force of contraction of the heart muscle) steadily increases with rising exercise intensity.
>
> *(23)*

Inotropic (systolic) function (as well as diastolic relaxation properties) of the ventricles are stimulated by exercise. This increased force and speed of contraction of heart muscle during systole can reflect a number of triggering factors, including sympathetic nervous system activation, decreased after-load (fall in peripheral vascular resistance), and tachycardia. Since all of these variables are at work during exercise it is difficult to decipher the relative contributions of each to the observed rise in contractile function.

When measured by Doppler ultrasound techniques, the rate of aortic flow and the systolic ejection rate (the stroke volume generated in the time of ejection from the ventricles) increase by a factor of approximately 1.5 over resting values. Estimations of the velocity of shortening of myocardial fibers indicate a twofold rise at maximal exercise. Since the left ventricular diastolic dimension remains relatively stable during progressive exercise, the rise in contractility is manifest by a steadily decreasing end-systolic size.

This increase in contractile function occurs as the time of ejection of blood from the ventricles falls from about 0.25 seconds at rest to 0.18 seconds at peak exercise. At maximal exercise the left ventricle of an adolescent is capable of ejecting blood at the remarkable rate of 400 ml per second.

Harmony in Complexity: A Synthesis

Given the recognized dynamics of its separate factions, the collective function created by the interactions of these elements, one with another, in this complex system can be appreciated. What emerges is, in fact, an extraordinarily elegant scenario which supports those critically important purposes of the cardiovascular system with exercise.

To start with, one is confronted with the difficulty of explaining how the end-diastolic size of the left ventricle can remain unchanged during a bout of exercise in which the systemic venous return of blood to the heart is increasing fourfold. The most reasonable—indeed, necessary—explanation is that the heart rate must increase commensurately during this rise in venous return such that the volume per beat of blood traversing the tricuspid valve into the right ventricle (and, as well, crossing the mitral valve into the left ventricle) during diastole remains constant. The best candidate for such a precise matching of heart rate with venous return can be found in the Bainbridge reflex, by which the heart rate increases by sympathetic stimulation in response to a rise in right atrial pressure. In the past, the existence of this reflex has been surrounded by controversy (9), but more recent studies in both humans and primates have substantiated its validity (5). Bainbridge himself proposed the effects of this reflex during exercise almost a century ago:

> If these conclusions are correct, the heart is provided a reflex mechanism whereby, when the venous filling is increased, the circulation can be maintained by the more rapid transference of blood from the venous to the arterial system and the risk of excessive dilatation and failure of the heat is lessened. This mechanism must play a part in the quickening of the heart during muscular exercise, which is accompanied by increased venous inflow to the heart and by a rise in venous pressure.
>
> *(1)*

In this statement, Bainbridge also hints at a reasonable "purpose" for this reflex, which must act to *defend* the left ventricle from expanding during exercise (10). As expressed by Laplace's law, an acute increase in the radius of the left ventricle would result in augmented wall tension, diminishing mechanical efficiency by increasing the workload of individual muscle fibers.

Support for the veracity of this mechanism for reconciling the major increase in systemic venous return with a constant ventricular filling volume can be found in studies in which sympathetic blockade, which prevents a rise in heart rate, results in increases in cardiac stroke volume with exercise. In 1964 Donald and Shepherd demonstrated this in dogs who had undergone a surgical cardiac sympathectomy (7). Compared to normal dogs, heart rate response to exercise was, as expected, markedly dampened, while stroke volume rose by 80% (without change in the control animals). Similarly, administration of medications which block beta-adrenergic sympathetic effects (i.e., propranolol) in human subjects results in a reduced heart rate during exercise with an increase in stroke volume (16,26).

Then one is faced with the apparent paradox that with increasing workload, the heart contracts more forcefully, resulting in a smaller left ventricular end-systolic size, yet stroke volume remains unchanged. This is explained by the necessity of the myocardium to eject the same amount of blood (the stable stroke volume) in a shorter ejection period as heart rate increases (Figure 8.2). Supporting this intuitively obvious interpretation are the findings of one study which found a 20% increase in ventricular shortening fraction (as a measure of myocardial contractility) between the first workload and maximal exercise while the average systolic ejection period fell by 14% (and meanwhile maintaining a stable stroke volume) (21). Increased myocardial contractility during the course of an

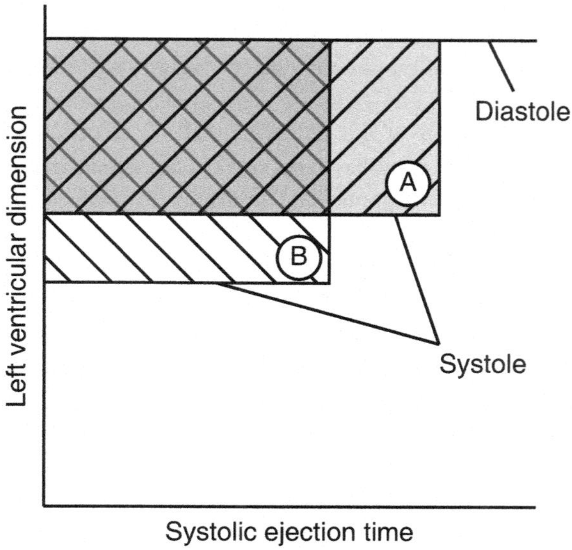

FIGURE 8.2 As exercise intensity increases, myocardial contractility rises and systolic ejection time shortens (because of the more rapid heart rate), yet stroke volume remains unchanged. The stroke volume (area of rectangle A) at low intensity exercise equals that indicated by rectangle B at higher work intensity despite greater ventricular emptying, because that reduction in ventricular end-systolic size occurs in a shorter time period.

Reprinted, by permission, from T. Rowland, *Children's Exercise Physiology, 2n ed.* (Champaign, IL: Human Kinetics, 2005), 122.

acute bout of progressive exercise thus serves to *maintain* rather than increase stoke volume.

All of that is convenient, since the shorter systolic ejection time is a necessary outcome of the faster heart rate, which is required to maintain the proper left ventricular size, and it is this same increased heart rate that is the sole factor responsible for the rise in cardiac output. Dizzying to visualize all these dynamics, yes, but it's a magically performed dance of the elements of the complex system, interacting with each other, to assure the system's obligatory emergent functional purpose, a rise in circulatory blood flow.

Conclusions

This chapter opened with the question of "what is the purpose of the cardiovascular system?", one which any alert high school biology student might be expected to easily handle. But beneath any simple answer it is abundantly clear that the issue is not quite as facile as it might appear. Indeed, one immediately encounters some rather heavy philosophical—and often-times controversial—issues that weigh on biological phenomena:

- "It is the organization of life rather than the *stuff* of life that makes life the unique phenomenon that it is" (15). That organization provides for self-replication and the capture and utilization of energy to maintain this organization.
- An identifiable purpose separates living from non-living matter, being ascribed to the evolutionary process of Darwinian natural selection (that "quintessential biologic principle") (15). That purpose can be considered as a natural, self-generating one requiring no superior directing agent.
- The function of biological systems can be defined only in the context of their hierarchical structures which underlie the inter- and intra-system interactions of complex systems.
- The purpose of the cardiovascular system, then, is provided not only by the interplay of its separate parts but also by functions defined within the hierarchical scaffolding of its underlying subsystems.

In this synthesis of cardiovascular function, one cannot fail to be awed by the sense of order, elegance, and balance at the level of its emergent properties. That such aesthetics are an essential nature of natural truth has long been—and continues to be—strongly debated (12,25). It would seem difficult to deny, however, the harmonic beauty evident in the interactions of the cardiovascular system in providing for its life-sustaining functions.

References

1. Bainbridge FA. The influence of venous filling upon the rate of the heart. *J Physiol.* 1915;50:65–84.
2. Bevegard S, Holmgren A, Johnsson B. The effect of body position on the circulation at rest and during exercise, with special reference to the influence on stroke volume. *Acta Physiol Scand.* 1960;49:279–298.
3. Bevegard BS, Shepherd JT. Regulation of the circulation during exercise in man. *Physiol Rev.* 1967;47:178–213.
4. Binak K, Regan TJ, Christensen RC, et al. Arteriovenous fistula: hemodynamic effects of occlusion and exercise. *Am Heart J.* 1960;60:495–502.
5. Boettcher DH, Zimpfer M, Vatner SF. Phylogenesis of the Bainbridge reflex. *Am J Physiol.* 1982;242:R244–R246.
6. Capra F. *The Tao of Physics.* Boston: Shambhala; 2010.
7. Donald DE, Shepherd JT. Sustained capacity for exercise in dogs after complete cardiac denervation. *Am J Cardiol.* 1964;14:853–859.
8. Guyton AC. Regulation of cardiac output. *N Engl J Med.* 1967;277:805–812.
9. Hakumaki MOK. Seventy years of the Bainbridge reflex. *Acta Physiol Scand.* 1987;130:177–185.

10. Linden RJ. The size of the heart. *Cardioscience*. 1994;5:225–233.
11. Nobel D. *Dance to the Tune of Life: Biological Relativity*. Cambridge: Cambridge University Press; 2017.
12. Orrell D. *Truth or Beauty: Science and the Quest for Order*. New Haven: Yale University Press; 2012.
13. Patterson SW, Starling EH. On the mechanical factors which determine the output of the ventricles. *J Physiol*. 1914;48:357–359.
14. Pokan R, von Duvillard SP, Hoffman P. Change in left atrial and ventricular dimensions during and immediately after exercise. *Med Sci Sports Exerc*. 2000;32:1713–1718.
15. Pross A. *What Is Life? How Chemistry Becomes Biology*. Oxford: Oxford University Press; 2012.
16. Reybrouck T, Amery A, Billiet L. Hemodynamic response to graded exercise after chronic β-blockade. *J Appl Physiol*. 1977;42:133–138.
17. Ross J, Linhart JW, Braunwald E. Effects of changing heart rate in man by electrical stimulation in the right atrium. *Circulation*. 1965;32:549–558.
18. Rowland T. Echocardiography and circulatory response to progressive endurance exercise. *Sports Med*. 2008;38:545–551.
19. Rowland T. Normal cardiovascular responses to progressive exercise. In: Rowland T, editor. *Cardiopulmonary Exercise Testing in Children and Adolescents*. Champaign, IL: Human Kinetics; 2018. pp. 41–49.
20. Rowland T, Blum J. Cardiac dynamics during upright cycle exercise in boys. *Am J Hum Biol*. 2000;12:749–757.
21. Rowland T, Potts J, Potts T, et al. Cardiac responses to progressive exercise in children: a synthesis. *Med Sci Sports Exerc*. 2000;32:253–259.
22. Rowland T, Unnithan V. Stroke volume dynamics during progressive exercise in healthy adolescents. *Pediatr Exerc Science*. 2013;25:173–185.
23. Rowland T, Unnithan V. Myocardial inotropic response to progressive exercise in healthy subjects: a review. *Curr Sports Med Rep*. 2013;12:93–100.
24. Tschakovsky ME, Shoemaker JK, Hughson RL. Vasodilation and muscle pump contribution to immediate exercise hyperemia. *Am J Physiol*. 1996;271:H1697–H1701.
25. Wilczek F. *A Beautiful Question. Finding Nature's Deep Design*. New York: Penguin Press; 2015.
26. Wilmore JH, Freund BJ, Joyner MJ, et al. Acute response to submaximal and maximal exercise consequent to beta-adrenergic blockade: implications for the prescription of exercise. *Am J Cardiol*. 1985;55:135D–141D.

9

WHAT CAUSES EXERCISE-INDUCED HYPOXEMIA IN ATHLETES?

Insights from Saratoga

Characters in the works of the author Charles Bukowski are some of the most foul, degenerate, and disgusting persons in all of literary history, and yet his regular readers (of which there were a great many) loved him. (In the spirit of full disclosure, this author admits to having himself several of Bukowski's works sitting on the bookshelf.) When not drinking, whoring, vomiting in public, and a host of other socially deplorable pastimes, his personages (and presumably Bukowski himself) spent much of their time and money at the horse track. To wit (from *Tales of Ordinary Madness*):

> then Pixie Dew came running on out from the outside, Ackerman giving the 20 to one shot all the string it needed and going to the whip . . . and that's the way they came down—O'Brien holding that space open, clucking to his horse, sailing by, smiling just a bit, as he does, and it was over . . . the two dollar win and two dollar show windows were filled with little old ladies on pension checks with half pints of gin in their purses.
>
> *(3)*

Bukowski was, for certain, no exercise physiologist, but he knew his horses and how to pick them. And he was no doubt aware that virtually all Thoroughbreds exhibit some degree of lung hemorrhage when they race, and that this bleeding impairs their performance, and that the diuretic furosemide, administered intravenously four hours before the race would counter this effect. And, too, this pre-race routine of drugging racehorses is very much legal—but only in the United States and Canada. Whether this practice, said to be utilized in about 90% of horses in such races, constitutes unethical drug-induced performance enhancement or instead a salutary intervention for the well-being of the horse remains contested.

(In some states, including California, where Bukowski lived, the astute track bettor can tell which of the equine contestants have received furosemide by consulting the track program. In others, one is left in the dark.) So that's one of the ways Bukowski and his characters improved their betting odds.

No one is quite certain as to the cause of this airway bleeding, which is usually not visually obvious except by direct endoscopic visualization and is not consistently associated with arterial hypoxemia. Sometimes such episodes are more dramatic, such as the 1987 Kentucky Derby favorite Demons Begone being pulled up by his jockey on the back stretch, bleeding profusely from the nose. Some have suggested that pulmonary hemorrhage might be incriminated in cases of sudden death of racehorses (21), but the fact that evidence that such bleeding is so common and the risk of sudden death so small (0.08–0.29 per 1,000 races) makes it very difficult to establish hemorrhage as the cause of death (15).

The prevailing opinion is that exercise-induced pulmonary hemorrhage in racehorses is caused by excessive pressures in the pulmonary circulation, the exact site and mechanistic explanation for which remain uncertain. West considered this phenomenon a classic case of pulmonary capillary stress failure, meaning an increase in the pressure gradient across the alveolar-capillary membrane from excessive blood pressure, with subsequent membrane rupture and entrance of hemorrhagic edema fluid into the alveolar space (38). In an early study, he and his colleagues tested this hypothesis in a post-mortem tissue study of three Thoroughbred horses with known exercise-induced pulmonary hemorrhage who were administered barbiturate euthanasia after galloping on a treadmill (39). Electron microscopy revealed disruption of alveolar epithelium and capillary endothelium—the combination of which provides the thin membranous barrier to gas exchange—with red blood cells and edema in the alveolar space.

In the discussion of this article, the authors referred to a) the report by Jones et al. of an elevated mean pulmonary artery pressure in galloping horses on a treadmill of an astounding 120 mm Hg and mean left atrial pressure of 70 mm Hg, indicating an estimated capillary pressure of 95 mm Hg (19), and b) their own previous studies which had indicated that a capillary pressure created in resting cats of >40 mm Hg was associated with similar disruptive findings of the blood gas barrier (35,40). The authors concluded from these combined findings that "Little wonder that galloping racehorses bleed into their lungs" (39). This conclusion was consistent with the finding of Manohar, who found a catheter-estimated maximal pulmonary capillary pressure of 73 mm Hg in horses galloping on a treadmill (24).

This was a reasonable conclusion. Successful racing and training of horses demands a high cardiovascular capacity, and limited physiological studies indicate that, pound for pound, the aerobic machinery of the trained Thoroughbred is about twice as powerful as that of the elite human male endurance athlete. On treadmill testing, the maximal oxygen uptake (VO_2max) of the Thoroughbred is typically 150 ml/kg/min (compared to 70–80 ml/kg/min in highly trained male humans), with a peak cardiac output of 300 liters/min (700 ml/kg/min) and 25 liters/min (340 ml/kg/min), respectively (5,11).

(One interesting aspect of equine exercise physiology that contributes to the horse's high VO_2max is a superior level of peripheral oxygen extraction by muscle cells (arterial venous oxygen difference) of approximately 20–25 ml/dl. That compares to expected values in humans of 16–20 ml/dl. The explanation appears to be the effect of the horse's release of erythrocytes from the spleen during exercise as well as a more complete extraction of oxygen by the exercising muscle [5,11].)

The maximal heart rate of a racing Thoroughbred is 220–240 bpm. It follows that high pressures in the left atrium (and thus in the entire pulmonary vascular circuit) will be necessary to create a sufficiently high trans-mitral valve gradient required for adequate filling of the large left ventricle in a progressively shorter time period as exercise intensity increases. However, such elevations in pressure, as documented in the above-mentioned studies, can cause the fragile alveolar-capillary membrane to rupture, causing filling of alveolar spaces with hemorrhagic edema fluid.

Birks et al. recognized that the actual capillary pressures which are necessary to cause capillary-alveolar membrane rupture in racehorses had not been documented (4). To address this issue, they perfused lung tissue from killed horses with blood producing different capillary hydrostatic pressures and examined the associated membrane structural characteristics. They found that significant disruption of capillary epithelium did not occur until transmembrane pressure gradients reached 75–100 mm Hg, which was substantially higher than similarly conducted previous studies of rabbits and cats (damage threshold >40 mm Hg) and dogs (>70 mm Hg). Still, they noted that the higher capillary rupture threshold pressures in racehorses were compatible with values normally achieved during racing. They concluded that their findings supported the model of capillary stress failure for explaining exercise-induced hemorrhage in racehorses and suggested that the blood gas exchange barrier in the lungs of these animals was "extremely strong."

Intuitively attractive as this model is, Manohar and Goetz raised the stubborn question of documentation of cause and effect when they demonstrated that the pressures in the pulmonary circuit during exercise of horses with exercise-induced pulmonary hemorrhage were not significantly different from those without hemorrhage (25). Overall peak estimated mean capillary pressure was 83 mm Hg in this study, as indicated by indwelling vascular catheters as the horses galloped at 14.5 m/sec up a 5% treadmill incline, reaching an average heart rate of 214 bpm. The authors did not interpret these findings as necessarily negating the capillary stress failure model, suggesting that their findings might be explained by differences in alveolar pressure and strength of the blood gas exchange barrier in the two groups of animals.

A number of other etiologies for pulmonary hemorrhage in racehorses have been proposed, although none have solid research support: chronic bronchiolitis, parasitic infection, coagulation defects, asphyxia, cardiac failure, mechanical stresses on lung parenchyma. However, if one accepts that an increase in the alveolar-capillary transmembrane pressure *gradient* is the core feature underlying this pulmonary hemorrhage, an alternative to augmented capillary blood pressure—a substantial fall in alveolar (i.e., "downstream") pressure—is plausible.

The hyperpnea during Thoroughbred racing is profound. Hackett et al., for instance, reported average breathing rates of 122 breaths per minute with maximal treadmill galloping (peak heart rate 208 bpm) (13). During such labored breathing, wide swings of alveolar pressure are evident, these being exaggerated by naturally occurring partial obstructions of the upper airway which are common in horses, such as palatal dysfunction, laryngeal collapse, epiglottic entrapment, and collapse of the crico-tracheal ligament (10,20).

Such obstructions serve to lower inspiratory alveolar pressures during strenuous exercise and augment the alveolar-capillary pressure gradient. For example, in the study by Hackett et al. the average inspiratory esophageal pressure (reflecting alveolar pressure) fell in Thoroughbred horses from a value of −5 mm Hg at rest to −36 mm Hg at peak exercise (13). Manohar cautioned that the true transmural pressure gradient across the blood gas barrier with high intensity exercise in horses may be significantly greater than the 70–75 mm reported capillary pressures, since the gradient will be augmented by the negative alveolar pressures associated with swings of pleural pressure (24).

The key study in this regard was performed by Ducharme et al., in which the effect of various applied obstructive loads on pulmonary capillary pressure was examined during treadmill exercise by horses galloping at 75, 90, and 100% of maximal heart rate (9). Important insights can be gained from this study, since it included not only the effects of airway obstruction but also estimates of both capillary pressure and alveolar pressures, i.e., the determinants of the true transmembrane pressure gradient. The seven horses in this study exercised in each of four conditions: a) control—no airway obstruction, b) inspiratory obstruction (left laryngeal hemiplegia, c) expiratory obstruction (one-way nostril valve), and d) a combination of inspiratory and expiratory loads. At peak exercise, average inspiratory esophageal pressures (indicative of alveolar pressure) in the four conditions were −31, −57, −49, and −34 mm Hg, respectively, indicating the effect of inspiratory airway obstruction of exaggerating the fall in pressure on the alveolar side of the blood gas barrier. The mean peak estimated pulmonary capillary-alveolar transmural pressures in each of these conditions were 57, 70, 77, and 49 mm Hg.

The collective findings in both *in vivo* and *in vitro* studies thus provide a reasonably consistent picture of alveolar-capillary membrane rupture causing pulmonary hemorrhage in racing horses as a consequence of high capillary hydrostatic pressures resulting from heightened cardiac output coupled with exaggerated negative alveolar pressures consequent to upper airway obstruction (Figure 9.1). The effectiveness of furosemide as a prophylactic agent for exercise-induced pulmonary hemorrhage presumably then relates to its action of decreasing blood volume

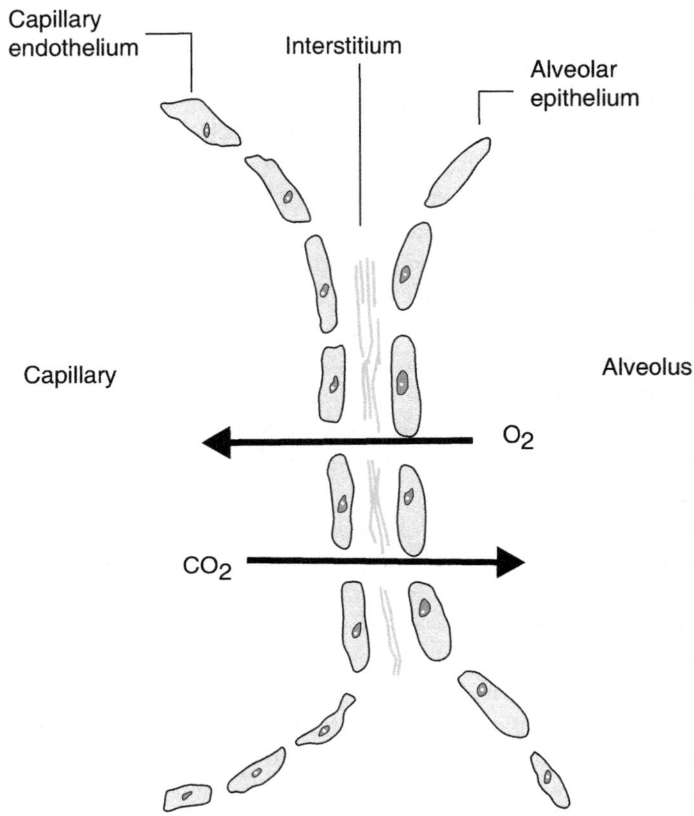

FIGURE 9.1 The membrane separating blood flowing in the capillaries from lung air space is a "sandwich" of capillary endothelial cells and alveolar epithelial cells with a center of connective tissue interstitium. Oxygen and carbon dioxide are exchanged in bidirectional diffusion through the membrane, which must be robust enough to prevent rupture due to increased capillary pressures and/or exaggerated negative pressures in the alveolar space. Exercise may, in fact, provoke pulmonary edema and hemorrhage through both of these mechanisms.

through diuresis, thereby reducing capillary hydrostatic pressure and transmembrane pressure gradient.

To biologists, whose foundations of belief are rooted in Darwinian principles, this almost ubiquitous pulmonary hemorrhage recognized in racehorses is a bit unsettling. That is, the "wisdom" of a biological system should not permit that the safe limits of functional response to exercise be exceeded (this is a concept that will be re-visited in Chapter 13 in a consideration of the control by a central governor of one's race pace). One's obvious response to this might be that in the selective breeding of racehorses for high circulatory responses to exercise, the line might be crossed beyond normal and expected natural constraints. This conclusion is supported by the observation that pulmonary hemorrhage is observed in racing greyhounds and camels, who are also bred for speed and agility. Too, exercise-induced hemorrhage appears to be less common in horses involved in slower, long duration activities and those less highly bred. Still, such hemorrhage is observed in other than Thoroughbred horses at Churchill Downs and—as we shall see in a bit—in human beings as well.

The somewhat striking conclusion, however, is that stress failure of pulmonary capillaries, a pathological process, is recognized to occur during a normal physiological state (i.e., intense exercise) (23). The only means of protecting against such membrane breakdown would be to increase the barrier thickness, a feature reported in diving birds, whose relatively thick barrier may have evolved to protect against damage from the high hydrostatic capillary pressures during dives (23).

The Alveolar-Capillary Membrane

In the lungs, the alveolar-capillary membrane (or the blood gas barrier) is a sandwich consisting of layers of capillary endothelial cells and alveolar epithelial cells between which is filled a sparse spread of interstitial connective tissue. It is extraordinarily thin—just 0.3–0.6 μm—yet it covers a vast area, in the human being equaling the surface area of a regulation tennis court. Its job is that of a gaseous exchanger, transferring by the process of passive diffusion oxygen from the alveoli to the passing capillary circulation and sending carbon dioxide in the reverse direction for exhalation from the lungs.

This membrane has an architectural problem. It must be thin enough to permit rapid gas diffusion transfer, yet at the same time must possess sufficient structural integrity to withstand the pressure gradient which exists between the capillary and the alveolus (23). As the foregoing discussion has already implied, there exist conditions—in this case the demands of high intensity exercise in racehorses—in which the limits of this compromise are exceeded, resulting in membrane damage and hemorrhagic edematous fluid passing in to the alveolar space. Yet in its efforts to provide a structural compromise, there is another side to the story, one of *time*.

(Such Faustian conflicts of purpose in living beings are not rare. Mother Nature is sometimes faced with the operational difficulty of satisfying two diametrically opposed goals, each by itself reflecting a Darwinian objective of self-preservation. As an example, thermoregulatory mechanisms of sweat production and shift of blood flow to the skin for convective loss serve to protect against hyperthermia, yet these responses engender loss of central blood volume and perils of dehydration.)

The efficiency of the blood gas barrier in facilitating gaseous diffusion depends on the alveolar-capillary partial pressure gradient of the gas, and, according to Fick's first law, is directly proportional to the cross-sectional area and inversely proportional to the thickness of the barrier. In the normal resting human this is achieved satisfactorily with the "compromise" structural thinness of the blood gas barrier, as oxygen flow occurs across the barrier at a rate of 2.3 X 10^{-5} cm^2/s over a time period of 250–500 ms (31). With intense exercise, however, there are new challenges. Even though the diffusion capacity of the membrane rises in direct proportion to increases in cardiac output, the decreased red blood cell transit time through the area of alveolar-capillary interface in the lungs threatens gaseous equilibrium between the two (28).

This difficulty has been cited to explain yet a separate pulmonary issue in racehorses of *arterial hypoxemia* at high exercise intensities. This is manifest as a decline in the difference between capillary arterial oxygen partial pressure and that of the juxtaposed alveolar gas ($AaDO_2$) as well as arterial PO_2 and hypercapnia (elevated PCO_2 levels) as high running speeds are approached (1,17,39). Typical of these reports, Wagner et al. demonstrated in five catheterized gelding horses that average $AaDO_2$ and arterial PO_2 remained stable during progressive treadmill exercise until high speeds were attained (39). At this point, mean $AaDO_2$ values increased abruptly from 20 to 30 mm Hg, while arterial PO_2 declined by 11%, from 90 to 80 mm Hg. Bayly et al. found that $AaDO_2$ increased 4–6 times at heavy exercise in Thoroughbred horses compared to resting values (1). In that study, no compensatory hyperventilation was observed, as retention of CO_2 was evidenced by a rise in arterial PCO_2 of 5–10 mm Hg during very heavy exercise.

In the study noted above, Wagner et al. sought to establish the mechanism underlying these abnormalities of gas exchange (39). Utilizing the multiple inert gas elimination technique, they ascertained that at the high treadmill speeds associated with horse hypoxemia, 76% of the $AaDO_2$ was accounted for by limitations in alveolar-arterial oxygen diffusion. The authors surmised that this could be accounted for by the shortening of pulmonary capillary transit times occurring with exercise. That is, with the greatly accelerated flow of blood through the lungs during intense exercise, there simply does not exist a sufficient time to permit gas exchange.

The thickness of the gas barrier is constructed wisely to accommodate gas exchange and resist capillary hydrostatic pressures within a wide range of normal conditions. Yet during intense exercise it fails on both counts, at least in racehorses—too thick to permit gas exchange in the limited time constraints of high blood flow while too thin to withstand the hydrostatic pressures that accompany such exaggerated pulmonary blood flow. The consequence is depression of exercise performance from a combination of a) hemorrhagic pulmonary edema and b) diffusion-limited hypoxemia.

Compounding these issues, racehorses suffer from anatomic and dynamic upper airway obstruction, and ventilatory work is augmented by their comparatively high breathing frequencies, which occurs as a consequence of a tight 1:1 coupling of strides to breaths when galloping. It comes as no surprise, then, that Franklin et al. concluded that "in [most mammalian species] performance is limited by cardiovascular or muscular performance whereas in athletic horses it is the respiratory system which appears to be rate limiting" (12). Think on this the next time you read Bukowski.

Human Endurance Athletes

The preceding discussion could be considered simply of veterinarian import, with side directives to the heavy bettors at Saratoga, if it weren't for the observation that both of these issues—hemorrhagic pulmonary edema and arterial hypoxemia—are witnessed as well during vigorous exercise in human elite athletes (a species not usually recognized for inbreeding practices). A considerable body of research evidence indicates that arterial hypoxemia is common at high exercise intensities, particularly in trained athletes, and some would argue for a similar occurrence of pulmonary edema—hemorrhagic or otherwise. This area of inquiry in human beings is replete with inconclusive and sometimes conflicting research findings, and there remains considerable uncertainty regarding these issues. Particularly, whether the lessons learned from racehorses outlined in the previous section can be transferred to humans remains to be seen. The architectural dilemma of the alveolar-capillary membrane remains the same—thick enough to resist the hydrostatic pressures on the capillary side yet sufficiently thin to permit gas exchange, particularly challenging as the transit time of red cells through the lungs decreases with exercise. Failure of the former speaks to membrane stress rupture with hemorrhagic pulmonary edema, while the latter, a lack of sufficient transmembrane diffusion of blood gases, would be manifest as an increasing alveolar-capillary oxygen difference as exercise intensified.

Pulmonary Edema

The occurrence of pulmonary edema with exercise in humans is the physiological analog of the conditions considered responsible for triggering pulmonary hemorrhage in galloping racehorses—marked increases in capillary hydrostatic pressure in highly trained animals coupled with exaggerated declines in inspiratory alveolar pressure, creating a stress failure in the gas exchange barrier. The difference, obviously, is that conditions on both sides of this membrane in even elite human athletes do not reach the extremes observed in racing Thoroughbreds.

At high exercise work the peak pulmonary capillary pressure in a trained human endurance athlete is approximately 20–30 mm Hg, far lower than that of a racing Thoroughbred (38). Thus, to start with, the occurrence of rupture of the blood gas barrier due to high hydrostatic pressure during exercise in humans might be expected to be less dramatic than that of equine competitors. Indeed, controversy persists as to whether or not exercise at high intensities by human athletes can truly trigger pulmonary edema (defined as the accumulation of plasma transudate within the interstitial layer of the gas exchange barrier or alveolar spaces). The

Journal of Applied Physiology has, in fact, published two literary debates in which supporters of both "yea" and "nay" arguments have expressed their viewpoints.

The controversy appears to stem from a report by McKechnie et al. in the *South African Medical Journal* of two competitors in the 90-km Comrades Marathon who developed clear evidence of pulmonary edema, with dyspnea, hemorrhagic frothy sputum, and abnormal chest x-rays (26). The question: Were these sentinel cases the tip of an iceberg, indicative of a more extensive occurrence of subclinical pulmonary edema in human athletes, cases that proved the point? Or, on the other hand, were these just isolated occurrences, the pulmonary effects of extreme exercise in pathologically predisposed individuals?

In advocating for the former point of view, Susan Hopkins suggested the following scenario: During maximal exercise, cardiac output and pulmonary capillary blood volume rise, increasing capillary hydrostatic pressure, which forces fluid leakage across the alveolar-capillary membrane (16). Animal research data indicate that in this process the resulting increase in fluid within the membrane interstitium is normally removed by lymphatic drainage, thereby preventing extravasation into the alveolar space and the occurrence of frank pulmonary edema. It is only when this lymphatic defense mechanism is overwhelmed by very high capillary pressures in rare cases of extreme exercise in humans that the clinical findings of pulmonary edema occur. She suggested, then, that interstitial edema is common in the exercising human and only in certain unusual conditions, such as very prolonged intense exercise, psychological stress, or moderate altitude exposure do human athletes exhibit overt pulmonary edema. Thus, she concluded that "the normal lung has a large safety margin preventing the development of alveolar flooding except in the most extreme cases. However, interstitial edema is more likely."

Sheel and McKenzie argued, however, that certain evidence failed to support this construct (32). For instance, in repeated bouts of exercise, gas exchange in humans is either unchanged or improved, the opposite finding one would expect with capillary stress failure. They contended that in reported cases of pulmonary edema in athletes, such as the two participants in the Comrades Marathon, the pulmonary artery pressures would not be expected to be sufficiently elevated to cause stress failure at the pulmonary capillary level. And if the proposed scenario of Hopkins was true, why would there not be frequently similar cases of overt clinical pulmonary edema in the many similar ultra-distance competitions?

Zavorsky and Anholm expressed some impatience with this discussion, contending that "We do not think there is much debate [on this subject]" (42). They note that in a review of 11 studies in the research literature, two-thirds of subjects demonstrated mild interstitial pulmonary edema with sustained maximal exercise efforts, as indicated by evidence of increased lung water on various imaging techniques (such as computed tomography, magnetic resonance imaging, and positron emission tomography) (41). The frequency of such positive findings was related to the type of exercise protocol employed in the study: Only 16% of the subjects demonstrated evidence of pulmonary edema during non-exhaustive but prolonged submaximal exercise (15 minutes to two hours at an intensity equivalent to 50–75% VO_2max), 65% with sustained maximal effort in quasi-race situations, but none in a standard progressive exercise test to exhaustion. "The real question is not whether mild interstitial pulmonary edema is triggered by heavy exercise," they concluded, "but whether this edema is meaningful. [Particularly] it is unclear what effect, if any, it may have on endurance exercise performance."

Insightful in this discussion is the study of Hopkins et al. that confirmed that at least in some exercise conditions true extravasation of hemorrhagic fluid into the alveolar space—capillary stress failure—can occur in highly trained athletes (18). They performed bronchoalveolar lavage immediately following an exercise challenge in six elite endurance cyclists and runners with a history "suggestive of lung bleeding after very intense short duration exercise" and compared findings with those of control non-athletic subjects performing similar exercise. (With this experimental approach, then, they mimicked that of studies which have utilized similar endoscopic findings to establish hemorrhagic pulmonary edema in racehorses.) The exercise challenge consisted of a 7-minute duration 4.0 km cycle steep hill climb with grades up to 12%. Post-exercise, red blood cells were detected in lavage fluid of all the athletes but only one control subject, and higher concentrations of total protein and albumin were detected in the lavages of athletes compared to the control group. These findings, the authors concluded, "support our hypothesis that the integrity of the blood-gas barrier in athletes is impaired by short-term exercise."

There is an interesting side story to this discussion—that of "swimming-induced pulmonary edema (SIPE)"—which may or may not bear importance to this mechanistic discussion of capillary stress failure with exercise. In 2016, Moon et al. indicated that nearly 300 cases of overt clinical pulmonary edema (dyspnea, cough, hypoxemia) had been described in humans while swimming or diving (27). These include competitors in triathlon events. For instance, Ma and Dutch described five athletes (among 1,594 competitors) who developed severe hemoptysis and dyspnea after the swimming leg of the 2012 triathlon in Victoria, Australia (22).

The pathophysiology of this condition is unclear. Beale et al. suggested that although increase in capillary hydrostatic pressure might be incriminated in these cases, it might be more likely that loss of integrity of the alveolar-capillary membrane occurs because of large negative inspiratory pressures unique to the process of swimming (2). That is, "some vigorous inspiratory efforts may be rapidly truncated when the athlete's face is submerged in a wave or the splashes of neighboring swimmers," in effect reducing alveolar pressure, increasing the gas exchange barrier gradient, and precipitating pulmonary capillary stress failure.

Arterial Hypoxemia

There exists no similar debate regarding the negative impact of exercise in humans on oxygen transfer across the pulmonary alveolar-capillary membrane. As Stickland et al. succinctly put it, "It is now accepted that most humans develop an impairment of pulmonary gas exchange with exercise, as demonstrated by a widening of the alveolar-arterial oxygen partial pressure difference" (33). Additionally, three corollaries are reasonably well-established: a) such responses of increased $AaDO_2$ with exercise are greater in elite athletes, b) in most human subjects the hyperventilation occurring normally with high intensity exercise serves to prevent arterial hypoxemia, and c) a combination of impaired diffusion and ventilation:perfusion (V_A/Q) mismatch are responsible for this impairment of gas exchange.

Given its potential for diminishing endurance performance, the phenomenon of exercise-induced arterial hypoxemia has attracted a good deal of research attention. Still, many questions surrounding its pathophysiology and influence on endurance performance remain. (The reader is referred to two comprehensive reviews of this topic for a more in-depth discussion [29,30].)

General Observations

At rest, the alveolar-capillary oxygen difference ($AaDO_2$) is small, approximately 5–10 mm Hg, the result of minor V_A/Q inequalities within the lung (occurring when areas of lung are perfused with blood but not ventilated or blood is not circulated through ventilated regions). At the commencement of progressive exercise, this difference increases and then steadily widens in a linear fashion as work intensity rises, indicating a progressive impairment of pulmonary gas exchange. Peak values at exhaustive exercise are directly related to athletic training status, reaching approximately 20–25 mm Hg in the nontrained subject but often exceeding 35 mm Hg in the elite endurance runner or cyclist (8).

During progressive exercise minute ventilation matches oxygen uptake (VO_2) until an intensity demanding about 60% VO_2max, when, stimulated by increased $[H_+]$ from buffering of lactic acid, the rise in ventilation exceeds that of VO_2. This hyperventilation serves to raise alveolar PO_2 and thereby compensates for the widening $DAaO_2$. As a consequence, in most nontrained individuals, despite the progressive rise in $AaDO_2$, arterial hypoxemia is avoided and PaO_2 remains stable to maximal exercise. In a certain percentage of highly trained elite endurance athletes, however, this hyperventilation response is dampened and insufficient in avoiding overt arterial hypoxemia (30). As a result of this relative hypoventilation, arterial PO_2 falls, sometimes reaching 20–35 mm Hg below resting values at peak exercise, associated with an arterial PCO_2 >35 mm Hg (7).

Just why the highly trained athlete should lack such an appropriate compensatory ventilatory response, which in a salutary fashion prevents arterial hypoxemia during exercise in nonathletes, is not at all clear. Mechanical features of the airways such as limitations to high air flow rates have been suggested. Too, for unexplained reasons, exercise training might be associated with blunted responses to factors which normally stimulate ventilation with exercise ($[H^+]$, PCO_2) (8).

Exercise-induced arterial hypoxemia in trained athletes can be accounted for, then, by a combination of a) an excessive widening of the $AaDO_2$ with exercise (>25–30 mm Hg), and b) an inadequate compensatory hyperventilation. An estimated 40–60% of highly trained endurance cyclists and runners will demonstrate an 8–35 mm Hg drop in arterial PO_2 with intense exercise (7,14,30), and exercise-induced hypoxemia has also been described in triathletes, swimmers, and rowers as well (29). Included in these reports are prepubertal, elderly, and both male and female athletes (29).

Dempsey et al. defined exercise-induced hypoxemia as mild with an arterial oxygen saturation of 93–95% (or 3–4% below resting values), moderate as 88–93%, and severe as <88%, the latter being associated with an arterial PO_2 at peak exercise approaching 30 mm Hg below resting values (8). According to this categorization, it takes little in the way of arterial hypoxemia to negatively affect VO_2max. Harms et al. demonstrated in experienced female competitive runners (mean VO_2max 57 ml/kg/min) that a decline in peak aerobic power is demonstrable when hemoglobin saturation is depressed by 3–4% (14). A direct relationship was observed between further reductions in saturation and fall in VO_2max such that for every 1% decrease in saturation peak aerobic power fell by 1–2%.

Etiology of Impaired Gas Exchange

Factors potentially responsible for the impairment of gas exchange with exercise have been examined in a number of studies. The multiple inert gas elimination technique has been utilized specifically to identify extent of V_A/Q inequality, and a deficiency in gas diffusion in the pathway of oxygen from alveolus, across the gas exchange barrier, through the capillary plasma, and into the red blood cell has been assumed to represent the remainder of the $AaDO_2$. In general, these reveal in the trained athlete a pattern of initial progressive rise in V_A/Q mismatch at low and moderate exercise intensities, supplemented by increasing gas diffusion limitations as peak exercise is approached. The extent of the contribution of limitations in diffusion to the $AaDO_2$ at peak exercise is related to level of aerobic fitness. In the nontrained individual little or no such diffusion abnormalities are observed, while in the elite endurance athlete, limitations of diffusion may account for one-third to one-half of the $AaDO_2$.

Ventilation:Perfusion Mismatch

The explanation for the increase in V_A/Q inequality with exercise remains obscure. A number of candidate factors have been proposed, including exercise-induced bronchospasm, enhanced pulmonary secretions, nonuniform changes in the modulation of airway and blood vessel tone, and the occurrence of interstitial edema described in the previous section as a result of stress failure in response to augmented capillary hydrostatic pressure (36). Contribution of increases in V_A/Q mismatch with exercise via the latter explanation was supported by the findings of Wagner et al. of a strong correlation between mean pulmonary artery pressure and ventilation:perfusion inequality during exercise by athletic subjects (36). However, Stickland et al. showed that mild increase in pulmonary artery and venous pressures (3.7 and 4.0 mm Hg, respectively) created by application of lower-body positive pressure had no effect on $AaDO_2$ (34).

Diffusion Limitations

Juxtaposition of the capillary and alveolar linings for gas exchange occurs across a discrete distance in the lung. (This being analogous to the distinct area on the track in which the baton may be passed from runner to runner in a relay race.) This anatomic length is not altered with exercise, but the time available for diffusion of oxygen across the alveolar-capillary membrane (as well as through the plasma and into the passing red blood cell) is diminished as a consequence of the increased pulmonary arterial flow rate. At rest, this transit time is approximately 0.75 seconds, providing a wide safety margin for attainment of complete gas equilibration, which occurs in about 0.30 seconds.

With the augmented pulmonary arterial flow rate during exercise in non-trained individuals, the transit time is diminished by one-half, which still provides adequate time for gas exchange. Typically, then, an untrained person demonstrates no limitations of diffusion with exercise. In elite endurance athletes, however, the high cardiac output during intense exercise may result in transit times that impinge on the minimal time necessary for full gas equilibrium. This negative effect of transit time shortening is counteracted by increases in capillary blood volume as new capillaries are recruited at heavy exercise, thereby increasing the surface area for diffusion and prolonging red cell transit time in the pulmonary capillaries.

Dempsey et al. postulated that pulmonary capillary transit time might be expected to fall to gas exchange-limiting levels if the limits of pulmonary capillary blood volume had been reached and pulmonary blood flow exceeded 26–28 L/min (7). This scenario would then explain the contribution of diffusion limitation to $AaDO_2$ in elite athletes at high exercise intensities.

In the final analysis, the mysteries surrounding the deficiencies of pulmonary gas exchange during exercise appear to be distilled down to the anatomic and functional limitations of the three-tiered gas exchange barrier which separates capillary blood flow from alveolar ventilation. And the story in racehorses appears to be mirrored in human beings as well. No studies have yet directly examined damage to the alveolar-capillary membrane with severe exercise in human beings.

But the argument that the pathophysiology surrounding such damage observed in racehorses—exaggerated by breeding practices—is reflected in a similar membrane stress failure in humans is compelling.

Humans share with other mammals a vulnerable barrier for gas exchange at the capillary-alveolar interface, one not designed for high levels of endurance athletic competition. The alveolar-capillary membrane faces the challenge of satisfying two directly conflicting goals of gaseous permeability and constraint of fluid extravasation. In its quest for a Goldilocks-like solution to this dilemma—not too thick, not too thin, but just right—the membrane's responses to the evolutionary pressures which have designed the pulmonary blood exchange barrier have been remarkably astute—at least for the resting mammal. But with intense exercise in the highly trained human the compromise strategy fails, and at both extremes. The membrane is not thin enough to permit complete gas exchange in short time intervals of rapid red blood cell transit and, at the same time, is insufficiently thick to maintain membrane integrity when capillary pressure rises with high pulmonary blood flows. And for highly elite athletes—as well as racing Thoroughbreds—the effect of consequent reduction of blood oxygenation and supply to exercising muscles on performance may be a problem.

Which leads to the question, stealing here from the title of Jerry Dempsey's classical article, is the lung really built for exercise (6)? During acute bouts of exercise, the lung of the elite athlete fails to meet the metabolic demands of high work intensities, with augmentation of the $AaDO_2$, relative hypoventilation, and arterial hypoxemia. Explaining the pulmonary adaptations—or lack thereof—to endurance training are equally problematic. In response to a period of endurance training, the body's systems respond in a predictable fashion with anatomic and functional adaptations that underpin associated increases in endurance performance. All systems, that is, except the lung. "The lung in physically trained humans or in athletic animals differs not at all or very little from the sedentary animal, and the physical training sufficient to increase VO_2max has no measurable effects on lung function or structure" (8). The explanations remain obscure.

References

1. Bayly WM, Hodgson DR, Schulz DA, Dempsey JA, Gollnick PD. Exercise-induced hypercapnia in the horse. *J Appl Physiol.* 1989;67:1958–1966.
2. Beale A, Gong FF. La Gerche A. Exercise-induced pulmonary oedema in endurance triathletes. *Int J Cardiol.* 2016;203:980–981.
3. Bukowski C. *Tales of Ordinary Madness.* San Francisco: City Light Books; 1983.
4. Birks EK, Mathieu-Costello O, Fu Z, Tyler WS. West JB. Very high pressures are required to cause stress failure of pulmonary capillaries in Thoroughbred racehorses. *J Appl Physiol.* 1997;82:1584–1592.
5. Butler PJ, Woakes AJ, Anderson LS, Smale K, Roberts CA, Snow DH. The effect of cessation of training on cardiorespiratory variables during exercise. In: Persson SEB,

Lindholm A, Jeffcott LB, editors. *Equine Exercise Physiology 3*. Stockholm: ICEEP Publications; 1991. pp. 71–76.

6. Dempsey JA. Is the lung built for exercise? *Med Sci Sports Exerc*. 1986;18:143–155.
7. Dempsey J, Hanson P, Henderson K. Exercise-induced arterial hypoxemia in healthy persons at sea level. *J Physiol*. 1984;355:161–175.
8. Dempsey JA, Wagner PD. Exercise-induced arterial hypoxemia. *J Appl Physiol*. 1999;87:1997–2006.
9. Ducharme NG, Hackett RP, Gleed RD, et al. Pulmonary capillary pressure in horses undergoing alteration of pleural pressure by imposition of various upper airway resistive loads. *Equine Vet J. Suppl* 1999;July:27–33.
10. Durando MM, Martin BB, Hammer EJ, Langsam SP, Birks EK. Dynamic upper airway changes and arterial blood gas parameters during treadmill exercise. *Equine Vet J. Suppl* 2002;Sep:408–412.
11. Evans DL, Rose RJ. Cardiovascular and respiratory responses in thoroughbred horses during treadmill exercise. *J Exp Biol*. 1988;134:397–408.
12. Franklin SH, Van Erck-Westergren E, Bayly WM. Respiratory responses to exercise in the horse. *Equine Vet J*. 2012;44:726–732.
13. Hackett RP, Ducharme NG, Gleed RD, et al. Do thoroughbred and standardbred horses have similar increases in pulmonary vascular pressures during exertion? *Can J Vet Res*. 2003;67:291–296.
14. Harms CA, McClaran SR, Nickele GA, Pegelow DF, Nelson WB, Dempsey JA. Effect of exercise-induced arterial O2 desaturation on VO2max in women. *Med Sci Sports Exerc*. 2000;32:1101–1118.
15. Hinchcliff KW, Couetil LL, Knight PK, et al. Exercise induced pulmonary hemorrhage in horses: American College of Veterinary Internal Medicine consensus statement. *J Vet Intern Med*. 2015;29:743–758.
16. Hopkins SR. Point: pulmonary edema does occur in human athletes performing heavy sea-level exercise. *J Appl Physiol*. 2010;109:1270–1275.
17. Hopkins SR, Bayly WM, Slocombe RF, Wagner H, Wagner PD. Effect of prolonged heavy exercise on pulmonary gas exchange in horses. *J Appl Physiol*. 1998;84:1723–1730.
18. Hopkins SR, Schoene RB, Henderson WR, Spragg RG, Martin TR, West JB. Intense exercise impairs the integrity of the pulmonary blood-gas barrier in elite athletes. *Am J Respir Crit Care Med*. 1997;155:1090–1094.
19. Jones JH, Smith BL, Birks EK, Pascoe JR, Hughes TR. Left atrial and pulmonary arterial pressures in exercising horses [abstract]. *FASEB*. 1992;6:A2020.
20. Lane JG, Bladon B, Little DR, Naylor JR, Franklin SH. Dynamic obstructions of the equine upper respiratory tract. Part 1: observations during high-speed treadmill endoscopy of 600 Thoroughbred racehorses. *Equine Vet J*. 2006;38:393–399.
21. Lyle CH. Sudden death in racing thoroughbred horses: an international multicenter study of postmortem findings. *Equine Vet J*. 2011;43:324–331.
22. Ma JLG, Dutch MJ. Extreme sports: extreme physiology: Exercise-induced pulmonary oedema. *Emerg Med Austral*. 2012;25:368–371.
23. Maina JN, West JB. Thin and strong! The bioengineering dilemma in the structural and functional design of the blood-gas barrier. *Physiol Rev*. 2005;85:811–844.
24. Manohar M. Pulmonary artery wedge pressure increases with high-intensity exercise in horses. *Am J Vet Res*. 1993;54:142–146.
25. Manohar M, Goetz TE. Pulmonary vascular pressures of exercising Thoroughbred horses with and without endoscopic evidence of EIPH. *J Appl Physiol*. 1996;81:1589–1593.

26. McKechnie JK, Leary WP, Noakes TD, Kallmeyer JC, MacSearraigh ET, Olivier LR. Acute pulmonary edema in two athletes during a 90-km running race. *S Afr Med J.* 1979;56:261–265.
27. Moon RE, Martina SD, Peacher DF, et al. Swimming-induced pulmonary edema: pathophysiology and risk reduction with sildenafil. *Circulation.* 2016;133:988–996.
28. Naeije R, Chesler N. Pulmonary circulation at exercise. *Comp Physiol.* 2012;2:711–741.
29. Powers SK, Martin D, Dodd S. Exercise-induced hypoxaemia in elite endurance athletes. Incidence, causes and impact on VO_2max. *Sports Med.* 1993;16:14–22.
30. Prefaut C, Durand F, Mucci P, Caillaud C. Exercise-induced arterial hypoxemia in athletes: a review. *Sports Med.* 2000;30:47–61.
31. Roughton FJW, Forster RE. Relative importance of diffusion and chemical reaction rates in determining rate of exchange of gases in the human lung, with special reference to true diffusing capacity of pulmonary membrane and volume of blood in the lung capillaries. *J Appl Physiol.* 1957;11:290–302.
32. Sheel AW, McKenzie DC. Counterpoint: pulmonary edema does not occur in human athletes performing heavy sea-level exercise. *J Appl Physiol.* 2010;109:1272–1273.
33. Stickland MK, Amann M, Katayama K, Dempsey JA. Pulmonary responses to exercise and limitations to human performance. In: Taylor NAS, Groeller H, editors. *Physiological Bases of Human Performance during Work and Exercise.* London: Elsevier; 2008. pp. 29–48.
34. Stickland MK, Welsh RC, Haykowsky MJ, et al. Effect of acute increases in pulmonary vascular pressures on exercise pulmonary gas exchange. *J Appl Physiol.* 2006;100:1910–1917.
35. Tsukimoto K, Mathieu-Costello O, Prediletto R, Elliott AR, West JB. Ultrastructural appearances of pulmonary capillaries at high transmural pressures. *J Appl Physiol.* 1991;71:573–582.
36. Wagner PD, Gale GE, Moon RE, Torre-Bueno JR, Stolp BW, Saltzman HA. Pulmonary gas exchange in humans exercising at sea level and simulated altitude. *J Appl Physiol.* 1986;61:260–270.
37. Wagner PD, Gillespie JR, Landgren GL, et al. Mechanism of exercise-induced hypoxemia in horses. *J Appl Physiol.* 1989;66:1227–1233.
38. West JB. Invited review: pulmonary capillary stress failure. *J Appl Physiol.* 2000;89:2483–2489.
39. West JB, Mathieu-Costello O, Jones JH, et al. Stress failure of pulmonary capillaries in racehorses with exercise-induced pulmonary hemorrhage. *J Appl Physiol.* 1993;75:1097–1109.
40. West JB, Tsukimoto K, Mathieu-Costello O, Prediletto R. Stress failure in pulmonary capillaries. *J Appl Physiol.* 1991;70:1731–1742.
41. Zavorsky GS. Evidence of pulmonary oedema triggered by exercise in healthy humans and detected by various imaging techniques. *Acta Physiol.* 2007;189:305–317.
42. Zavorsky GS, Anholm JD. Comments on Point:Counterpoint: pulmonary edema does/does not occur in human athletes performing heavy sea-level exercise. *J Appl Physiol.* 2010;109:1776.

10

IS THERE A BIOLOGICAL BASIS FOR CHILDREN'S REDUCED AEROBIC TRAINABILITY?

The increased research attention to children and exercise in recent decades can be attributed to three developments: a) the rise in participation in sport training and competition by young athletes at levels once considered intense even for adult athletes, b) an awareness of the link between exercise during childhood and salutary health outcomes, and c) recognition of the therapeutic potential of exercise in youth with chronic disease. These investigations have revealed that the physiological responses to exercise in children are often-times dissimilar to those in adults. This chapter addresses one of those: following a period of endurance exercise training, the physiological adaptation of augmented aerobic capacity (maximal oxygen uptake) is dampened in children compared to mature individuals.

Adaptive improvement in response to repetitive function is a hallmark of all living organisms, including humans. The stresses imposed by repeated usage—applied within certain limits—predictably trigger increases in functional capacity within a multitude of widely discrepant physical, physiological, and mental domains. Intriguingly, such adaptive responses which eventuate in improved performance are in each case achieved via unique mechanisms—memorization of a Shakespearean sonnet (neuronal), learning to play the clarinet (neuromuscular), acclimatization to heat stress (physiological), increased muscular strength (anatomic and neuromuscular), and so forth.

In the realm of endurance exercise, repeated sustained contractions of sufficient intensity involving large muscle groups over time stimulate a complex of adaptive responses, prominent of which is an augmented capacity for aerobic metabolism. This training effect is readily measured by an increase in a person's maximal oxygen uptake (VO_2max), reflecting improvements in oxygen delivery, cellular extraction, and utilization by exercising muscle. Increased aerobic capacity, in turn, translates into improvements in mid- and long-duration physical performance capacity.

The current body of research data has provided a compelling argument that improvements in VO_2max in response to a period of endurance exercise training in pre- and early-pubertal children is dampened compared to that of mature individuals (3,50,52,61). These reports have consistently revealed that, on average, children's VO_2max rise following such programs is approximately one-third that observed in previously sedentary young and middle-aged adults. The causal factors—be they methodological or biological—remain enigmatic. The quandary is an important one, since understanding the reasons for this difference might well shed light on the basic mechanisms responsible for the aerobic training effect. Moreover, such an understanding bears potential importance in the training of young athletes as well as in recognizing how endurance exercise might be appropriately employed in the management of children with chronic disease.

Based on both adult human and animal models, considerable progress has been achieved in revealing the mechanisms which underlie the aerobic fitness effect. In view of these contemporary insights, this chapter will examine the potential factors which might provide a biological basis for the curtailed VO_2max response to endurance training in children compared to adults. No definitive answer is currently at hand; however, each of these candidate explanations possesses sufficient credibility as to identify research paths which might yield insights into this issue.

Aerobic Responses to Endurance Training

In normally active young adults, a 2–3 month period of endurance exercise training of sufficient duration (>30 minutes), intensity (60–90% maximum heart rate), and frequency (3 times/week) typically evokes a rise in VO_2max of approximately 15–20% (67). A considerable inter-individual variability exists in the magnitude of this response. An oft-cited example is the training study of Lortie et al. (46), who found individual increases ranging from 5% to 88% after a 20-week endurance training program. The degree of training-induced improvement in studies of adults is typically inversely related to the pre-training VO_2max level. That is, individuals with low initial values often demonstrate larger increases (+20–30%), while those with high initial values (such as trained athletes) are expected to exhibit little or no rise (72). No sex differences have been documented, as females and males appear to possess similar plasticity in VO_2max response to endurance training (62).

It has long been recognized that increases in VO_2max following endurance training in non-athletic 8–13-year-old children are less than those expected in comparably trained adults. In 1993, a 23-study review by Payne and Morrow indicated an average +5% VO_2max training response in children (61). Seven years later, in reviewing 22 studies with optimal research protocols, Baquet et al. found a mean improvement in children's VO_2max of 5–6% (3). In 2008 Mahon tabulated the results of 19 endurance training studies with 23 intervention groups of 8–13-year-old boys and girls which complied with adult training guidelines (50). Nine of the 23 groups (39%) did not manifest a statistically significant rise in VO_2max with training. Armstrong and Barker (2), in their later review of 14 published training studies in children up to age 11 years, confirmed that 35% failed to trigger a significant rise in VO_2max. Among those investigations, the average overall increase was 6.7%.

As in adults, considerable inter-individual variability in aerobic-training response has been observed in children. In the study of Rowland and Boyajian (70), following a 12-week exercise program the range of VO_2max increases in 11–13-year-old children ranged from 3% to 21%. Abundant evidence indicates no sex-dependency in magnitude of training-induced VO_2max increases in this age group (2). An inverse relationship between initial VO_2max and degree of training response has not been clearly established in children. However, a modest negative association was observed ($r = -0.43$, $p = 0.015$) in the studies reviewed by Armstrong and Barker (2) with pre-training VO_2max values ranging from 40 to 58 ml kg^{-1} min^{-1}.

A number of explanations for this developmental difference in aerobic trainability have been offered. Some have felt that the discrepancy between children and adults in aerobic trainability is a manifestation of methodological issues (1,2,50,52). Might prepubertal children, for instance, be less motivated to sustain sufficiently intense training programs and hence train less effectively than adults? Are definitions of maximal effort in VO_2max testing consistently the same in child and adult studies? Are adult-derived training criteria of intensity and duration comparably appropriate for children? As Mahon (50) has noted, "other considerations include the randomization of subjects to training or non-training groups, comparable pubertal status within and between groups, specificity of exercise training and testing, and limiting the involvement of the subjects in other physical activity regimens that might influence the training response. However, in many instances some or all of these considerations are lacking in the design or not reported, thereby limiting the conclusions that can be drawn."

Then, too—in an "apples and oranges" argument—the characteristics of participants recruited for adult and child endurance training studies may not be comparable. For example, "previously sedentary" adults with low initial VO_2max values would be expected to demonstrate greater training-induced VO_2max changes than "normally active" children with higher pre-training levels of aerobic fitness. Based on the current research literature it is difficult to substantiate or refute the importance of these methodological issues. Still, they hover in the backdrop of all discussions regarding pediatric-adult differences in aerobic trainability.

The suggestion that child-adult trainability differences might reflect true developmental biological differences was first introduced in 1983 by Katch (40). He proposed that

> There is one critical time period in a child's life (termed the "trigger point") which coincides with puberty in most children, but may occur earlier in

> some, below which the effects of physical conditioning will be minimal, or will not occur at all. This trigger phenomenon is the result of modulating effects of hormones that initiate puberty and influence functional development and subsequent organic adaptations.

Ten years later, Rowland (68) provided an assessment of this hypothesis based on then-current knowledge of the mechanisms underlying the fitness effect. While no definitive proof was presented, it was concluded that "current research data provide some tantalizing clues" for a physiological explanation for child-adult differences in aerobic trainability.

Mechanisms Underlying the Aerobic Training Effect in Adults

While a multitude of factors contribute to establishing maximal aerobic power, values of VO_2max are critically determined by the parallel function of two specific systems: 1) the cellular biochemical processes which define the aerobic metabolic capacity of exercising muscle, and 2) the facility to augment oxygen supply to the same muscle, principally by increasing maximal cardiac output, in satisfying requirements for oxidative metabolism. The last two decades have witnessed considerable progress in deciphering the genetic and molecular mechanisms underlying these adaptations in adults, but many mysteries remain to be solved. For example, conceptually both of these functions should rise in a parallel fashion during exercise testing when determining a person's VO_2max, and both should demonstrate a similar magnitude of rise in response to endurance training. Indeed, such training responses should be expected to conform to the principle of *symmorphosis*, which holds that no individual element within a biological function should exceed that of another (82). That is, it would make no biological "sense" if increases in aerobic metabolic capacity to provide energy for endurance exercise rose with training in excess of the magnitude of rise in oxygen supply via muscle flow needed to satisfy that metabolic capacity. Surprisingly, as will be described below, this disparity in the extent of training-induced responses appears to be the case, unique to human beings.

Aerobic Metabolic Capacity and Mitochondrial Biogenesis

The aerobic metabolic machinery comprises a series of enzyme-driven oxidative events involving the Krebs cycle and the mitochondrial respiratory chain which generates high-energy phosphates to drive the contractile elements of skeletal muscle. This complex of biochemical activity resides in the mitochondria, organelles located in both the nucleus and cytoplasm of the muscle cell. The functional capacity of this metabolic complex can be assessed, then, by quantifying aerobic enzyme activity, mitochondrial number, and—more specifically—mitochondrial density from muscle biopsy specimens.

As would be expected, adult individuals with greater aerobic metabolic capacity generally demonstrate higher levels of VO_2max (33), yet such metabolic fitness does not always correspond closely with maximal oxygen uptake (10,30). For this reason, as Holloszy and Coyle (30) concluded (in respect to endurance athletes), "the greater capacity of their cardiovascular system to deliver O_2 to the muscles, rather than their elevated muscle respiratory capacity, is the primary factor responsible for the extremely high VO_2max."

This becomes evident in a consideration of training/detraining studies which indicate that a period of endurance training in adult humans triggers at least a 40–50% increase in mitochondrial marker aerobic enzymes (such as citrate synthetase and succinate dehydrogenase), components of the cytochrome respiratory chain, and mitochondrial content and density within the skeletal muscle (termed "mitochondrial biogenesis") (15,29,32,47). At the same time, VO_2max in these training studies typically increases by only 14–18%.

Evidence indicates, then, that at least as adults, human beings in this way peculiarly violate the principle of symmorphosis, at least in respect to endurance training of large muscle groups (10). In this they may be alone in the animal kingdom. In accord with symmorphosis, animals ranging in mass from 20 g to 500 kg demonstrate such an extraordinarily tight correspondence of VO_2max and mitochondrial volume ($r^2 = 0.97$) that it can be predicted that a non-human organism will consume ~ 4–5 ml O_2 for each ml of mitochondrial volume (75).

The explanation for the excessive aerobic metabolic training response in *Homo sapiens* is not clear. Indeed, Lundby and Jacobs (47) posed the question, "given that the capacity for skeletal muscle oxidative respiration outstrips the capacity of O_2 transport, one may wonder why the mitochondria adapt to exercise training at all." Perhaps there exist "possible evolutionary differences in the oxygen cascade in humans" (10). Or, the excess of mitochondrial adaptation may relate to endurance performance rather than VO_2max (34).

Considerable progress has been achieved in identifying gene loci responsible for mitochondrial biogenesis with endurance training in adults as well as the translational agents which serve to control expression of these genes. Particularly critical is the action of PGC-1α (peroxisome-proliferator-activated receptor γ coactivator-1α), which serves to stimulate transcription factors that control function of target genes, which, in turn, are responsible for mitochondrial biogenesis and increased activity of oxidative enzymes in response to exercise (see these references for reviews: 29,31,38). These adaptive biochemical events appear to be triggered by at least two stimulating factors occurring during exercise: (1) the consumption of high-energy adenosine triphosphate, and (2) increases in cytosolic calcium ion concentration that occur as calcium is released from the sarcoplasmic reticulum during excitation-contraction coupling (29).

Specific gene loci have been identified which regulate the separate elements of aerobic metabolic capacity, supporting the argument that inter-individual variability in VO_2max response to training depends on one's genetic endowment. There is growing evidence, as well, that non-genetic intra-cellular agents serve to control gene expression, and that these *epigenetic factors* can provide a means by which environmental influences can affect gene action. Predominant among such regulators are the processes of DNA methylation, histone acetylation, and microRNAs (miRNAs) (60). Epigenetic effects have been proposed for a wide diversity of influences on human health and disease, including prenatal effects on cardiovascular risk factors, brain function, and immunological reactivity (39).

Augmented activity of epigenetic factors have been described in adult subjects in response to both resistance (16) and endurance training (18,86). Voisin et al. (86) recently reviewed 25 publications describing the effect of physical activity on DNA methylation, concluding that "both acute and chronic exercise significantly impact DNA methylation in a highly tissue- and gene-specific manner." This effect of exercise includes not only muscle tissue but also extends to cardiovascular, bone, immunologic, and brain functions, suggesting a mechanism by which exercise-triggered epigenetic modifications might influence not only aerobic trainability but also salutary health outcomes (56).

Oxygen Availability

Although aerobic metabolic capacity in skeletal muscle is a critical contributor to VO_2max, it is clear from the above that adaptations in oxygen supply to exercising muscle should be expected to serve as the principal "arm" defining the magnitude of response of VO_2max with endurance training. The delivery chain which delivers oxygen to contracting muscle is multifactorial, but the critical element in a healthy individual is the ability of the circulatory system to augment blood flow to the skeletal muscle cell. Past research in adult subjects has often provided a considerable discrepancy of results and conflict of opinion in how this is accomplished. While there would be detractors (e.g., 65), the following represents a construct that the majority of research data would support.

According to the Fick equation the peak delivery and utilization of oxygen is dependent on the product of maximal values of heart rate, cardiac stroke volume, and cellular oxygen extraction (arteriovenous oxygen difference). As maximal heart rate and arteriovenous oxygen difference are not significantly altered following a period of endurance training, the ability of the heart to generate stroke volume stands as the critical factor in maximizing blood flow and oxygen delivery to exercising muscle (54). Maximal stroke volume, in turn, is determined principally by ventricular preload, as myocardial systolic and diastolic function are not influenced by endurance training in non-athletic individuals (71).

Changes in ventricular preload with training are effected by enlargement of the diastolic dimension (with eccentric hypertrophy) of the cardiac ventricles. Among seven training studies of previously sedentary adults, the average reported increase in left ventricular diastolic dimension at rest was approximately 2 mm (range 1–4 mm), or +4% (43,73,87). It is often explained that this remodeling of the ventricles with training is a consequence of wall stretch caused by the volume overload on the heart during endurance exercise (78). However, recent studies indicate that the left ventricular diastolic dimension remains unchanged during the course of an acute bout of exercise (64). Instead, a combination of two other factors—a fall in resting heart rate and augmented plasma volume—are most likely responsible for increased left ventricular diastolic dimension, and, by extension, maximal stroke volume as a consequence of endurance training (63).

Resting heart rate following endurance training in non-athletic adult subjects typically falls by approximately 10 bpm (~ −15%) (11,87). While traditionally this decline has been considered due to a rise in parasympathetic tone (12), recent evidence suggests that intrinsic alterations in sinus node function are more likely causal (11). By permitting a longer diastolic filling period, this bradycardia provides for a larger ventricular cavity dimension. DeMaria et al. (17) examined the relationship of heart rate to left ventricular diastolic dimension in adults and found that for a 10-beat fall in heart rate, diastolic dimension would be expected to increase by 2.7%. Given an expected 4% rise in end diastolic dimension with training (see above), it can be suggested that the resting bradycardia triggered by endurance training serves as a significant contributor to the concomitant augmentation of ventricular diastolic size.

It is widely accepted that an increase in plasma volume is a key element driving expansion of the circulatory system in response to endurance training (13). Increases of approximately 5–10% are generally reported in previously sedentary adult cohorts after short-term training (<4 months), with a similar magnitude of change observed in men and women. Abundant experimental and observational evidence exists that such increases in plasma volume are tightly linked to VO_2max, left ventricular size, stroke volume, and cardiac output (7,14,25). Since serum osmolality and protein concentrations remain unchanged, this hypervolemic response is contingent on an increase in amount of total circulating plasma proteins. This does not necessarily imply an augmented production (in the liver) but could also reflect a decline in protein leakage from the intravascular space (80).

Biological Candidates for Child-Adult Aerobic Trainability Differences

To summarize, in adults a period of endurance training triggers improvements in aerobic metabolic capacity by stimulating gene action through repetitive depletion of high-energy phosphates (ATP) and rise in sarcoplasmal calcium concentration. Gene expression, modified by epigenetic factors, triggers synthesis of aerobic enzymatic potential and mitochondrial biogenesis, the end result culminating in a 40–50% increase in aerobic metabolic capacity. Concomitant expansion of the circulatory system via augmented plasma volume, coupled with a fall in resting heart rate, increases left ventricular diastolic dimension, and, by extension, maximal stroke volume and cardiac output. As a consequence, oxygen delivery to exercising muscle is augmented to facilitate aerobic metabolism. In light of this scheme developed in adult subjects, training responses in children and potential candidates among recognized child-adult physiologic differences can now be examined to assess their potential role in defining maturational differences in aerobic trainability.

The physiologic and anatomic effects of endurance training in children have often been studied by cross-sectional comparisons of child athletes and nonathletes, an inappropriate endeavor since the effects of training in such cases are confounded by the influences of genetic pre-selection and progressive choices by coaches of more talented players. In fact, few training studies have examined cardiovascular or metabolic contributions to VO_2max response to endurance training in non-athletic children, and none have provided direct child-adult comparisons. In the only investigation of training responses in aerobic metabolic capacity, Eriksson et al. (21) reported a 3– increase in the aerobic enzyme succinate dehydrogenase in boys ages 11–13 years. The relative magnitude of reduction in resting heart in training studies of children has generally mimicked that observed in adult studies (7–10 bpm) (22,24,58). Neither maximal heart rate nor myocardial function in youth is influenced by endurance training (57,58).

Obert et al. (58) described an average 1.4 mm (+4%) increase in left ventricular dimension in children after a 13-week running program. In a later study, Obert et al. (57) reported echocardiographic features in 10–11-year-old children before and after a 13-week endurance training program compared to non-training control subjects. On the average, maximal stroke volume rose with training from 52 to 60 ml per square meter body surface area in the boys and from 47 to 52 in the girls, with no change in maximal arteriovenous difference in either group. Mean resting left ventricular end diastolic dimension increased by 5.6% and 5.1% in the boys and girls, respectively. However, George, Gates, and Tolfrey (24) could detect no "biologically meaningful increases" in left ventricular diastolic dimension, myocardial contractility, or VO_2max after 12 weeks of training in 10–11-year-old prepubertal children. In the single study which examined changes in blood volume with aerobic training, Eriksson and Koch (22) described a 12% rise after 4 months of training in nine males ages 11–13 years.

The most one can conclude from these findings is that children's mechanistic responses to aerobic training generally appear to be consistent with the schema outlined above for adults. However, there are insufficient data to permit any quantitative analysis of child-adult differences nor to define any factor which accounts for developmental differences in aerobic trainability. Nonetheless, it is possible to propose the potential influence of three determinant biological mechanisms which might explain such differences: quantitative differences in action of sex hormones, inadequate opportunity for expansion of cellular mitochondrial mass, and developmental suppression of gene expression.

Sex Hormones and Plasma Volume

If a) an increase in oxygen delivery by the cardiovascular system is the driving factor in defining magnitude of aerobic trainability, and b) this mechanism is contingent on augmentation of plasma volume, it is reasonable to address the possibility that developmental differences in expansion of plasma volume might explain child-adult differences in VO_2max responses to endurance training. As noted above, there currently exist no data by which such an effect might be examined. Still, a possible explanation for such differences rests in the virtual absence of circulating levels of sex hormones in prepubertal children. In fact, both testosterone and estrogen—at minimal blood levels prior to a multifold increase at puberty—are recognized to trigger increases in plasma volume.

Testosterone, as an anabolic steroid, acts to increase plasma volume, hemoglobin and red cell mass, and blood volume. Broulik et al. (9) initially confirmed this effect in castrated mice. Lundh and Gardner (48) demonstrated a 10% rise in plasma volume following 6 weeks of testosterone administration to men with sexual impotence, and Johannsson et al. (37) confirmed an increase in extracellular water in men with hypopituitarism treated with testosterone. Kraus et al. (42) described increased blood volume and hemoglobin content (but not plasma volume) after testosterone treatment for erectile dysfunction.

There are several other observations which might bear importance in defining the role of testosterone in male child-adult differences in endurance training effects:

- Zajac et al. (88) found that injections of testosterone (combined with growth hormone) over a 12-week period (without training) triggered a 12% increase in VO_2max in middle-aged men.
- Manttari et al. (51) demonstrated that testosterone administration to mice causes significant increases in muscle myoglobin content which they speculated "may have an influence on the aerobic capacity of mouse skeletal muscle." Muscle myoglobin content is recognized to increase in adult humans with endurance training (85).
- By its traditional genomic action, testosterone serves to stimulate muscle protein synthesis, size, and strength. Evidence is growing that testosterone may also influence muscle function by non-genomic (epigenetic) mechanisms, particularly in facilitating calcium availability to myofilaments, a recognized stimulant to mitochondrial biogenesis (19).

Estrogen, as well, is recognized to promote increases in plasma volume in females. Ueda et al. (84) reported a 27% increase in plasma volume after a 3-week infusion of 17 beta-estradiol in ewes. In adult women, Stachenfeld (80) described a rise in plasma volume after administered estrogen, which was caused by a reduction in capillary protein leakage. There exists evidence, as well, that estrogen, acting as an antioxidant, may stimulate muscle repair and act in a protective role against exercise-induced muscle damage (20). Estrogen also appears to share with testosterone the non-genomic action of increasing calcium release from the sarcolemma (19).

There exists sufficient evidence, then, to hypothesize that prepubertal boys and girls, lacking the stimulating effects of sex hormones on plasma volume expansion (as well as other actions), might thereby be impaired in their ability to increase VO_2max with training compared to adults. This concept would support Katch's original proposition in 1983 that a threshold period surrounding hormonal influences at the time of puberty serves to differentiate the magnitude of aerobic training responses in pre- and post-pubertal subjects. Still, no particular chronological or biological age has been identified that clearly demarcates such a training capacity, causing Armstrong and Barker to contend that "the existence of a maturational threshold below which children are not trainable remains to be proven" (2).

Resting Oxidative Capacity and Cellular Overcrowding

Maintenance of a constant size and volume is critical to a cell's functional and anatomic integrity (45). The body employs a number of mechanisms for sustaining this constancy (44), defending against maladaptive consequences that are recognized to accompany transgressions of cell size: disruption of rate and equilibrium of biochemical reactions, osmotic stress, disturbed diffusion rates, unintended macromolecule interactions, and threats to protein stability and conformation (53,55). Importantly, too, evidence exists that overcrowding of cells may negatively impact gene function (66).

As Foffi et al. (23) have noted, "biological macromolecules live and operate in an extremely structured and complex environment within the cell, [which is] a most crowded and confining one." Considerable research interest has been focused on the prevention and consequences of cellular overcrowding, a field of investigation that "is now emerging as one of the most thriving in molecular and cell biology," having been the focus of two recent international conferences.

In this context it has been proposed that limitations imposed by cell size might explain child-adult differences in aerobic trainability. According to what has been termed the "crowded cell hypothesis," increases in the volume of metabolic elements in response to endurance training (mitochondrial biogenesis) may be constrained by limitations of cell space (69). As children possess a greater relative resting metabolic rate than adults, the magnitude of increase in the volume of elements of the aerobic metabolic machine with training would therefore be necessarily reduced in comparison to that of adults.

This story unfolds as follows: the well-established biological tenet holds that an inverse relationship exists between mass-specific basal metabolic rate and animal size (74). For example, the metabolic rate expressed per kg body mass in a 20-gm mouse is 10-fold that of a 200-kg horse. This relationship can be expressed mathematically as

$$\text{Metabolic rate} \sim \text{Mass}^{0.75}$$
$$\text{Metabolic rate/kg} \sim \text{Mass}^{-0.25}$$

Similarly, during the childhood years the basal metabolic rate (related to body surface area) steadily falls with age, declining between the ages of 6 and 18 years by 31% in males and 18% in females (41). Holliday et al. (28) reported an exponent relating mass to resting metabolic rate of 0.58 in children who have a body mass between 10 and 60 kg.

That this greater relative whole-body metabolic rate in children compared to adults is due, at least in part, to higher levels of cellular metabolic function is supported by findings of higher aerobic enzymatic activity in prepubertal subjects. In biopsies of vastus lateralis muscle, Berg et al. (5) reported activities of citrate synthetase in youth 6.4 and 17 years old of 28.3 ± 6.8 and 22.1 ± 8.2 ɥmoles min^{-1} g^{-1}, respectively, with fumerase activities of 57.6 ± 9.5 and 41.0 ± 13.4 ɥmoles min^{-1} g^{-1}. Haralambie (26) described citrate synthetase activity in vastus lateralis muscle to be 50% greater in children ages 5–7 years than mature subjects. In the single study which directly compared mitochondrial densities in children and adults, Jerusalem et al. (36) found a 42% greater density in biopsies of four female children ages 1 month to 12 years than in adults aged 28–55.

The elements of mitochondria and aerobic enzymes associated with this greater metabolic activity in children are space-occupying. And in the skeletal muscle cell obligatory room must be reserved for the contractile apparatus (actin-myosin filaments) and the sarcoplasmic reticulum, critical for regulating calcium flux which dictates contractile speed. The space remaining for metabolic machinery may serve as a critical determinant of the limits of adaptive responses to endurance training. Hochachka et al. (27) expressed this idea when considering if one could train a hummingbird, which possesses an extremely high resting metabolic rate, to improve aerobic fitness: "It is probable that any further increase in oxidative enzyme capacity (i.e., mitochondrial volume densities) would be counterproductive because it would simultaneously require reductions in either SR [sarcoplasmic reticulum] or myofilaments. Thus there seems to be very little room left for adaptation (at least expressed as upward regulation of mitochondrial abundance)."

According to this construct, a ceiling of mitochondrial density exists in response to training because of constraints posed by the need to maintain cell size and volume. Since children have a greater metabolic capacity at rest, goes the hypothesis, there will be consequently less space available for training adaptations (i.e., mitochondrial biogenesis) and limited rise in VO_2max compared to adults.

In an animal study that nicely supports this idea, Simoneau et al. (79) found that increases in aerobic enzyme activity and mitochondrial density were directly related to animal size in response to 28 days of chronic electrical stimulation of tibialis anterior muscle. The activity of citrate synthetase activity rose by a factor of 3.0 in rabbits, 2.5 in rats, 2.3 in guinea pigs, and 1.2 in mice. Moreover, the "pretraining" levels of oxidative enzymes were inversely related to animal size (being almost four times greater in the mouse than the rabbit). So, consistent with the "crowded cell hypothesis," the magnitude of rise in metabolic capacity with repetitive muscle contractions was indirectly related to the size-relative resting metabolic rate.

This concept is consistent with the observations in groups of humans that the magnitude of rise in VO_2max with endurance training is inversely related to the initial pre-training value. Saltin et al. documented this relationship in adults (72). In children this correlation has been less strong (1), but this may reflect the homogeneity of fitness levels in subjects typically recruited for pediatric training studies.

Developmental Tempo of Gene Expression

In examining the myriad of variables that contribute to the aerobic fitness effect, it is apparent that, ultimately, all act under the dictates of one's genetic information. It is the genome that triggers mitochondrial biogenesis, stimulates protein synthesis causing enlargement of blood volume and expansion of the circulatory system, and initiates changes in sinus node function and/or parasympathetic influences that lowers resting heart rate. *Current research is now making it clear that the genetic direction of such training responses involves capacities defined by not only a) one's intrinsic genetic blueprint, but also b) non-genomic (epigenetic) factors which influence the extent of gene expression and its timing.* The former mechanism has been used to account for inter-individual differences in VO_2max responses to training in adults (8) while the latter, as described above, have been recently documented to equally participate in training adaptations (18,86).

It is not illogical to suggest that differences in the magnitude of VO_2max improvements with training between children and adults might reflect normal suppression of this genetic expression in biologically immature individuals. The how, why, and when of such a limitation in gene expression in children are currently problematic. Still, recent research indicates a number of examples of developmental restriction of gene action in children that might serve as mechanistic models in the course of ontogenetic changes. (In fact, the entirety of the course of growth and development during childhood can be viewed as a progressive unmasking of genetic information which codes for the mature adult state.)

The past decade has witnessed a surge of research efforts to understand the genomic, transcriptional, and epigenetic factors that dictate the tempo and magnitude of developmental processes during the childhood years (49,77). These initial studies have revealed the critical roles of both genomic and non-genomic influences on osteal (35), neurologic (81), and cardiovascular (6) developmental changes, focusing mainly on the fetal and early childhood periods.

The most obvious parallel to a potential for timing of genetic expression for aerobic trainability exists in the complex of events that surround puberty (59,76,83). After over a decade of dormancy, neurons located in the hypothalamus trigger the pulsatile increase in gonadotrophin hormone, which provides for the acquisition of reproductive capacity and appearance of secondary features of sexual maturation. All of this is under the control of a complex network of multiple gene regulation. These factors directing both the advent and timing of pubertal events which were obviously present but suppressed during the first decade of life. As Ojeda et al. (59) have commented, "Though not yet proven, emerging evidence is beginning to surface suggesting that puberty may not occur earlier because it is held in check by a developmental program involving transcriptional/posttranscriptional repression of genes that are stimulatory to the pubertal process."

By a similar genetic developmental program, the timing of gene expression of the aerobic training response could be similarly controlled. It is not unreasonable, as well, to suggest that other exercise features which distinguish children from their adult counterparts might be similarly explained—lower rates of sweating, limited glycolytic capacity, differing patterns of habitual physical activity, and differences in metabolic substrate utilization.

Research Directions

The basis for the reported inferior aerobic trainability of children is far from being clarified. However, this chapter has provided several credible (albeit speculative) means—methodological and biological—by which this child-adult difference might be explained. Newer insights into this issue bear importance for athletes, medical caregivers, and exercise physiologists alike. To this end, a number of research avenues might be approached:

1. Creative study designs could help establish the extent that methodological issues are responsible for the lower increase in VO_2max with training in children. For example, the great majority of pediatric training studies have involved "normally active but not athletic" youth, resulting in a homogeneous pre-training fitness level. A study involving groups of children with low, moderate, and high levels of pre-training values of VO_2max would be revealing as to the effect of initial aerobic fitness on children's aerobic trainability. Similarly, a side-by-side child-adult training study in which the two groups were equated (utilizing an appropriate scaling approach) by initial size-relative VO_2max would be illuminating.
2. A comparison of responses to an endurance training program in a group of prepubertal subjects to those *in the same individuals* in an identical program performed in the late teen years would shed light on the role of pubertal hormonal influences on aerobic trainability. Such insights could also be gained by examining the influence on aerobic trainability of testosterone and/or estrogen administered to immature animals.
3. A major gap in understanding developmental differences in aerobic trainability surrounds the lack of information regarding plasma volume responses in children. Ethical uncertainties and lack of familiarity with measurement methods may be largely responsible. Such issues need to be addressed and resolved.

4. Lack of biopsy tissue continues to serve as a major roadblock to understanding the process of mitochondrial biogenesis in children. Alternative surrogate methods for assessing cellular metabolic capacity that can be safely applied to children need to be developed. Work in this area using magnetic resonance spectroscopy has illustrated how new technologies can be developed to this end (4).

References

1. Armstrong N. Aerobic fitness and training in children. *Pediatr Exerc Science.* 2015;27:8–12.
2. Armstrong N, Barker AR. Endurance training and elite young athletes. *Med Sport Science.* 2011;57:59–83.
3. Baquet G, Van Praagh E, Berthoin S. Endurance training and aerobic fitness in young people. *Sports Med.* 2003;33:1127–1143.
4. Barker AR, Armstrong N. Insights into developmental muscle metabolism through the use of 31P-magnetic resonance spectroscopy: a review. *Pediatr Exerc Science.* 2010;22:350–368.
5. Berg A, Kim SS, Keul J. Skeletal muscle enzyme activities in healthy young subjects. *Int J Sports Med.* 1986;7:236–239.
6. Blech-Hermoni Y, Ladd AN. RNA binding proteins in the regulation of heart development. *Int J Biochem Cell Biol.* 2013;45:2467–2478.
7. Bonne TC, Doucende G, Fluck D, Jacobs RA, Nordsborg NB, Robach P, Walther G. Phlebotomy eliminates the maximal cardiac output response to six weeks of exercise training. *Am J Physiol.* 2014;306:R752–R760.
8. Bouchard C, Malina RM, Perusse L. *Genetics of Fitness and Physical Performance.* Champaign, IL: Human Kinetics; 1997. pp. 341–342.
9. Broulik PD, Kochakian CD, Dubovsky J. Influence of castration and testosterone propionate on cardiac output, renal blood flow, and blood volume in mice. *Proc Soc Exper Biol Med.* 1973;144:671–673.
10. Boushel R, Gnaiger E, Calbet JAL, Gonzalez-Alonso J, Wright-Paradis C, Sondergaard H, Ignacio A. Muscle mitochondrial capacity exceeds maximal oxygen delivery in humans. *Mitochondrion.* 2011;11:303–307.
11. Boyett MR, D'Souza A, Zhang H, Morris GM, Dobrzynski H, Monfredi O. Viewpoint: is the resting bradycardia in athletes the result of remodeling of the sinoatrial node rather than high vagal tone? *J Appl Physiol.* 2013;114:1351–1355.
12. Carter JB, Banister EW, Blaber AP. Effect of endurance exercise on autonomic control of heart rate. *Sports Med.* 2003;33:33–46.
13. Convertino VA. Blood volume response to training. In: Fletcher GF, editor. *Cardiovascular Response to Exercise.* Mount Kisco, NY: Futura Publishing Company; 1994. pp. 207–221.
14. Coyle EF, Hopper MK, Coggan AR. Maximal oxygen uptake relative to plasma volume expansion. *Int J Sports Med.* 1990;11:116–119.
15. Coyle EF, Martin WH, Sinacore DR, Joyner MJ, Hagberg JM, Holloszy JO. Time course of adaptations after stopping prolonged intense endurance exercise. *J Appl Physiol.* 1984;57:1857–1864.
16. Davidson PK, Gallagher IJ, Hartman JW, et al. High responders to resistance exercise training demonstrate differential regulation of skeletal muscle microRNA expression. *J Appl Physiol.* 2011;110:309–317.

17. DeMaria AN, Neumann A, Schubart PJ, Lee G, Mason DT. Systematic correlation of cardiac chamber size and ventricular performance determined with echocardiography and alterations in heart rate in normal persons. *Am J Cardiol.* 1979;43:1–9.
18. Denham J, Marques FZ, O'Brien BJ, Charchar FJ. Exercise: putting action into our epigenome. *Sports Med.* 2014;44:189–209.
19. Dent JR, Fletcher DK, McGuigan MR. Evidence for a non-genomic action of testosterone in skeletal muscle which may improve athletic performance: implications for the female athlete. *J Sports Sci Med.* 2012;11:363–370.
20. Enns DL, Tiidus PM. The influence of estrogen on skeletal muscle: sex matters. *Sports Med.* 2010;40:41–58.
21. Eriksson BO, Gollnick PD, Saltin B. Muscle metabolism and enzyme activities after training in boys 11–13 years old. *Acta Physiol Scand.* 1973;87:485–487.
22. Eriksson BO, Koch G. Effect of physical training on hemodynamic response during submaximal and maximal exercise. *Acta Physiol Scad.* 1973;87:27–29.
23. Foffi G, Pastore A, Piazza, Temussi PA. Macromolecular crowding: chemistry and physics meet biolgy (Asona, Switzerland, 10–14 June 2012). *Phys Biol.* 2014;10:1–7.
24. George KP, Gates PE, Tolfrey K. The impact of aerobic training upon left ventricular morphology and function in pre-pubescent children. *Ergonomics.* 2005;48:1378–1389.
25. Gledhill N, Warburton D, Jamnik V. Haemoglobin, blood volume, cardiac function, and aerobic power. *Can J Appl Physiol.* 1999;24:54–65.
26. Haralambie G. Activities enzymatiques dans le muscle squelettique des enfants de divers ages [Enzymatic activity in the skeletal muscle of children of various ages] In: *Les sports et l'enfant.* Montpellier: Euromed; 1980. pp. 243–258.
27. Hochachka PW, Emmett B, Suarez RK. Limits and constraints in the scaling of oxidative and glycolytic enzymes in homeotherms. *Can J Zool.* 1988;66:1128–1138.
28. Holliday MA, Potter D, Jarrah A, Bearg S. The relationship of metabolic rate in body weight and organ size. *Pediatr Res.* 1967;1:185–195.
29. Holloszy JO. Regulation of exercise of skeletal muscle content of mitochondria and GLUT4. *J Physiol Pharmacol.* 2008;59 Suppl 7:5–18.
30. Holloszy JO, Coyle EF. Adaptations of skeletal muscle to endurance exercise and their metabolic consequences. *J Appl Physiol.* 1984;56:831–838.
31. Hood DA, Irrcher I, Ljubicic V, Joseph A-M. Coordination of metabolic plasticity in skeletal muscle. *J Exper Biol.* 2006;209:2265–2275.
32. Hoppeler H, Howald H, Conley K, et al. Endurance training in humans: aerobic capacity and structure of skeletal muscle. *J Appl Physiol.* 1985;59:320–327.
33. Jacobs RA, Lundby C. Mitochondria express enhanced quality as well as quantity in association with aerobic fitness across recreationally active individuals up to elite athletes. *J Appl Physiol.* 2013;114:344–350.
34. Jacobs RA, Rasmussen P, Siebenmann C, et al. Determinants of time trial performance and maximal incremental exercise in highly trained endurance athletes. *J Appl Physiol.* 2011;111:1422–1430.
35. Jensen ED, Gopalakrishnan R, Westendorf, JJ. Regulation of gene expression in osteoblasts. *Biofactors.* 2010;36:25–32.
36. Jerusalem FA, Engel AG, Peterson HA. Human muscle fiber fine structure: morphologic data on controls. *Neurology.* 1975;25:127–134.
37. Johannsson G, Gibney J, Wolthus T, Leung K-C, Ho KKY. Independent and combined effects of testosterone and growth hormone on extracellular water in hypopituitary men. *J Clin Endocrin Metab.* 2005;90:3989–3994.

38. Joseph A-M, Pilegaard H, Litvintsev A, Leick L, Hood DA. Control of gene expression and mitochondrial biogenesis in the muscular adaptation to endurance exercise. *Essays Biochem.* 2006;108:13–29.
39. Kanherkar RR, Bhatia-Dey N, Csoka, AB. Epigenetics across the human lifespan. *Front Cell Develop Biol.* 2014;2:49.
40. Katch VL. Physical conditioning of children. *J Adol Health Care.* 1983;3:241–246.
41. Knoebel, LK. Energy metabolism. In: Selkurt EE, editor. *Physiology*. Boston: Little Brown; 1963. pp. 564–579.
42. Kraus DJ, Taub HA, Lantiga LJ, Dunsky MH, Kelly CM. Risks of blood volume changes in hypogonadal men treated with testosterone enanthate for erectile impotence. *J Urol.* 1991;146:1566–1570.
43. Landry F, Bouchard C, Dumesnil J. Cardiac dimension changes with endurance training. *JAMA.* 1985;254:77–80.
44. Lang F, Busch GL, Ritter M, et al. Functional significance of cell volume regulatory mechanisms. *Physiol Rev.* 1988;78:247–306.
45. Lang F, Ritter M, Volkl H, Haussinger D. The biological significance of cell volume. *Renal Physiol Biochem.* 1993;16:48–65.
46. Lortie G, Simoneau JA, Hamel P, Boulay MR, Landry F, Bouchard C. Responses of maximal aerobic power and capacity to aerobic training. *Int J Sports Med.* 1984;5:232–236.
47. Lundby C, Jacobs RA. Adaptations of skeletal muscle mitochondria to exercise training. *Exper Physiol.* 2016;101:17–22.
48. Lundh B, Gardner FH. The effect of testosterone in pharmacological doses on plasma volume and on some serum proteins in patients with sickle cell anemia and in sexually impotent men. *Scand J Clin Lab Invest.* 1971;28:72–78.
49. MacNicol MC, MacNicol AM. Developmental timing of mRNA translation—integration of distinct regulatory elements. *Molec Reprod Develop.* 2010;77:662–669.
50. Mahon AD. Aerobic training. In: Armstrong N, van Mechelen W, editors. *Paediatric Exercise Science and Medicine. Second Edition.* Oxford: Oxford University Press; 2008. pp. 513–529.
51. Manttari S, Anttila K, Jarvilehto M. Testosterone stimulates myoglobin expression in different muscle of the mouse. *J Comp Physiol.* 2008;178:899–907.
52. McNarry M, Jones A. The influence of training status on the aerobic and anaerobic responses to exercise in children: a review. *Eur J Sport Science.* 2014;14:S57–S68.
53. Mittal S, Chowhan RK, Singh LR. Macromolecular crowding: macromolecules friend or foe. *Biochim Biophys Acta.* 2015;1850:1822–1831.
54. Montero D, Diaz-Canestro C, Lundby C. Endurance training and VO_2max: role of maximal cardiac output and oxygen extraction. *Med Sci Sports Exerc.* 2015;47:2024–2033.
55. Mourao MA, Hakim JB, Schnell. Connecting the dots: the effects of macromolecular crowding on cell physiology. *Biophys J.* 2014;107:2761–2766.
56. Ntanasis-Stathopoulos J, Tzanninis J-G, Philippou A, Koutsilieris M. Epigenetic regulation on gene expression induced by physical exercise. *J Musculoskel Neuronal Interact.* 2013;13:133–146.
57. Obert P, Mandigout S, Nottin S, Vinet A, N'Guyen LD, Lecoq AM. Cardiovascular responses to endurance training in children: effect of gender. *Eur J Clin Invest.* 2003;33:199–208.
58. Obert P, Mandigout S, Vinet A, N'Guyen LD, Stecken F, Courteix D. Effect of aerobic training and detraining on left ventricular dimensions and diastolic function in prepubertal boys and girls. *Int J Sports Med.* 2001;22:90–96.

59. Ojeda SR, Lomniczi A, Loche A, et al. The transcriptional control of female puberty. *Brain Res.* 2010;1364:164–174.
60. Pareja-Galeano H, Sanchis-Gomar F, Garcia-Gimenez JL. Physical exercise and epigenetic modulation: elucidating intricate mechanisms. *Sports Med.* 2014;44:429–436.
61. Payne VG, Morrow JR. The effect of physical training on prepubescent VO_2max: a meta-analysis. *Res Q Exerc Sport.* 1993;64:305–313.
62. Perrault H. Cardiorespiratory function. In: Bar-Or O, Lamb DR, Clarkson PM, editors. *Perspectives in Exercise Science and Sports Medicine. Vol. 9: Exercise and the Female: A Life Span Approach.* Carmel, IN: Cooper Publishing; 1996. pp. 215–247.
63. Perrault HM, Turcotte RA. Do athletes have the "athlete's heart"? *Progr Pediatr Cardiol.* 1993;2:40–50.
64. Pokan R, von Duvillard SP, Hofman P, et al. Change in left atrial and ventricular dimensions during and immediately after exercise. *Med Sci Sports Exerc.* 2000;32:1719–1728.
65. Poole DC, Kelley GA, Musch TI. Training increases muscle O_2 diffusing capacity intrinsic to the elevated VO_2max (letter). *Med Sci Sports Exerc.* 2016;48:762–763.
66. Richter K, Nessling M, Lichter P. Macromolecular crowding and its potential impact on nuclear function. *Biochim Biophys Acta.* 2008;1873:2100–2107.
67. Rowell LB. *Human circulation regulation during physical stress.* New York: Oxford University Press; 1986. p. 259.
68. Rowland T. The 'trigger hypothesis' for aerobic trainability: a 14-year follow-up. *Pediatr Exerc Science.* 1997;9:1–9.
69. Rowland T. Aerobic (un)trainability of children: mitochondrial biogenesis and the "crowded cell" hypothesis. *Pediatr Exerc Science.* 2009;21:1–9.
70. Rowland T, Boyajian A. Aerobic response to endurance training in children: magnitude, variability, and gender comparisons. *Pediatrics.* 1995;96:654–658.
71. Sadaniantz A, Yurgalevitch S, Zmuda JM, Thompson PD. One year of exercise training does not alter resting left ventricular systolic or diastolic function. *Med Sci Sport Exerc.* 1996;28:1345–1350.
72. Saltin B, Hartley LH, Kilbom A, Astrand I. Physical training in sedentary middle-aged and older men. II: oxygen uptake, heart rate, and blood lactate concentration at submaximal and maximal exercise. *Scand J Clin Lab Invest.* 1969;24:323–334.
73. Schaible TF, Scheuer J. Cardiac adaptations to chronic exercise. *Progr Cardiovasc Dis.* 1985;27:297–324.
74. Schmidt-Nielsen K. *Scaling: Why Is Animal Size So Important?* Cambridge: Cambridge University Press; 1984. pp. 56–74.
75. Schwerzmann K, Hoppeler H, Kayar SP, Weibel ER. Oxidative capacity of muscle and mitochondria: correlation of physiological, biochemical and morphometric characteristics. *Proc Nat Acad Science.* 1989;86:1583–1587.
76. Semaan SJ, Kauffman AS. Emerging concepts on the epigenetic and transcriptional regulation of the *Kiss1* gene. *Int J Develop Neurosci.* 2013;31:452–462.
77. Shah AA, Meese E, Blin N. Profiling of regulatory microRNA transcriptomes in various biological processes: a review. *J Appl Genetics.* 2010;51:501–507.
78. Shapiro LM. The morphologic consequences of systemic training. *Cardiovasc Clin.* 1997;15:373–379.
79. Simoneau J-A, Hood DA, Pette D. Species-specific responses in enzyme activities of anaerobic and aerobic energy metabolism to increased contractile activity. In: Taylor AW, Gollnick PD, et al., editors. *Biochemistry of Exercise VII.* Champaign, IL: Human Kinetics; 1990. pp. 95–104.

80. Stachenfeld NS. Sex hormone effects on body fluid regulation. *Exerc Sports Science Rev.* 2008;36:152–159.
81. Swaminathan A, Kumar M, Halder Sinha S, Schneider-Anthony A, Boutillier AL, Kundu TK. Modulation of neurogenesis by targeting epigenetic enzymes using small molecules: an overview. *ACS Chem Neurosci.* 2014;5:1164–1177.
82. Taylor C, Weibel E. Design of the mammalian respiratory system. I: problem and strategy. *Resp Physiol.* 1981;44:1–10.
83. Tena-Sempere M. Keeping puberty on time: novel signals and mechanisms involved. *Curr Topics Develop Biol.* 2013;105:299–329.
84. Ueda S, Fortune V, Bull BS, Valenzuela GJ, Longo LD. Estrogen effects on plasma volume, arterial blood pressure, interstitial space, plasma proteins, and blood viscosity in sheep. *Am J Obst Gynecol.* 1986;155:195–201.
85. Vogelaere P, S'Jongers JJ, Quiron A. Review of the literature on myoglobin in the development of exertion and aerobic training. *Can J Appl Sports Sci.* 1980;5:236–238.
86. Voisin S, Eynon N, Yan X, Bishop DJ. Exercise training and DNA methylation in humans. *Acta Physiol.* 2015;213:39–59.
87. Younis L, Poelnitz AV, Sturbois X, Detry J-M. Effects of exercise training on left ventricular function in healthy young men: a longitudinal echocardiographic study. *J Cardiopulm Rehab.* 1987;278:278–284.
88. Zajac A, Wilk M, Socha T, Maszczyk A, Chycki J. Effects of growth hormone and testosterone therapy on aerobic and anaerobic fitness, body composition and lipoprotein profile in middle-aged men. *Ann Agric Environ Med.* 2014;21:156–160.

11

HOW CAN MUSIC ENHANCE PHYSICAL PERFORMANCE?

It's a universal experience, of course, that music can charge the emotions, can motivate, can stimulate. If the movie begins with low sonorous tones from the cellos, it's for certain going to be a dark psychological thriller. If one hears the chirpy sounds of the staccato clarinet and flute, be prepared for a farce. There is music specifically designed to crown new heads of state, open festivals, get married, bury a beloved uncle, dance, make love, rock a baby asleep, ride in elevators, enjoy a bistro meal, ride a flying trapeze, open baseball games, protest social injustice, file into a high school commencement, march in a parade, and so on and so on. Music is everywhere, powerfully molding our emotional responses to events in our daily lives.

For many listeners, though, music bears a more profound meaning than simply emotional pleasure, offering an essential, transcendental harmony that "engenders some kind of psychosomatic resonance" which is inherent in the very nature of life itself (40). A goodly number of authors have waxed poetically on this soulful nature of music. A few examples here just for the emphasis:

> *Without music life would be a mistake.*
>
> —*Friedrich Nietzsche, 1889*

> *Music was born free, and to win freedom is its destiny.*
>
> —*Ferruccio Busoni, 1907*

> *Music is our myth of the inner life.*
>
> —*Susanne Langer, 1942*

And perhaps apropos to the chapter at hand

> *Nothing is more futile than theorizing about music.*
>
> —*Heinrich Heine, 1837*

(Note that not all have considered this effect in a positive light. The French essayist Milan Kundera once wrote that "despite Stravinsky's denial that music expresses feeling, the naïve listener cannot see it any other way. That is music's curse, its mindless aspect. All it takes is a violinist playing the three long opening notes of a largo, and a sensitive listener will sigh, 'ah, how beautiful!' In those three notes that set off the emotional response, there is nothing, no invention, no creation, nothing at all: it's the most ridiculous 'sentimental hoax.' But no one is proof against that perception of music, or against the foolish sigh it stirs" (24).

The role of music in enhancing exercise performance, too, has long been appreciated. Indeed, there is no lack of supportive experimental evidence that listening to music during exercise improves physical performance. In two reviews in 1997 and again in 2012, Karageorghis and his colleagues examined a total of 75 research publications which, for the most part, indicated that music is a true ergogenic aid, enhancing variables such as aerobic fitness, muscle strength, and muscular endurance (20–22). Such findings have been typically accompanied by evidence for a positive psychological influence of music on exercise performance as well, including positive alterations of mood, affect, motivation, and perception of effort. "In this sense," these authors concluded, "music can be thought of as a type of legal performance-enhancing drug" (20).

These studies have involved a plethora of research designs and study protocols, many of which suffer from methodological weakness that hamper confident conclusions. Too, the literature is confounded by the large number of variables that one might expect would influence the music-performance association: the timing (music before, during, or after exercise); type of music (vigorous, sedative); familiarity of the test subjects with the music presented; sex, age, fitness level, and personality of the subjects; reporting tools for assessing psychological responses; physiological measures employed; and so on.

Such difficulties notwithstanding, these reviews have highlighted certain take-away lessons gained from the extant literature:

1. Music appears to be more effective in enhancing exercise performance in physical tasks involving low-to-moderate work intensities. The effect of music is reduced or even eliminated when performing exercise at intensity levels above the *anaerobic threshold* (when blood lactate level begins to rise and a disproportionate rise in ventilation to oxygen consumption is observed—typically about 60% of the level of exhaustive exercise).

   Examples: Miller et al. found that participants reported lower ratings of perceived exertion (RPE) during a submaximal 20-minute treadmill test while listening to music (30). Szmedra and Bacharach described a 10% reduction in RPEs when subjects listened to classical music compared to non-music during a moderate treadmill running intensity (42), mimicking similar findings by Nethery (32). Meanwhile, a number of studies have indicated no effect of listening to music on endurance time on a progressive treadmill test to exhaustion (e.g.,10,28,43).

2. Athletically trained individuals may be less susceptible to the ergogenic effects of exercise than those individuals who are untrained.

   Examples: Mohammadzadeh et al. reported that music listening increased treadmill endurance time in a graded treadmill test to exhaustion in both trained and untrained persons (31). However, the untrained had lower Rating of Perceived Exertion (RPE) scores (indicating they were less physically stressed). Brownley et al. found that untrained subjects experienced "more positive affect" with stimulatory music compared to trained runners during both low and high intensity treadmill exercise (7). Young et al. reported that self-selected music had no effect on maximal treadmill endurance or RPE in a group of trained female soccer players (47).

3. Exercise performance may be enhanced when listening to music whose rhythm is synchronous with body movements (i.e., stride frequency).

   Examples: Karageorghis et al. had 30 participants walk to exhaustion on a treadmill while listening to synchronous motivational music (popular music tracks from self-selected artists), nonmotivational synchronous music, or no music (19). Endurance was augmented in both music conditions compared to non-music, and was enhanced to a great extent when listening to motivational music. RPE was not influenced by experimental condition.

   Bacon et al. reported lower oxygen uptake during cycle exercise with music in synchronous compared to asynchronous pedaling (2). This was interpreted as indicating greater energy efficiency when cycle exercise is performed matched to music tempo. However, Lim et al. could not duplicate this finding, describing no significant differences for oxygen uptake with synchronous and asynchronous cycle exercise to music in a group of active young men (27).

4. When examining the collective research data, no consistent effect of music type (upbeat or slow, familiar or unfamiliar) has been observed which influences magnitude of enhanced exercise performance. Instead, personality traits may influence the exercise-music link. Extroverts, for example, are more likely to respond to stimulant music. In general, faster and louder music may be preferred at high work intensities.

   Example: Edworthy and Waring found that during 10-minute treadmill exercise sessions, loud music (in contrast to quiet or none) was linked to running speed and heart rate, although no effects on RPE were observed (11). The authors concluded that fast, loud music might be optimal to enhance exercise performance.

5. Studies in which participants self-selected their exercise pace have shown more consistently to improve performance but without altering perception of effort.

   Examples: Lee and Kimmerly found that listening to fast tempo music in 12 subjects resulted in a faster self-selected speed (10.8 [1.7] vs. 9.9 [1.4] km hr^{-1}) and higher peak heart rate than with slow music but no differences were evident in RPE between the two conditions (25). Bigliassi et al. described greater improvements in 5 km running performance among 15 well-trained long-distance runners with music (both fast and slow) than with pre-event music alone (4).

Explanations

But—the topic of this chapter's mystery—how can this pervasive effect of music on how long one can run or pedal or generate force of muscle contraction be explained? The answer is not yet in, but this chapter will examine the information at hand. Attempts to gain insights on etiologic mechanisms have been hampered by a number of practical obstacles (brain imaging studies are prohibitive during exercise, for instance). Karageorghis and Priest noted, too, that the social context in which music is experienced is not readily mimicked in the experimental setting (20). And simply requesting subjects' ratings of perceived exertions—their psychological sense of work effort when exercising while listening to music—might alter their exercise focus. Nonetheless, several possible explanations for the music-exercise performance link have been proposed (20), none of which is universally accepted.

Effect of Arousal?

Some have considered the ergogenic effect of music in enhancing motor performance and delaying fatigue as a straightforward example of the effect of *arousal* on the central nervous system. By this interpretation, music acts to stimulate action of the sympathetic nervous system, which, as part of the "flight or fight" response to stress, enhances muscular function and promotes alertness. To put it simply, by this account the right kind of music simply causes one to become excited.

A number of studies, in fact, have demonstrated that listening to music during exercise increases heart rate, the traditional easily measured marker of central nervous system arousal (e.g., 5,7,44). Levels of circulating biochemical markers of sympathetic nervous system activity, such as norepinephrine and cortisol, have also been found to rise during music listening compared to a non-listening condition (7,46).

Further evidence comes from the study of Urakawa and Yokoyama, who examined changes in heart rate variability before and after exercise in music and non-music conditions (45). Beat-to-beat changes in the interval between successive heart beats can follow either low or high frequency patterns, and the ratio of the two is considered a marker of sympathetic nervous system activity. In this study the ratio of low frequency to high frequency components of such variability following exercise was significantly greater than pre-exercise values when twelve female college students listened to their preferred music. However, no such response was observed in the non-music condition. The authors concluded that during "exercise in which sympathetic nerve activity is dominant, preferred music synchronizes with the activated physical response, further promoting the response and increasing sympathetic nerve activity."

In a similar investigation, Archana and Mukilan found that the post-exercise low frequency:high frequency ratio of heart rate variability of students 20–25 years old was significantly increased by listening to preferred music during a 15-minute bout of cycle exercise (1). No similar responses were seen following in a non-music exercise.

Or is it Distraction?

Others would see music as serving as a *distraction* from the discomforts of exercise effort (20). In this proposed scenario, afferent signals to the brain of music and sensations of fatigue (breathlessness, leg fatigue, etc.) compete with each other for the "attention" of brain centers. At low-to-moderate intensities the former may win out, blocking out unpleasant fatigue signals, while at high levels of work the input from fatigue signals overwhelms that of music (13). This idea fits nicely with the experimentally observed findings noted above that music is more effective as an ergogenic agent at low rather than high exercise intensities.

A Matter of "Harmonization"?

Alternatively, the ergogenic and positive emotional responses to exercise might somehow reflect a "harmonization" between musical rhythms and that observed in all physiological systems. This idea was perhaps popularized by the legendary composer and conductor Leonard Bernstein, who once impressively opened one of his television shows with a video recording of the human heart beating, placed in juxtaposition with an identical rhythm heard in the first movement of Beethoven's Seventh Symphony. "Beat, beat, beat—the fundamental pulse of all life, whether it be our blood or our breath, a pile driver, a galloping horse, or a leaky faucet," he said. "Pulse is everywhere in our lives" (3).

Schneider et al. noted that the commonality of a reported frequency of 3 Hz in the longitudinal axis of leg movement during running was similar to the frequency exhibited by physiological systems (such as heart rate and brain cortical activity) (39). They examined oscillations during exercise in 18 runners compared to brain electrical activity before and after exercise as well as of the frequency spectra of the subjects' favorite pieces of music. A peak frequency of 2.7–2.8 Hz for vertical accelerations during running corresponded closely to similar frequencies in post-exercise electroencephalographic findings as well as the preferred musical pieces.

Interestingly, similar *entrainment* is observed between breathing frequency and stride rate in highly trained runners (as well as racehorses and a variety of other animals), hypothesized to be manifestation of an intrinsic biological clock (35). That is, a fixed ratio often exists between taking a breath and strides. For most experienced runners a common ratio is 2:1 (strides to breaths), but at slow running speeds this often changes to 4:1.

Not all have found this explanation linking musical and physiological rhythms appealing. For example, Jourdain contended that "This is one of those observations that, like the flatness of the earth, is blatantly obvious and blatantly wrong" (17). He pointed out that many human activities are rhythmic (heart beat, walking, "sexual thrusting") and automatic but bear no relationship to timing and tempo of music: "If there were, short musicians would tend to play faster than tall musicians, since they move their legs more quickly when they walk."

All of the foregoing leaves a number of very key questions unanswered. If music triggers emotions, how much do such alterations in mental state also dictate changes in physical performance? Are both effects outcomes of a similar mechanism? Does music simply inspire alterations in perception of exercise effort, thereby improving performance?? Or, are there direct physiological alterations that are triggered by the brain's response to music? What neurophysiologic/biochemical processes in the brain might underlie these responses? Or, alternatively, are we dealing here with culturally acquired features of music perception that drive central nervous system changes? And, perhaps most critically, what is there about the nature of this thing we call music that has the ability to so powerfully influence our feelings and physical behavior?

Heavy issues, these. Not surprisingly, the answers to such questions are largely shrouded in mystery. Still, a number of recent advances in brain imaging technology and studies of biochemical changes in the central nervous system of animals have begun to provide some insights. Before delving into these bits of progress, however, it is important to take a step back and ask a more fundamental question: when addressing the effects of music on our psyche and physical capacities, just what are we dealing with here? Specifically, what is it about the nature of music that stimulates such remarkable effects? Most particularly, to start with, quite simply, what *is* music?

Defining Music

If one stopped random persons on the street and asked them this question they might respond by saying "some kinds" but they would, nonetheless, all have a clear idea of what you meant. There is, indeed, a popular perception of just what constitutes "music." Still, one would undoubtedly obtain a different response if one would address the question to a physicist, or a neurobiologist, or a composer of avant-garde minimalist music. The latter, for instance, who would have long tired of tackling this essential question with his colleagues, might insist that his single C note played continuously for two hours truly constituted music. It could hardly be argued that John Cage's composition entitled *Silence 4′33″* (which is just that, the "music" for over four minutes being the ambient sounds in the auditorium) would inspire one to pick up the pace in a 10K road race.

This is not to claim that a precise definition of music is not elusive. If one consults the *Oxford English Dictionary* one finds "The art or science of combining vocal or instrumental sounds with a view to beauty or coherence of form and expression of emotion," perhaps a not entirely satisfying definition. It would seem that, akin to the essential natures of matters like "love" and "time," music is more easily appreciated than its definition can be articulated. (One is tempted here to cite Justice Potter Stewart, who famously said "I can't define pornography, but I know it when I see it.") "The fact is that when we come to the fundamental question of what music really is, we are all—composers, critics, and public alike—very much in the dark," wrote Philip Heseltine. "Music's a rum go" (14).

Elsewhere, attempts at a definition have involved words that encircle the phenomenon of music such as "harmony," "rhythm," "melody," and "tone"—all which prove to describe certain of its essential characteristics. As each might bear importance in the triggering of emotions and stimulating physical capacities, we will discuss these separately later on.

By whatever definition, it is clear that music has played a role in human societies for literally hundreds of thousands of years. It is called the "universal language" for a reason. Every existing human culture includes music, indicating that music originated far into the distant past of evolving humanoids, before the time when our primitive ancestors were dispersed around the globe.

Just how and why music developed in human society remains obscure. A convincing Darwinian explanation—that there should be some survival value to music—has not been forthcoming. Any suggestion for a "biological utility" for the origins of music in human societies remains speculative. In fact, arguments have been put forward that, instead, music is simply a "non-adaptive pleasure-seeking behavior," devoid of an evolutionary advantage (26).

Some have viewed human music as an imitation of animal sounds—birds, of course, but also others, such as the humpback whale, which seems to able to perform a repertoire of musical numbers. These obviously bear importance in animal courtship and aggression, perhaps, it might be suggested, not too far-removed from the basis for many of the melodies produced by *Homo sapiens*. Others have considered that music might have evolved from human speech, but there is ongoing controversy as to which preceded which.

The Nature of Music

We embark now on a brief, admittedly superficial foray into music theory, as presented by standard texts (16,17). The purpose here is to examine each of the major elements of music in an effort to identify those that serve to trigger responses in central nervous system function. Consider these traditional components:

Sound

Stripped down to its bare essentials, a piece of music is composed of *sounds*. That would seem obvious—we say a melody "sounds beautiful." But here is expressed an important concept. To a physicist, sound originates as a set of vibrations—alternate compression and rarefication of molecules in the air—which our hearing apparatus transforms from a mechanical action to an electrical signal transmitted to the brain. Only there, among hundreds of millions of nerve cells and their connections in the cerebral cortex, does this become a "sound." The message here is that sound, rather than a tangible reality, is correctly understood as a neurophysiologically based *perception*. (Indeed, the brain does not have to "hear" sounds to perceive music. Witness a completely deaf Beethoven composing some of the world's greatest music entirely within the confines his central nervous system.)

By some means this perception, this interpretation, of music can be colored by unique individual experiences, triggering some altogether potent emotional reactions. The strains of "Where or When" elicit sharp memories of a first love—one ending in a devastating break-up. "Over the Rainbow" creates mental images of a beloved grandmother who took you to see *The Wizard of Oz* when you were six years old. When you hear Henry Mancini's "Moon River" you are again dancing with the bride at your daughter's wedding. (The reader is invited to make up his or her own list.)

Still, the construction of the ear, the neurons and their wiring connections in the brain, and the chemical transmitters that flit across synapses are all pretty much configured the same from one individual to the next. So, are such nostalgic emotions that arise on hearing a particular piece of music a *subjective* or *objective* phenomenon? One might suppose that the answer is, it must be both.

This gets us as far as thinking about the power of music to evoke emotions based on personal experience. But it falls short of providing any insights into just why a certain piece of music strikes us pleasurably as "beautiful" while another doesn't. We need to look further into the inherent nature of music in an attempt to address this issue and its corollary, how such an influence might translate into improved physical performance.

Tone

If you pluck a string on a violin or cello, it sets up vibrations in the air that occur at a particular frequency (cycles per second, or Hz) that produce oscillations in the tympanic membrane (ear drum), which are transmitted to the tiny bones of the middle ear and then to the cochlea, which converts this mechanical response into electrical nerve impulses. These travel to the *primary auditory cortex* in the temporal lobes of the brain, where it is interpreted as a certain musical note. Let's say that you selected a string such that this frequency was 110 Hz (cycles per second)—that's called an "A." Now if you shorten the string by one-half and pluck again, the frequency of the vibrations will double to 220 Hz, and the note—still an "A"—will have a higher *pitch*. Repeat the action again. The vibrations are now occurring at 440 Hz—still an "A" but sounding even higher in pitch to the ear. All of these notes are still an "A" but each pair—the sound perceived—is an *octave* higher.

Between any two notes of an octave there exist other notes, or frequencies. In Western music there are a total of 12, labeled as A♭ (or A flat), A, B♭, B, C, C♯ (or C sharp), D, E♭, E, F, F♯, and G. One can begin by creating the frequency of vibrations on a violin string which correspond to any of these notes, and then by shortening the string by one-half, or one-quarter, or one-eighth, produce notes which are octaves higher in pitch for that note. Some of these played together at the same time sound beautiful, or *concordant*. Others played simultaneously are grating, or even painful—they're *discordant* (more on this later).

When you plucked the string at a length that created an A note at 110 Hz there were produced, as well, a whole set of other vibrations, or notes, above this frequency. This group of *overtones* was composed mainly of notes which are higher octaves of A but also of other frequencies that correspond to notes that sound concordant, or harmonious, with each other. There are generally about 20 overtones that are produced above the fundamental frequency when a single note is played on a musical instrument. They become weaker as they ascend above the fundamental frequency; thus, the brain detects principally the sound of the fundamental note.

Even the existence of these overtones—just mathematical multiples of the fundamental note—can provoke a pleasurable emotional response when listening to a single note. Just why, nobody knows. If that note were made up of just a single frequency, like one that would be created by a computer, it would sound entirely banal (17).

The particular set of overtones of a note, or tone, provide its musical "color," or *timbre*, and distinguish how we perceive the sounds created by one musical instrument compared to that of another. That is, a saxophone and a clarinet both playing an identical A note are producing in their cylinders vibrations of 440 Hz but to the ear they "sound" different—possess a different "quality"—because each produces a different set of higher frequencies—the overtones—for that particular note.

The timbre of a clarinet is different from that of a flute, or trumpet, or double bass. And as such, those differences can serve to create a certain "personality" for a particular piece of music. Pertinent to the point of our discussion here, differences in timbre can influence the effect that certain music has on psychological reactions within the central nervous system. For example, tune into your emotional response when you listen to the dark, hauntingly soulful voice of the alto or tenor saxophone playing the jazz classic "Harlem Nocturne." Now imagine (you'll have to imagine, since this isn't available) how insipid the same song would be played on a clarinet or a flute. Timbre, the particular set of overtones produced by a single musical tone, plays on our emotions.

Chords and Harmony

As noted above, in Western music there exist 12 notes between each of the octaves in what is termed the *chromatic* scale. The intervals between each are sometimes half-steps, however, so that in the *diatonic scale* there are eight full steps between the notes that define an octave. When played simultaneously with the fundamental, certain combinations of these notes sound harmonious, others not. If C is the fundamental note (let's label it as the number 1), the combination of steps 1, 3, and 5 (that's a C, an E, and a G) played together sound beautiful (that's termed a C chord). You can try this on the piano. But then play a different combination, like 1, 2, and 5—a C, a D, and a G—and the chord sounds jarringly discordant. If an E is the fundamental note, then the beautiful 1–3–5 chord is E-G-B. If A is the fundamental, it's A-C#-E.

Why should this be so? Why does the brain love a 1–3–5 chord but provide discomfort with a 1–2–5? Or a 1–4–7? One is tempted to respond that there must be something in the brain's wiring that resonates sympathetically (or not) with the sound produced by a given musical chord that determines this kind of harmony (or disharmony). That sounds reasonable, but exactly how would this work (i.e., what is that "something"?)? And just when one might be convinced that the harmonious nature of a 1–3–5 chord has a biological basis one is confronted with the fact that this is not invariably true in the music of other societies around the world. Hindu music, for instance, includes scales (or step-wise progression of notes) between octaves that can include as many as 22 different notes. So maybe we are duped into accepting the familiar as beautiful, a conclusion based on our societal culture rather than our biology.

As an historical note, the Greek philosopher Pythagoras (he of right triangle-hypotenuse fame) was among the first to recognize that harmony existed in particular intervals of pitches of musical sounds. Little is known for certain, since he left no written records, but the story goes that he noted that the musical sounds emanating from a blacksmith's anvil produced certain intervals in ratios, based on the weight of the anvil. But beyond distinguishing concordant from discordant combinations of notes to the human ear, instead of relating octaves and steps so produced to their effect on the human ear, he insisted to his followers that such numerical ratios served as the basis for universal laws, such as the motion of the heavenly bodies. (He also reportedly forbade among the members of his cult the eating of beans, for reasons left open to speculation.) As the American mathematician Alfred Posamentier has noted, despite the erroneous foray of Pythagorean thinking into the nature of physical laws, "the foundations of the modern tonal system maintain a debt to the Pythagorean insight that discerned some hidden order behind the phenomenon of the consonance. In a very real sense, when it comes to music, we are all still Pythagorean" (33).

Chord Progression and Melody

The melody of a piece of music (the "tune") is the pattern by which notes are organized to follow each other in a piece of music. Each is a combination of certain rules of harmony and composition and the undiscernible, mysterious process of its composer's creative genius. As Jourdain has put it, "As is true of so many clever inventions, the workings of a great melody are inexplicably simple yet not at all obvious" (17).

Certain aspects of melody, though, remain traditionally established. The fundamental note of a scale forms the centering point, or basis, for the melody. If the piece starts with a fundamental note of A, we say that it is "in the key of A." The melody wanders among the notes of this scale but usually, in most pieces of music, it returns to, or resolves, "comfortably" back to the fundamental note as the music finishes. Importantly, certain notes within the scale of a particular key sound harmonious, while others are discordant. The melody in most Western music is built around a triad of the first, fourth, and fifth steps of the diatonic scale which are particularly consonant within a melody. In the key of C, that subsequent progression of notes would bounce among the notes C, F, and G, typically with "filler notes" in between. In the key of G, the harmonic triad would be G-C-D. In the key of E it's E-A-B. Take for example

(C) I've been workings on the railroad
(F) All the live long day.
(C) I've been working on the railroad
(G) To pass the time away.

The reader will have no difficulty recognizing this standard progression of notes or chords in rock, blues, country, and most other genres of music.

Composers throw in dissonant notes within the scale to create a sense of tension which can then be resolved by returning to the more comfortable 1–4–5 progression. Indeed, such departures from the anticipated harmonious chordal progression can serve to amplify one's emotional responses when listening to a piece of music.

> The deepest pleasure in music comes with deviations from the expected: dissonances, syncopations, kinks in melodic contours, sudden breaks and silences. Isn't this contradictory? Not if the deviation serves to set up an even stronger resolution.
>
> *(17)*

Why should this particular 1–4–5 chord progression in a melody, which serves as the basis for most Western music, provide listening pleasure? One gets into the same quandary here as was confronted in trying to explain the harmonious nature of certain notes that compromise a chord. Certainly there is a temptation, based on its ubiquitousness to human experience, to label it as—by some unexplained means—biological. However, there is little information to support this, and, again, abundant evidence exists that such harmonious perceptions of certain chord progressions are culturally based:

- Much non-Western music is based on different scales and chord progressions than are described above. Music of countries such as India, the Middle East, and the Orient often sounds "strange" to our ears but not to their inhabitants.
- Young children and untrained listeners display no preference for particular chord intervals (except for octaves) (17).
- Melodies comprised of chord progressions once considered disharmonious have become appreciated as pleasurable over time even within the confines of Western society. There is no shortage of examples. Audiences were so shattered on hearing the jarring, powerful rhythms of Stravinsky's *Rite of Spring* for the first time in 1913 at the Théâtre des Champs-Élysées in Paris that they rioted. Over time the Western ear has been become habituated to such startling juxtapositions of unusual rhythms and chord progressions such that the same piece of music is now accepted as a mainstay of the concert repertoire. Familiarity is a strong determinant of the amount of pleasure one receives from listening to a piece of music (26).

As difficult as it might be for the average listener tuned into his favorite country music station to believe, then, that soul-satisfying 1–4–5 progression bemoaning a true love lost would seem to be a learned phenomenon, a matter of cultural habituation. It is not easy to avoid the conclusion that when it comes to eliciting explanations for their emotional impact, "there is no real science of chordal relations" (17).

Rhythm

Rhythm, defined as a regular pulse or tempo, accompanied by accentuated beats, is considered an essential component of enjoyable music (17). And there is no question that the rhythmic aspect of a piece of music can be central to its emotional impact (think about Ravel's *Boléro*, in which its hypnotic effect depends on a driving rhythmic repetitiveness). Why this should be so remains uncertain. We've already discussed above the controversial idea that the rhythms of bodily functions might somehow account for the pleasure or a sense of harmony when tuning in to the pulse of music.

In considering the importance of rhythm, we now for the first time in this story see how emotional responses to music can be transmitted into motor activity. We tap our feet to the rhythm. We get up and dance ("It had a great beat that I could dance to" was the universal sentiment of those judging a new piece of rock music on *American Bandstand*). We fight off the urge to get up from our seat in symphony hall and march around during the "March to the Scaffold" in Hector Berlioz's *Symphonie Fantastique*. There is clearly a drive to satisfy a "kinesthetic pleasure" that is obtained by matching a rhythm of muscular contractions in time with the tempo of music. That link becomes even more globally expressed in dance, such as ballet, in which physical actions are evoked by lyrical music. Here is evidence that incoming auditory pathways to the brain manifesting a steady pulse are linked to centers in the central nervous system, called *central pattern generators*, clock-like oscillators which control the sequence and pace of muscle contraction which permit motor activities. That such controllers originated deeply in human evolutionary history is evidenced by the fact that these regulators of muscular rhythmicity are observed throughout the animal kingdom (35).

"This is really very odd," Jourdain once noted (17). Not only is there no clear-cut explanation for a link between auditory sensory centers and those that regulate motor activity in the brain, "there is no obvious evolutionary reason why the intricate patterns of sound that make up music should simultaneously unfold in our musculatures." However, more recently Chen et al. utilized brain imaging techniques to illustrate that interactions occurred between the auditory and dorsal motor cortex of the brain when subjects tapped their feet to rhythmic music (9). Too, the pleasurable association of musical and physical rhythms must have a long evolutionary history, as indications of dance in response to music date back as far as written records. And, as every parent knows, even human toddlers will happily dance to music as soon as they become ambulatory.

In summary, we've seen that while we cannot confidently specify the origins—or even a good definition—of music, we can identify certain of its elements that contribute to the strong influences that music holds on the central nervous system, at least those affecting emotional responses. Associations to personal experience, differences in timbre, the effect of chord structure and progression, the role of rhythm—they all can modify psychological state. But we're still left with unanswered questions. Do such changes in emotional state serve to improve exercise performance simply by enhancing motivation or reducing attention to fatigue? That is, do we perform better because we are simply more emotionally excited when we listen to a particular piece of music? Or are there biological explanations as well for the music-performance link? Can we point to specific physiological functions that are enhanced by exercising while listening to music?

Neurophysiological Research

Up to this point the discussion has largely ignored the other half—the receiving end—of the music-brain link. In effect, how does the central nervous system register and process incoming patterns of organized sound we call music, and how do these signals become transformed into something one can call emotional or physical responses? Clearly, an understanding of what occurs in cerebral function when listening to music might be expected to provide key insights into just how music might enhance physical performance.

In this regard, prior to the 1980s there was little to write about. Before that time, ideas surrounding function-specific anatomic localization within the brain were largely limited to the behavioral effects observed in humans suffering from traumatic or disease-related brain damage (37). Since that time, however, an explosion in the development of new technologies has provided major steps forward in understanding brain function in response to external stimuli (i.e., music). Most particularly these have involved technologies such as positron emission tomography (PET scan) and functional magnetic resonance imaging (fMRI) which identify regions of the brain exhibiting a rise in metabolic rate, assumed to reflect increased function, in response to listening to music.

Perhaps not surprisingly, the picture that has emerged from the use of these techniques is one of extraordinary complexity, far beyond that which had previously been envisaged. This information has, in fact, not resolved the mysteries underlying the brain's perception and responses to music but has only served to magnify an awareness of the limitations of our understanding of these processes.

Music is initially interpreted in the brain by the auditory cortex in the temporal lobes. But that's just the beginning. From there, a series of neural connections to various parts of the brain provides for specialized interpretations of musical sounds (26,48). The rhythm of the music is appreciated by dorsal pathways to the premotor cortex. Pitch is discerned by separate cortical regions. Emotions are generated by lower, more primitive regions of the brain, such as the limbic system and the amygdala. Areas in the cerebellum are concerned with rhythmic movement in response to music (such as foot tapping). The memory for music and its associations with past experience are the provenance of the hippocampus. And so on. Even dissonance and consonance of music appear to be assessed by independent brain sites. One's overall perception of a piece of music thus reflects the intercommunication of a tangled network of musical interpreters. There exists, as well, evidence that the brain "listens" to music by means of all this anatomic-functional specificity in a particular order, so that an incoming piece of music is appraised in a specific cascade of these various aspects of music interpretation (26).

Pertinent insights have been achieved, as well, into a biochemical basis of music's impact on brain function that bears relevance to both emotional responses and influences on physical performance. Much of this has centered on a key role of the neurotransmitter dopamine, which facilitates transmission of electrical impulses across synapses between neurons in the central nervous system (36). This agent has attracted attention in a number of domains, as it appears to be responsible for a variety of excitatory functions, such as falling in love, enjoying your morning coffee, and the cravings of narcotic addiction. Among these actions, dopamine has been demonstrated in animal studies to account for motivation for exercise, particularly that which provides pleasurable rewards.

In this regard are the actions of dopamine biochemical pathways *felt* by human emotions? Does such a chemically generated function, triggered by music, create a shared sense of pleasure through motor activity in human beings? Such an action has been supposed but not yet documented by direct evidence. As Knab and Lightfoot have concluded, "evidence is still lacking as to whether the dopamine system is actually working in an independent role in influencing voluntary physical activity (e.g., can dopaminergic differences *cause* changes in motivated physical activity in humans?)" (23).

Music has been recognized to increase brain dopamine activity in animal models (29,41). Sutoo and Akiyama, for instance, found that exposing (presumably highly discriminating) rats to music of Mozart significantly increased their neostriatal levels of dopamine (41). In humans, Salimpoor et al. utilized PET scans and an agent that competes with dopamine receptors to demonstrate that pleasurable emotional responses to music were accompanied by increased dopamine release in the mesolimbic striatum of the brain (38). And Kanduri et al. reported that genes responsible for secretion and transport of dopamine were more frequently upregulated when subjects listened to classical music compared to no music (18).

The Bottom Line

All of this information provides a rudimentary—but far from comprehensive—schema by which music might trigger emotional and motivational responses in the brain. And it is not difficult to conceive that this neurological network that surrounds the psychological responses to music might serve as a driving motivating factor responsible for increased muscular effort. This is a particularly attractive idea considering the evidence that dopamine function is augmented by listening to music, and this biochemical response appears to be responsible, at least in animals, for motivation-for-reward that increases motor activity (as witnessed by obsessional wheel running in rodents) (6).

The slate of how listening to music can directly enhance physical performance, on the other hand, is virtually blank. Still, what we now know about the neurophysiological responses in the brain to music provides some clues as to how such a link might exist. The most obvious means by which the brain effects—and controls the limits of—physical effort is the transmission from the motor cortex of efferent signals down the spinal cord to activate motor neurons which trigger the contraction of skeletal muscle. The limits of this process define "central fatigue," which has traditionally been considered as a major determinant in defining an exercise fatigue threshold. Could listening to music impact this central nervous system-generated effect and thus serve to alter physical performance? It's an attractive idea. A key piece of evidence, yet to be obtained, would be identification of a neurological link between brain centers processing incoming music and those responsible for establishing level of central fatigue.

Besides serving as a motivational agent for exercise, dopamine may have a direct effect of enhancing endurance capacity. Foley et al. found elevated levels of dopamine receptor mRNA in rodents that had been bred for a high level of endurance performance (12). Indeed, these authors suggested that this neurotransmitter might contribute to altering the fatigue threshold defined by central fatigue. Others have supported this concept, reporting that experimental manipulations that increase dopamine action improve exercise performance in animal models (e.g., 15).

It has been suggested that dopamine might physiologically influence exercise performance by its actions of inhibiting hyperthermia-induced fatigue (34,49). Dopamine affects regulation of core temperature in the hypothalamus during exercise, so as to indicate that this agent might serve to block inhibitory signals in the brain in response to hyperthermia that can limit exercise performance.

Concluding Thoughts

We've now come to the end of this analysis, and a critic could claim—and rightly so—that the Big Questions we've been asking have not at all been resolved. Specifically, the means by which music augments one's capacity for physical work remains obscure. But in closing, perhaps it should be noted that maybe the author hasn't been all that fair to the mystique of music and its influence on the human psyche. This dissection of the nature of music has been unapologetically served up in a reductionist fashion, attempting to tease out the individual elements that constitute music and how they influence human emotions and behavior. But, in reality, music is made up of more than the sum of its parts. It has an *emergent* quality that transcends a simple understanding of its composite characteristics. And that quality, which defies analysis, is what defines music. The author Sarah Caldwell has expressed this most eloquently:

> [Music is more than] a set of string vibrations and mathematical note relationships on which I have pinned personal emotion. Melancholy music *is* melancholy; a sweet air *is* a sweet air; those descriptions are fundamental to what music is. . . . Even if I describe a sequence of notes as going "up" or "down," this has less to do with what the sound waves are doing (which is becoming more or less frequent, and longer or shorter) than with how the music plays out in my mind. I hear the notes climbing up an invisible ladder. I almost physically rise in my chair as I listen to Ralph Vaughan Williams' "The Lark Ascending"; my very soul takes flight. That's not just me: it is what the music is.
>
> *(8)*

References

1. Archana R, Mukilan R. Beneficial effect of preferential music on exercise induced changes in heart rate variability. *J Clin Diagn Res.* 2016;10:9–11.
2. Bacon CJ, Myers TR, Karageorghis CI. Effect of music-movement synchrony on exercise oxygen consumption. *J Sports Med Phys Fitness.* 2012;52:359–365.
3. Bernstein L. *The Infinite Variety of Music.* New York: Simon and Schuster; 1966. p. 83.
4. Bigliassi M, Leon-Dominguez U, Buzzachera CF, Barreto-Silva V, Altimari LR. How does music aid 5 km of running? *J Strength Cond Res.* 2015;29:305–314.
5. Birnbaum L, Boone T, Huschle B. Cardiovascular responses to music tempo during steady state exercise. *J Exerc Physiol.* 2009;12:50–57.
6. Boso M, Politi P, Barale F, Emanuele E. Neurophysiology and neurobiology of the musical experience. *Func Neurobiol.* 2006;21:187–191.
7. Brownley KA, McMurray RG, Hackney AC. Effects of music on physiological and affective response to graded treadmill exercise in trained and untrained runners. *Int J Psychophysiol.* 1995;19:193–201.
8. Caldwell S. *At the Existentialist Café.* New York: Other Press; 2016.
9. Chen JL, Zatorre RJ, Penhume VB. Interactions between auditory and dorsal premotor cortex during synchronization to musical rhythms. *Neuro Image.* 2006;12:1771–1781.
10. Crust L. Effects of familiar and unfamiliar asynchronous music on treadmill walking endurance. *Percept Mot Skills.* 2004;99:361–368.
11. Edworthy J, Waring H. The effects of music tempo and loudness level on treadmill exercise. *Ergonomics.* 2006;49:1597–610.
12. Foley TE, Greenwood BN, Day HE, Koch LG, Britton SL, Fleshner M. Elevated central monoamine receptor mRNA in rats bred for high endurance capacity: implications for central fatigue. *Behav Brain Res.* 2006;174:132–142.
13. Hernandez-Peon R. The efferent control of afferent signals entering the central nervous system. *Ann NY Acad Science.* 1961;89:866–882.
14. Heseltine P. The idea of a song. In: Barzun J, editor. *Pleasures of Music.* Chicago: University of Chicago Press; 1977. p. 39–40.
15. Heyes MP, Garnett ES, Coates G. Central dopaminergic activity influences rats ability to exercise. *Life Sci.* 1985;36:671–677.
16. Jones GT. *Music Theory.* New York: Barnes & Noble Books; 1974.
17. Jourdain R. *Music, the Brain, and Ecstasy.* New York: Harper Collins; 1997.
18. Kanduri C, Raijas P, Ahvenainen M, et al. The effect of listening to music on human transcriptome. *PeerJ.* 2015;3:e830.
19. Karageorghis CI, Mouzourides DA, Priest DL, Sasso TA, Morrish DJ, Walley CJ. Psychophysical and ergogenic effects of synchronous music during treadmill walking. *J Sport Exerc Psychol.* 2009;31:18–36.
20. Karageorghis CI, Priest D-L. Music in the exercise domain: a review and synthesis (Part I). *Int Rev Sport Exerc Psychol.* 2012;5:44–66.
21. Karageorghis CI, Priest D-L. Music in the exercise domain: a review and synthesis (Part II). *Int Rev Sport Exerc Psychol.* 2012;5:67–84.
22. Karageorghis CI, Terry PC. The psychophysical effects of music in sport and exercise: a review. *J Sport Behav.* 1997;20:54–68.
23. Knab AM, Lightfoot JT. Does the difference between physically active and couch potato lie in the dopamine system? *Int J Biol Sci.* 2010;6:133–150.

24. Kundera K. *Encounter Essays*. New York: Harper Collins; 2009.
25. Lee S, Kimmerly DS. Influence of music on maximal self-paced running performance and passive post-exercise recovery rate. *J Sports Med Phys Fitness*. 2016;56:39–48.
26. Levitin DJ. *This is Your Brain on Music. The Science of a Human Obsession*. New York: Penguin Books; 2006.
27. Lim HB, Karageorghis CI, Romer LM, Bishop DT. Psychophysiological effects of synchronous versus asynchronous music during cycling. *Med Sci Sports Exerc*. 2014;46:407–413.
28. Macone D, Baldari C, Zelli A, Guidetti L. Music and physical activity in psychological well-being. *Percept Mot Skills*. 2006;103:285–295.
29. Mavridis IN. Music and the nucleus accumbens. *Surg Radio Anat*. 205;37:121–125.
30. Miller T, Swank AM, Manire JT, Robertson RJ, Wheeler B. Effect of music and dialog on perception of exertion enjoyment, and metabolic responses during exercise. *Int J Fitness*. 2010;6:45–52.
31. Mohammadzadeh H, Tartibyan B, Ahmadi A. The effects of music on the perceived exertion rate and performance of trained and untrained individuals during progressive exercise. *Facta Universitatis: Series Physical Education & Sport*. 2008;6:67–74.
32. Nethery VM. Competition between internal and external sources of information during exercise: influence on RPE and the impact of the exercise load. *J Sports Med Phys Fitness*. 2002;42:172–178.
33. Posamentier AS. *The Pythagorean Theorem*. Amherst, NY: Prometheus Books; 2010.
34. Roelands B, Meeusen R. Alterations in central fatigue by pharmacological manipulations of neurotransmitters in normal and high ambient temperature. *Sports Med*. 2010;40:229–246.
35. Rowland T. *The Athlete's Clock*. Champaign, IL: Human Kinetics Publishers; 2011. pp. 56–58.
36. Rowland T. *Biologic Regulation of Physical Activity*. Champaign, IL: Human Kinetics; 2017. p. 43–47.
37. Sachs O. *Musicophilia*. New York: Vintage Books; 2012.
38. Salimpoor VN, Benovoy M, Larcher K, Dagher A, Zatorre RJ. Anatomically distinct dopamine release during anticipation and experience of peak emotion to music. *Nat Neurosci*. 2011;14:257–262.
39. Schneider S, Askew CD, Abel T, Struder HK. Exercise, music, and the brain: is there a central pattern generator? *J Sports Sci*. 2010;28:1337–1343.
40. Steiner G. *Errata*. New Haven: Yale University Press; 1998.
41. Sutoo D, Akiyama K. Music improves dopaminergic neurotransmission: demonstration based on the effect of music on blood pressure regulation. *Brain Res*. 2004;1016:255–262.
42. Szmedra L, Bacharach DW. Effect of music on perceive exertion, plasma lactate, norepinephrine and cardiovascular hemodynamics during treadmill running. *Int J Sports Med*. 1998;19:32–37.
43. Tenenbaum G, Lidor R, Lavyan N, et al. The effect of music type on running perseverance and coping with effort sensations. *Psychol Sport Exerc*. 2004;5:89–109.
44. Thakare AE, Mehrotra R, Singh A. Effect of music tempo on exercise performance and heart rate among young adults. *Int J Physiol Pathophysiol Pharmacol*. 2017;9:35–39.
45. Urakawa K, Yokoyama K. Music can enhance exercise-induced sympathetic dominancy assessed by heart rate variability. *Tohoku J Exp Med*. 2005;206:213–218.

46. Yamamoto T, Ohkuwa T, Itoh H, Kitoh M, Terawasa J, Tsuda T, Kitagama S, Sato Y. Effects of pre-exercise listening to slow and fast rhythm music on supramaximal cycle performance and selected metabolic variables. *Arch Physiol Biochem.* 2003;111:211–214.
47. Young SC, Sands CD, Jung AP. Effect of music in female college soccer players during a maximal treadmill test. *Int J Fitness.* 2009;5:31–36.
48. Zatorre RJ, Salimpoor VN. From perception to pleasure: music and its neural sub-strates. *PNAS.* 2013;10 suppl 2:10430–10437.
49. Zheng X, Hasegawa H. Central dopaminergic neurotransmission plays an important role in thermoregulation and performance during endurance exercise. *Eur J Sport Sci.* 2016;16:818–828.

12

WHEN IS IRON SUPPLEMENTATION INDICATED FOR ATHLETES WITH IRON DEFICIENCY?

Given the near-sanctity conferred on sports success, it comes as no surprise that an ardent controversy surrounds the influence of depleted body iron stores on athletic performance. Indeed, it's a question, as the hematologist Randy Eicher has written, "that recurs regularly and seems to endure forever" (20). The controversy is this: There is no question that performance in those with overt iron deficiency—enough to cause anemia—is likely to be impaired, and all are in agreement that these athletes should be identified and treated. However, whether the same holds true for those with milder degrees of depletion of body iron—nonanemic iron deficiency—lies clouded in a good deal of dispute and uncertainty.

Theoretical considerations would hold that such athletes might also experience depressed athletic performance, given the importance of iron in metabolic processes critical for muscular work. Indeed, such seems to be the case in animal models. However, the research evidence supporting this conclusion in humans is unclear and far from compelling. Consequently, the justification and guidelines for screening and treating athletes with low body iron stores remain controversial (12,50). The question is confounded by the observation that nonanemic iron deficiency is common among competitive athletes, particularly females. Add to this the considerable evidence that sports participation itself can increase losses of body iron and provoke iron deficiency.

While this debate rages, a good number of people would like to know the answer. Athletes, coaches, parents, athletic directors, nutritionists—even physiologists—are tuned into this controversy, the outcome of which has very pragmatic bearing on decisions regarding the use of iron supplements during sports training and competition. Herein lies the story.

The Basic Facts

This chemical controversy involves the physiological role of a well-known element (Fe, atomic number 26), one whose meager contribution to body content belies its biological significance. The total quantity of iron in an adult male is only 4 g, in a female 2.5 g (about the quantity in three 2-inch finishing nails). The average daily adult diet contains approximately 12 mg of iron, of which only 2 mg are absorbed via the intestinal mucosa. Two-thirds of this absorbed iron is incorporated in hemoglobin, 10% resides in myoglobin, 5% serves as a component of iron-containing enzymes, and about 20% is transported by transferrin to the liver and reticuloendothelial system to be stored in the form of ferritin.

Ferritin levels measured in the blood are indicative of the amount of this storage iron and provide an easily accessible means of detecting iron deficiency. The average serum ferritin value in post-pubertal males is approximately 90 ng/ml and in females 25–30 ng/ml during their reproductive period. A number of different "normal" values to define a lower limit of ferritin concentration—and identify an individual as having iron deficiency—have been utilized in the research literature. Generally, however, a value of serum ferritin of <12–20 ng/dl is considered to reflect deficient iron stores. (It is important to recognize that ferritin is an "acute phase reactant," meaning that serum levels rise in response to an inflammatory process, which includes vigorous exercise. Thus, ferritin determinations in athletes need to be delayed for at least 24–48 hours after a bout of training or competition and in those with an acute febrile illness.) Serum iron levels fluctuate markedly over the course of a day and do not serve as an accurate indicator of body iron stores.

How Iron Affects Exercise Performance

Iron plays a role in exercise performance by three possible—and independent—functions. In order of descending certainty, these involve a) oxygen transport by hemoglobin, b) enzymatic activities that control metabolic pathways for energy availability, and c) mental processes that may influence motivation.

Oxygen Delivery

Sometime around 500 million years ago, the primitive single-celled organisms that populated the Earth "devised" the means, via Darwinian processes, to utilize the oxygen in the surrounding air for obtaining their required energy derived from aerobic metabolism. As multicellularity gave way over time to increasingly complex organisms, a variety of functional means developed for obtaining this oxygen (by lungs and gills) and transporting it in circulatory systems (a heart pumping into branching vessels of blood flow) to the individual cells within the body. All well and good, except for one challenging problem: The amount of oxygen that could be dissolved in the blood—just 3 ml oxygen in each liter—was far too meager to support life. In fact, the amount of oxygen dissolved in all the blood of the average adult human would be consumed by his or her metabolic machinery in just a few seconds.

(The only way to effectively increase the amount of dissolved oxygen in the blood is to augment the pressure in the surrounding air. This is accomplished today by means of a "hyperbaric chamber," which can raise environmental oxygen pressure at least three-fold. As such, it has therapeutic value for administering oxygen when treating patients with burns, gangrene, and carbon monoxide poisoning. But such a device did not become commercially available until the early 1900s, so from the perspective of animal evolution this was a bit late.)

The difficulty became resolved by the evolutionary advent of *hemoglobin*, a large iron-containing molecule with the capacity to bind substantial amounts of oxygen in the lung, transport it in red blood cells (erythrocytes) in the blood throughout the body, and then release it at the capillary level to diffuse into the cells (28). There oxygen participates in the aerobically based metabolic machinery that provides an energy supply for cellular functions, including, most importantly to the topic at hand, skeletal muscle contraction for human locomotion. Here was the ideal solution to the problem of oxygen delivery, since hemoglobin increases the amount of oxygen delivered to the cells 70 times that compared to just dissolved oxygen.

Hemoglobin is a complex molecule composed of a central porphyrin ring, to which four atoms of iron are attached, surrounded by a group of globulin proteins. This complex—or one of its variants—serves as the oxygen transport mechanism for almost all vertebrates. (It should be noted, to correct a common misconception, that the source of the red color of blood is not its iron content but rather resides in the characteristics of the porphyrin moiety.) In the face of significant iron deficiency, hemoglobin formation is impaired, resulting in *anemia*. It is not difficult to envisage the scenario, then, of an athlete in which iron deficiency → diminished hemoglobin formation → impaired oxygen delivery to skeletal muscle fibers → interference with normal cellular aerobic metabolism → diminished muscular function → decreased athletic performance.

Threshold values for defining normal hemoglobin concentrations are typically noted as >13.0 gm/dl in adult males and >12.0 gm/dl in non-pregnant females (13). However, it is important to recognize that "these limits are not absolute and refer only to the likelihood (around 95%) of anaemia being present; in some individuals hemoglobin concentrations above the threshold are still lower than those normally maintained, while in others individual hemoglobin concentrations may normally be below the threshold" (6). This observation will be re-visited later when the issue is raised of identifying those athletes with true anemia despite possessing expected "normal" values.

In addition to depressed hemoglobin concentration, microcytic and hypochromic red blood cells are characteristic findings in persons with iron deficiency anemia. The former indicates a shrunken erythrocyte size (<78μ^3), while the latter reflects a smaller amount of hemoglobin per cell (mean corpuscular hemoglobin <27 μμg and mean corpuscular hemoglobin concentration <30%) (56).

Cellular Aerobic Metabolism

Iron is a key component of the enzymatic system of the respiratory chain which forms ATP (adenosine triphosphate), the energy source for muscular contraction. The iron-containing cytochromes, situated primarily in the mitochondria, form the electron transport chain which is essential in the oxidative production of cellular energy. Enzymes critical to cellular energy transfer also depend on iron content, including succinic dehydrogenase, aconitase, and xanthine oxidase. Iron also acts to store and transfer oxygen within the cell as a component of the myoglobin molecule.

It can be assumed intuitively that iron deficiency which interferes with this intramuscular energy-providing process will eventuate in diminished physical performance, and, as will be described below, there is good evidence, at least in animal models, that this is in fact so. The difficulty in assessing the possible role of impaired oxidative metabolism from depressed iron availability in humans is hampered by the absence of any biochemical marker by which such an effect might be confirmed. That is, serum ferritin levels provide recognition of extent of depletion of body iron stores, and hemoglobin concentration reveals the effect of iron deficiency on oxygen carrying capacity of the blood. But there is no clinical means—short of muscle biopsy—of determining if any particular level of iron depletion is acting to depress aerobic metabolic pathways in the cell. As a consequence, too, it becomes impossible to establish threshold levels of low levels of ferritin (hypoferritinemia) that need to be reached before such an influence might become physiologically important (i.e., decreased athletic performance) in a given individual.

Psychological Function

Two observations here are pertinent: First, mental resilience, concentration, and motivation are all psychological attributes critical for athletic success. And, second, iron is considered important to factors controlling central nervous system functions underlying emotional health and cognitive function. It is not unreasonable, then, to suspect that athletes who suffer from iron deficiency might display a decline in performance based on a depreciation of certain mental attributes.

The evidence for a role of iron deficiency in depressing cognitive function comes almost exclusively from studies in children with iron deficiency anemia (35). Even here conclusions are rather speculative, given conflicting results as well as the number of associated variables that could influence mental function (lower socioeconomic status, poor nutrition status, effect of anemia itself, etc.) (6). Still, studies in animals have indicated that depressed brain iron content can interfere with the function of neurotransmitters in the central nervous system (3). In 2014 Kim and Wessling-Resnick provided a review of "Iron and Mechanisms of Emotional Behavior," pointing out that psychological disturbances caused by depressed brain iron can be manifestations of poor myelination, impaired neurotransmitter metabolism, and a downregulation of dopamine receptors (32).

Limited investigations in older subjects with nonanemic iron deficiency have provided support for its speculative impact on psychological function. Bruner et al. found that iron treatment resulted in improved performance on tests of verbal learning and memory (but not mood or attention) in 81 teenage girls who initially had normal hemoglobin levels and ferritin <12 ng/ml (7). Murray-Kolb and Beard demonstrated a 5- to 7-fold improvement in eight tests of cognitive function along with a rise in ferritin levels following iron treatment in a large group of 18–35-year-old females (37). The authors concluded that "iron status is a significant factor in cognitive performance in women of reproductive age."

It has been noted, too, that those with iron deficiency anemia frequently express difficulties with memory, energy, and mood (60). "Mental toughness" is clearly a characteristic which often separates the "elite" from the "good" athlete. Whether iron deficiency might alter mental function and thereby depress sports performance currently remains a speculative idea, but it's one that deserves further research attention.

The Scenario of Progressive Iron Deficiency

Inadequate dietary iron intake and/or ongoing excessive iron losses are manifest by laboratory findings signaling body iron depletion. Initially this is indicated by a reduction of serum ferritin level to <12–18 ng/dl. In this early stage of iron deficiency, formation of hemoglobin and red blood cell production are not affected—serum hemoglobin level remains normal and red blood cells have normal morphology, being neither microcytic nor hypochromic. This stage is termed *nonanemic iron deficiency*. As iron depletion becomes more severe, however, hemoglobin production is impaired, resulting in overt *iron deficiency anemia*. Now both ferritin and hemoglobin levels are depressed, and under a microscope a slide of the blood will reveal microcytic and hypochromic red blood cells.

As discussed previously, the latter stage of progressive iron deficiency is marked by an impairment of oxygen delivery to exercising muscle cells consequent to the reduction in hemoglobin level. This is not true in the earlier stage of nonanemic iron deficiency, but the critical question here is, at what point in this progression of iron depletion are the important metabolic contributions of iron compromised, which would bear consequence in depressing muscular performance? To emphasize, the question is rendered highly problematic since there is no biochemical marker, such as blood ferritin and hemoglobin concentrations, one can measure that provides an indication of such function.

To summarize to this point: the maintenance of normal body iron stores is important for athletes, as iron plays a critical role in physical performance, particularly in providing for oxygen delivery and facilitation of cellular aerobic metabolism. Consequently, in the presence of inadequate dietary iron intake and/or excessive iron losses from the body, iron stores become depleted, posing a risk for impairment of athletic performance. Progressively severe levels of iron depletion are exhibited by a fall in serum concentration of ferritin, a marker of body iron stores. At low levels of iron deficiency, hemoglobin production is not impaired (nonanemic iron deficiency), but with a continued fall in ferritin level eventuates in low hemoglobin concentrations (iron deficiency anemia). Body iron status can thus be categorized as

	Hemoglobin	*Ferritin*
Normal body iron content	>12 gm/dl females >13 gm/dl males	>12–20 ng/ml
Nonanemic iron deficiency	>12 gm/dl females >13 gm/dl males	<12–20 ng/ml
Iron deficiency anemia	<12 gm/dl females <13 gm/dl males	<12–20 ng/ml

Iron Deficiency in Athletes

With these basic precepts in mind, we can now turn to the relevance of this information to competitive athletes, particularly those involved in endurance events. Given that adequacy of iron stores is critical for physical performance, oral iron supplementation is indicated for athletes with depleted stores. Yet the degree of such iron deficiency critical for impairing performance is unclear, creating uncertainty as to who deserves iron treatment. The immediacy of this issue is underscored by the observation that nonanemic iron deficiency is common in athletes, particularly females, and that sports training itself may act to deplete iron stores.

Frequency of Iron Deficiency in Athletes

The frequency of overt iron deficiency anemia (low ferritin level with hemoglobin concentration <12 gm/dl in females and <13 gm/dl in males) is very small in athletic populations. Most studies, involving a variety of sports, have revealed a frequency no greater than 2–7%, with higher values typically in females (17,43,47). In fact, Pate et al. could find no athletes with iron deficiency among 46 competitors in five varsity college teams (44). It is likely that the occurrence of such anemia in athletic populations is no greater than that in the general population (24,27). The important point here has been often raised that because of its rarity, "athletes found to have iron deficiency anemia, particularly males, should be considered for evaluation of disease processes that accelerate iron losses" (50).

On the other hand, nonanemic iron deficiency (low ferritin concentrations with preserved normal hemoglobin levels) is commonplace in athletes, predominantly in females. One review of 11 studies involving endurance athletes revealed an average of 34% of females and 7% of males with a serum ferritin value <12–20 ng/ml (50). Most recently, Parks et al. performed a retrospective medical review of laboratory values obtained in athletes at a single university between the years 2002 and 2014 (43). Among 1,059 females, 31% were found to have nonanemic iron deficiency, compared to 3% of 411 males. These data indicate, then, that in any group of young female athletes, one out of three can be expected to demonstrate evidence of iron deficiency without overt anemia. Indeed, it is just this surprisingly high frequency that has added to the dilemma surrounding the appropriate management of these athletes, as will be described later. At the same time, it is important to recognize that nonanemic iron deficiency is uncommon in males.

The sex difference in frequency of nonanemic iron deficiency has traditionally been attributed to the effect of iron losses via menstrual flow in females. This conclusion was supported by the finding of Rowland and Kelleher of a negative relationship between serum ferritin levels and estimated menstrual flow in a group of high school swimmers (53). Dietary practices may be involved as well, with some data indicating that female athletes generally consume less iron than their male counterparts. For example, Nickerson et al. described average daily intake of iron of 8.5 mg and 12.9 mg in female and male cross-country runners, respectively (39). Rowland and Kelleher described a similar sex gap in daily iron consumption in high school swimmers (7.8 mg in females and 12.1 mg in males), reflecting 43% and 67%, respectively, of the recommended daily intake (53).

Are the frequencies of nonanemic iron deficiency in athletes greater than those among their non-athletic peers? The data on this point are mixed. A number of authors have failed to identify differences in levels of nonanemic iron deficiency between athletes and nonathletes (5,18,54). Rowland et al. found no significant differences in average ferritin concentrations in female adolescent swimmers (18 ng/ml), cross-country runners (22 ng/ml), and non-athletic teenagers (22 ng/ml) at the beginning of a competitive season (54). The swimmers had no significant change in ferritin levels at the end of a 10-seek season (20 ng/ml). Similarly, Braun et al. reported no significant differences in average ferritin concentrations in training collegiate female swimmers and non-athletic control women (20 ng/ml and 17 ng/ml, respectively) (5). Di Santolo et al. found the percentage with low ferritin levels (<12 ng/ml) to be similar in 70 young Italian women characterized as non-professional athletes compared to 121 sedentary controls (27.1% and 29.8%, respectively) (18).

These findings would suggest that the high frequency of nonanemic iron deficiency in young female athletes is not unique to this group but rather reflects that observed among menstruating females of the same age in the general population. For instance, a prevalence study of non-training 15–16-year-old Swedish boys and girls revealed a frequency of those with a serum ferritin value <16 ng/ml to be 15% and 40%, respectively (29).

However, that athletes are at higher risk for iron deficiency is supported by reports of progressive declines in ferritin concentrations during the course of a period of sports training. In one study of high school distance runners, ferritin levels fell from a mean of 27 ng/ml to 14 ng/ml in girls and 29 ng/ml to 24 ng/ml in boys during 11 weeks of training (51). In another investigation female runners exhibited a fall in average ferritin values from 14 to 9 ng/ml over the course of a season (52).

Nickerson et al. reported that 34% of a group of female high school cross-country runners developed iron deficiency during the course of a competitive season (average ferritin falling from 12.5 to 7.3 ng/ml) (39). Spodaryk found that an 8-month training program in male 10–12-year-old championship-level swimmers caused a significant decrease in serum ferritin that was not observed in nontrained age-matched subjects (58). Similar findings were reported by Escanero et al. in Spanish professional soccer players (22).

Some authors have described negative correlations between training volume and serum ferritin levels (48), but such a relationship could not be confirmed by others (42). In addition, ferritin levels have been reported to be stable during a course of training in swimmers (31,53), soccer players (41), and gymnasts (24). In short, the question of whether athletic training promotes iron loss—and whether this phenomenon might be sport-specific—remains unresolved.

Several mechanisms have been suggested which could explain abnormal iron losses triggered by sports training (10). Fecal blood loss has not uncommonly been recorded in athletes following vigorous bouts of exercise. Nickerson et al. found that among 20 female high school runners, nine demonstrated iron losses via gastrointestinal bleeding, and seven of these nine had iron deficiency (39). It has been supposed that such iron loss might reflect transient ischemia from gut hypoperfusion during exercise.

Hematuria from bladder trauma during running, iron losses in heavy sweating, and rhabdomyolysis (muscle tissue breakdown) with myoglobin excretion in the urine have all been suggested in training athletes, but iron losses via these routes would seem to be minor. "Foot strike hemolysis" (destruction of red blood cells) has been described in military recruits after extended marches, and some have proposed that a similar effect might occur in distance runners and cyclists (36). However, hemolysis, unless severe, will not lead to iron deficiency, since the iron released from damaged erythrocytes will be utilized for new red cell production.

The Effect of Iron Deficiency on Performance

"Iron" has conjured up images of strength and toughness since antiquity (2), reflecting the observation that a large sledgehammer swung on a sheet of this element will create little impression. (The English language is replete with such examples. One competes in an Ironman triathlon. Or rules with an iron fist. Certainly, this requires an iron will, especially if one is in need of an iron-clad defense. "An iron curtain has descended across the Continent," said Winston Churchill. And then there's the Iron Maiden [Thatcher] and the Iron Duke [Wellington].)

In the physiological realm, however, the substantial nature of iron lies instead in the weakened physical capacities observed subsequent to depletion of body iron content. Reduction of body iron stores of sufficient severity to interfere with the formation of hemoglobin will impair endurance athletic performance. But the uncertainty that surrounds iron deficiency in athletes—and the focus of this chapter—involves these key questions: What is the physiological significance of nonanemic iron deficiency? And, specifically, does the condition of low ferritin level with normal hemoglobin concentration interfere with physical performance?

There is at least a theoretical backing for such to be the case, since depression of iron-containing cellular enzymes in skeletal muscle critical for energy-providing metabolism could occur at lower levels of iron deficiency than that required for hemoglobin formation. In fact, the experimental data in animal models indicate that the answer to the second question is "yes." Iron-deficient mice with normal hemoglobin levels suffer from lack of endurance exercise capacity. But, despite a good deal of research attention, investigators have yet to convincingly demonstrate that the same is true in human beings. Many, in fact, are dubious. Meanwhile, that group of one-third of female endurance athletes who have nonanemic iron deficiency and their coaches are seeking guidance, uncertain of appropriate approaches to routine screening and, importantly, oral iron supplementation.

Iron Deficiency Anemia

It is well-recognized that any pathological condition (such as cardiac or pulmonary disease) or environmental situation (e.g., high altitude) that reduces oxygen delivery via circulatory blood flow will depress work physical capacity. That the lowered arterial oxygen content associated with a reduction in hemoglobin concentration will impair athletic performance therefore comes as no surprise. The negative effect of iron deficiency on physical performance and measurement of the body's capacity to utilize oxygen (maximal oxygen uptake) has been well documented in both human and animal studies (59). A linear relationship between decline in hemoglobin concentration and treadmill endurance time has been documented in human volunteers who have undergone repeated phlebotomies (21). In fact, it takes little fall in hemoglobin concentration to diminish physical performance. Gardner et al. described an average 20% reduction in treadmill exercise endurance time when subjects demonstrated a decrease in hemoglobin level from >13 gm/dl to 11.0–11.9 gm/dl (26).

Nonanemic Iron Deficiency

As noted above, endurance performance depends on energy availability not only via oxygen delivery but also from iron-dependent intracellular metabolic pathways. That the latter might be compromised by low levels of iron depletion insufficient to disturb hemoglobin formation has been supported by animal studies, but the critical question of whether nonanemic iron deficiency similarly impairs exercise performance in humans is yet to be convincingly demonstrated.

Animals

The key study in animals was performed by Finch et al., who described reduced treadmill endurance times in nonanemic iron-deficient rats, after which performance was improved with iron treatment (23). The study was comprised of four groups of animals, all of which were free of anemia throughout, since normal hemoglobin levels were maintained by removal or addition of blood via a venous catheter. The rats in Group A consumed an iron-deficient diet for four weeks before the start of exercise testing, while those in Group B were fed a normal diet. The animals in Group C ate an iron-deficient diet but this was supplemented with iron. The animals in Group D consumed an iron-deficient diet but began oral iron supplementation only when exercise testing began. On treadmill running, the animals in groups B and C, those with normal iron stores, could sustain exercise for 15–20 minutes, while those in groups A and D, who had nonanemic iron deficiency, could only last four minutes. Following four days of iron treatment, however, the group D animals increased run endurance times equivalent to those in groups B and C. Compared to those in groups B and C, the groups with nonanemic iron deficiency had not only depressed exercise performance but also biopsy evidence of depressed muscle concentrations of cytochromes, myoglobin, and iron-containing enzymes. This study, then, indicated that nonanemic iron deficiency—at least in rats—is functionally significant in reducing physical performance. In addition, the results imply that interference of normal iron-dependent cellular metabolism from body iron depletion accounted for this negative effect on endurance.

Subsequent studies by Davies et al. demonstrated that iron treatment of rats with severe iron deficiency anemia resulted in a rise in hemoglobin concentration and maximal oxygen uptake (14,15). However, no improvement in treadmill endurance time was observed until several days later when concentration of muscle oxidative enzymes began to rise.

Age of these animals may influence the effects of nonanemic iron deficiency on intracellular metabolism. Galan et al. described several reports indicating a 20%

to 50% decrease in intracellular myoglobin concentration in iron-deficient growing rats (25). However, no such depletion of myoglobin was observed in mature animals, even in the face of severe iron deficiency.

Humans

Conceptually, it should not be difficult to design a study that would definitively determine if nonanemic iron deficiency reduces physical performance in human beings. Randomly and blindly assign female endurance athletes in a particular sport with low ferritin levels but normal hemoglobin concentrations into iron-treated and untreated groups. Assure that the two groups are matched for initial ferritin and hemoglobin levels, habitual dietary iron intake, menstrual history, and training volume. Assess performance in the two groups by a competition-realistic performance task (if not a competitive event itself). Following a period of at least several weeks, during which the training regimen is similar in the two groups, retest for performance and analyze differences in pre- and post-test values. Examine pre- and post-measures of ferritin (as an indicator of compliance to the iron supplement) and hemoglobin levels (an increase would suggest pre-treatment anemia).

Needless to say, such an idealized study has yet to be performed. Among the many interventional studies which have attempted to answer the question, one observes a large variety of sports, subject groups, different criteria for threshold ferritin values, mixed training experience, different competitive levels, inadequate consideration of confounding variables, various regimens of iron dosage and duration, inadequate documentation of supplement compliance, possible individual differences in gastrointestinal iron absorption, and so forth. It is not possible to "blind" the study to the athletes—those who are receiving iron treatment will know so by the black coloration of their stools.

Particularly problematic is the marker employed for assessment of "physical performance." At a given time, so many variables contribute to any form of athletic performance (environmental conditions, competing athletes, time of day, recent diet, motivation, fatigue from previous exercise, psychological state) that assigning differences to a particular influence (i.e., iron deficiency) becomes formidable. The measure of performance in these interventional studies has sometimes been measured on exercise tests in the laboratory, and those in the field have not often mimicked a true competitive situation. Some investigations of athletes with nonanemic iron deficiency have utilized peak oxygen utilization (maximal oxygen uptake) as a "performance" marker (8). This is problematic, since studies in animals suggest that VO_2max reflects oxygen delivery (i.e., via hemoglobin) rather than skeletal muscle enzyme activity (14,15).

Too, there is the difficulty of interpreting small differences in performance between experimental groups that are statistically insignificant but which might be critically important in a competitive setting. That is, a 5-second advantage in endurance treadmill time in respect to iron status which fails to reach statistical significance might prove highly important in a competitive mile run.

It is evident that it has been—and will continue to be—a difficult challenge to experimentally answer the question of the physiological and functional significance of nonanemic iron deficiency. Considering these obstacles, it is perhaps not surprising that such investigations have revealed various and sometimes conflicting results.

One study attempted to mimic the design of the animal studies which supported a critical role of nonanemic iron deficiency on performance. Celsing et al. created iron deficiency anemia in human volunteers by serial phlebotomies over a 9-week period (9). The subjects, who demonstrated a predictable decrement of treadmill exercise performance, were then transfused to create normal hemoglobin levels, leaving them in a condition of nonanemic iron deficiency (mean ferritin 9 ng/ml). In this state, the exercise endurance returned to normal, indicating that nonanemic iron deficiency did not impair performance.

Newhouse et al. treated adult female recreational runners who had nonanemic iron deficiency with ferrous sulfate (320 mg daily) for 8 weeks (38). This regimen resulted in no differences in maximal treadmill velocity, maximal oxygen uptake, or Wingate test performance (short-burst fitness) compared to a control, non-treated group. A number of other studies have failed to support a negative effect of nonanemic iron deficiency on performance, as indicated by tests of treadmill endurance (33,45), cycle endurance time (55), 15-km cycling time trial (62), and shuttle run (4). In these studies, athletes with nonanemic iron deficiency failed to augment performance with oral treatment (20–135 mg elemental iron per day) or intramuscular iron injections for a period of 2–8 weeks.

On the other hand, a number of studies have supported the negative impact of nonanemic iron deficiency on performance in humans. Yoshida et al. described an improvement of 3,000-m run velocity from 281 to 291 m/min in female collegiate runners with initial ferritin <20 ng/ml and normal hemoglobin concentration after oral iron treatment for eight weeks (61). Six of seven of the female cross-country runners with nonanemic iron deficiency studied by Rowland et al. improved treadmill endurance time following four weeks of treatment with high doses of oral iron (975 mg daily ferrous sulfate) compared to untreated controls (52). Mean ferritin levels in the treated runners rose from 11 to 23 ng/ml. Hinton et al. (30) and LaManca and Haymes (34) demonstrated similar effects in 15-km cycle time trial and submaximal treadmill duration, respectively.

It has been suggested, on reasonable grounds, that many of the athletes whose performance improved after iron treatment for nonanemic iron deficiency in these studies may have actually had mild anemia, even with hemoglobin levels in the lower acceptable range (19). Evidence for this is suggested by a rise in hemoglobin level with iron therapy. That is, there is some chance that a female with a ferritin level of 5 ng/ml and a hemoglobin concentration of 12.2 mg/dl actually suffers from mild iron-deficiency anemia and, on that basis, would be expected to show improved performance on iron therapy. As evidence for this, interventional studies of athletes categorized as having nonanemic iron deficiency sometimes include those who demonstrate increases in hemoglobin concentration with iron therapy (i.e., references 8,27).

To summarize, "the research literature in human subjects suffers from numerous methodological weaknesses, and among the many studies cited, no two studies have used the same investigative approach. Confident conclusions consequently are problematic. Nevertheless, it is difficult to mount a compelling argument from these data that nonanemic iron deficiency impairs endurance performance in athletes" (50).

Points of Agreement

The confusion surrounding the meaning of nonanemic iron deficiency—commonplace among female athletes but of questionable physiological or performance significance—leaves those responsible for practical guidance to athletes in a difficult situation. Still, there are some aspects of the issue of iron deficiency in athletes that might be generally accepted by the majority:

- All athletes with recognized iron deficiency anemia should undergo a medical evaluation for determining cause of iron depletion and should receive therapeutic doses of oral iron.
- "Blind" iron supplementation of athletes (that is, without laboratory determination of iron status) is not advisable. Increased iron intake poses a risk for those with unrecognized hemochromatosis, a serious genetic disorder characterized by organ damage due to excess body stores of iron (63). In some athletes oral iron may cause gastrointestinal upset (cramping, diarrhea) and can theoretically interfere with absorption of other minerals such as copper and zinc. Despite this admonition, there exists evidence that some athletes do in fact routinely consume oral iron. A survey study in the United Kingdom indicated that 30% of highly competitive athletes routinely take iron supplements (46).
- Any athlete who demonstrates progressive deterioration of performance deserves determination of serum ferritin level and hemoglobin concentration. If nonanemic iron deficiency is detected, treatment should be provided with a daily dose of 100 mg of elemental iron daily for 2–3 months with a follow-up laboratory determination of iron status (two 325-mg ferrous sulfate tablets contain 130 mg elemental iron) (39). It should be noted that vitamin tablets with iron do not contain sufficient iron (typically about 18 mg) for this purpose.
- Athletes should be encouraged to consume an iron-adequate diet (1). Foods rich in iron (red meat, liver, lima beans, shellfish, green vegetables) are not typically popular components of the athlete's carbohydrate-laden diet. Athletes should

be counseled to regularly consume lean red meat (rich in heme iron) as well as iron-enriched breakfast cereals. However, improving iron status once deficiency develops is usually not effective by dietary manipulation alone (11,39).

Points of Discord

Other questions remain to be resolved. Should nonanemic iron deficiency (in an athlete who is performing well) automatically be treated? YES: Some studies have shown that mild iron deficiency does in fact impair performance in humans, as it clearly does in animals. By treating, the development of overt iron deficiency anemia is prevented (40). Moreover, the athlete may actually have a subtle degree of iron deficiency anemia, which would depress performance. NO: There exists no convincing evidence that exercise performance is compromised in humans. "Based on the literature, supplementation for the iron-depleted nonanemic athlete does not appear to be justified to solely improve performance" (49). And yet ANOTHER OPINION: The treatment decision depends on the level of hemoglobin. "Low ferritin with hemoglobin in the mid- to upper normal range is at best a relative indication for iron supplementation: low ferritin with hemoglobin in the low normal range is a stronger, yet still relative, indication for iron supplementation in athletes" (27).

Should endurance athletes, particularly females, undergo routine screening for detection of nonanemic iron deficiency? NO: If there are no indications for treatment (i.e., no loss of performance), why routinely screen? And the cost of determining ferritin and hemoglobin levels, particularly if these need to be serially repeated, may be prohibitive. A review of routine laboratory screening of athletes in a single university revealed an annual cost of over $20,000 (43). YES: "Given the high prevalence of iron depletion . . . screening for low iron stores at the start of a training program in female athletes involved in an endurance sport may be clinically useful" (16). Regular assessment of iron status may be particularly important for those at risk for iron deficiency, such as athletes consuming a vegetarian diet and those with a previous history of iron deficiency (50). The American Academy of Pediatrics has supported assessment of iron status in females "with a serious commitment to exercise performance" (57).

References

1. Alaunyte I, Stojceska V, Plunkett A. Iron and the female athlete: a review of dietary treatment methods for improving iron status and exercise performance. *J Int Soc Sports Nutr.* 2015;12:e38
2. Aldersey-Williams H. *Periodic Tales: A Cultural History of the Elements, from Arsenic to Zinc.* New York: Harper Collins; 2011. pp. 43–55.
3. Beard JL, Connor JR. Iron status and neural functioning. *Annu Rev Nutr.* 2003;23:41–58.
4. Blee T, Goodman C, Dawson B, Stapff A. The effect of intramuscular iron injections on serum ferritin levels and physical performance in elite netballers. *J Sci Med Sport.* 1999;2:311–321.

5. Braun WA, Flynn MG, Carroll KK, Brickman T, Lambert CP. Iron status and resting immune function in female collegiate swimmers. *Int J Sport Nutr Exerc Metab.* 2000;10:425–433.
6. British Nutrition Foundation. *Iron. Nutritional and Physiological Significance: The Report of the British Nutrition Foundation Tasks Force.* London: Chapman & Hall; 1985.
7. Bruner AB, Joffe A, Duggan AK, Casella JF, Brandt J. Randomised study of cognitive effects of iron supplementation in non-anemic iron-deficient adolescent girls. *Lancet.* 1996;348:992–996.
8. Burden RJ, Morton K, Richards T, Whyte GP, Pedlar CR. Is iron treatment beneficial in iron-deficient but nonanemic (IDNA) endurance athletes? A systematic review and meta-analysis. *Br J Sports Med.* 2015;49:1389–1397.
9. Celsing F, Blomstrand E, Werner B, Pihlstedt P, Ekblom B. Effects of iron deficiency on endurance and muscle enzyme activity in man. *Med Sci Sports Exerc.* 1986;18:156–161.
10. Chatard J-C, MujikaI, Guy C, Lacout J-C. Anaemia and iron deficiency in athletes. *Sports Med.* 199;27:229–240.
11. Clement DB, Sawchuck LL. Iron status and sports performance. *Sports Med.* 1984;1:65–72.
12. Clénin GE, Cordes M, Huber A, Schumacher YO, Noack P, Scales J, Kriemler S. Iron deficiency in sports—definition, influence on performance and therapy: consensus statement of the Swiss Society of Sports Medicine. *Swiss Med Weekly.* 2015;145:w14196.
13. Cook JD, Skikne BS. Iron deficiency: definition and diagnosis. *J Intern Med.* 1989;226:349–355.
14. Davies KJA, Donovan CM, Refino CJ, et al. Distinguishing effects of anemia and muscle iron deficiency on exercise bioenergetics in the rat. *Am J Physiol.* 1984;246:E535–E542.
15. Davies KJA, Maguire JJ, Brooks GA. Muscle mitochondrial bioenergetics, oxygen supply, and work capacity during dietary iron deficiency and repletion. *Am J Physiol.* 1982;242:E418–E426.
16. DelaValle DM, Haas JD. Impact of iron depletion without anemia on performance in trained endurance athletes at the beginning of a training season: a study of female collegiate rowers. *Int J Sports Nutr Exerc Metab.* 2011;21:501–506.
17. DeWijn JF, DeLongste JL, Mosterd W, et al. Haemoglobin, packed cell volume, serum iron, and iron binding capacity of selected athletes during training. *J Sports Med.* 1971;11:42–49.
18. Di Santolo M, Stel G, Banfi G, Gonan F, Cauci S. Anemia and iron status in young fertile non-professional athletes. *Eur J Appl Physiol.* 2008;102:703–709.
19. Eichner ER. Iron deficiency anemia. *Curr Sports Med Rep.* 2010;9:122–123.
20. Eichner ER. Perennial questions: on fatigue, on iron, and on anemia. *Curr Sports Med Rep.* 2012;11:274–275.
21. Ekblom B, Goldbarg AN, Gullbring G. Response to exercise after blood loss and reinfusion. *Acta Med Scand.* 1970;188:361–374.
22. Escanero JF, Villanueva J, Rojo A, Herrera A, del Diego C, Guerra M. Iron stores in professional athletes throughout the sports season. *Physiol Behav.* 1997;62:811–814.
23. Finch CA, Miller LR, Inamdar AR, et al. Iron deficiency in the rat. Physiological and biochemical studies of muscle dysfunction. *J Clin Invest.* 1976;58:447–452.
24. Fogelholm M, Rankinen T, Isokaanta M, Kujala U, Uusitupa M. Growth, dietary intake, and trace element status in pubescent athletes and school children. *Med Sci Sports Exerc.* 2000;32:738–746.
25. Galan P, Hercberg S, Touitou Y. The activity of tissue enzymes in iron deficient rat and man: an overview. *Comp Biochem Physiol.* 1984;77:647–552.

26. Gardner GW, Edgerton VR, Barnard RJ, et al. Cardiorespiratory, hematological and physical performance responses of anemic subjects to iron treatment. *Am J Clin Nutr.* 1975;28:982–989.
27. Garza D, Shrier I, Kohl HW, Ford P, Brown M, Matheson GO. The clinical value of serum ferritin tests in endurance athletes. *Clin J Sports Med.* 1997;7:46–53.
28. Goodman MN, Moore EW, Matsuda G. Darwinian evolution in the genealogy of haemoglobin. *Nature.* 1975;253:603–608.
29. Hallberg L, Hulten L, Lindstedt G, et al. Prevalence of iron deficiency in Swedish adolescents. *Pediatr. Res.* 1993;34:680–687.
30. Hinton PS, Giordano C, Brownlie T, Haas JD. Iron supplementation improves endurance after training in iron-depleted, nonanemic women. *J Appl Physiol.* 2000;88:1103–1111.
31. Kabasakalis A, Kalitsis K, Nikolaidis MG, et al. Redox, iron, and nutritional status of children with swimming training. *J Sci Med Sport.* 2009;12:691–696.
32. Kim J, Wessling-Resnick M. Iron and mechanisms of emotional behavior. *J Nutr Biochem.* 2014;25:1101–1107.
33. Klingshirn LA, Pate RR, Bourque SP, Davis JM, Sargent RG. Effect of iron supplementation on endurance capacity in iron-depleted female runners. *Med Sci Sports Exerc.* 1992;24:819–824.
34. LaManca J, Haymes F. Effects of iron repletion on VO_2max, endurance, and blood lactate in iron-depleted female runners. *Med Sci Sports Exerc.* 1993;24:819–824.
35. Lozoff B, De Andraca I, Castillo M, et al. Behavioral and developmental effects of preventing iron-deficiency anemia in healthy full-term infants. *Pediatrics.* 2003;112:846–854.
36. Miller BJ. Haematological effects of running. *Sports Med.* 1990;9:1–6.
37. Murray-Kolb IE, Beard JL. Iron treatment normalizes cognitive function in young women. *Am J Clin Nutr.* 2007;85:778–787.
38. Newhouse IJ, Clement DB, Taunton JE, et al. The effect of prelatent/latent iron deficiency on physical work capacity. *Med Sci Sports Exerc.* 1989:21:263–280.
39. Nickerson HJ, Holubets MC, Weiler BR, et al. Causes of iron deficiency in adolescent athletes. *J Pediatr.* 1989;114:657–661.
40. Nielsen P, Nachtigall D. Iron supplementation in athletes: current recommendations. *Sports Med.* 1998;26:207–216.
41. Ostojic SM, Ahmetovic Z. Indicators of iron status in elite soccer players during the sports season. *Int J Lab Hematol.* 2008;31:447–452.
42. Ostojic SM, Ahmetovic Z. Weekly training volume and hematological status in female top level athletes of different sports. *J Sports Med Phys Fitness.* 2008;48:398–403.
43. Parks RB, Hetzel SJ, Brooks MA. Iron deficiency and anemia among collegiate athletes: a retrospective chart review. *Med Sci Sports Exerc.* 2017;49:1711–1715.
44, Pate RR, Maguire M, VanWyke J. Dietary iron supplementation in women athletes. *Phys Sportsmed.* 1979;7:81–89.
45. Peeling P, Blee T, Goodman C, et al. Effect of iron injection on aerobic exercise performance of iron-depleted female athletes. *Int J Sport Nutr Exerc Metab.* 2007;17:221–231.
46. Petroczi A, Naughton DP, Mazanov J, Holloway A, Bingham J. Performance enhancement with supplements: incongruence between rationale and practice. *J Int Soc Sports Nutr.* 2007:4:19–28.
47. Risser WL, Lee EJ, Poindexter HBW, et al. Iron deficiency in female athletes: its prevalence and impact on performance. *Med Sci Sports Exerc.* 1988;20:116–121.
48. Robertson JD, Maughan RJ, Milne AC, Davidson RJ. Hematological status of male runners in relation to the extent of physical training. *Int J Sports Nutr.* 1992;2:366–375.

49. Rodenberg RE. Gustafson S. Iron as an ergogenic aid: ironclad evidence? *Curr Sports Med Rep*. 2007;6:258–264.
50. Rowland T. Iron deficiency in athletes: an update. *Am J Lifestyle Med*. 2012;6:318–326.
51. Rowland T, Black SA, Kelleher JF. Iron deficiency in adolescent endurance athletes. *J Adol Health Care*. 1987;8:322–326.
52. Rowland T, Deisroth MB, Green GM, Keller JF. The effect of iron therapy on the exercise capacity of non-anemic iron deficient adolescent runners. *Am J Dis Child*. 1988;142:165–169.
53. Rowland T, Kelleher JF. Iron deficiency in athletes. Insights from high school swimmers. *Am J Dis Child*. 1989;143:197–200.
54. Rowland T, Stagg L, Kelleher JF. Iron deficiency in adolescent girls: are athletes at increased risk? *J Adol Health Care*. 1991;12:22–25.
55. Schoene RB, Escourrou P, Robertson HT, Nilson KL, Parsons JR, Smith NJ. Iron repletion decreases maximal exercise lactate concentrations in female athletes with minimal iron deficiency anemia. *J Lab Clin Invest*. 1983;102:306–312.
56. Smith CH. *Blood Diseases of Infancy and Childhood*. St. Louis: Mosby; 1972. pp. 205–221.
57. Smith NJ. *Sports Medicine: Health Care for the Young Athlete*. Evanston, IL: American Academy of Pediatrics; 1983. P. 1.
58. Spodaryk K. Iron metabolism in boys involved in intensive physical training. *Physiol Behav*. 2002;75:201–206.
59. Woodson RD. Hemoglobin concentration and exercise capacity. *Ann Rev Resp Dis*. 1984;129 (Suppl):S72–S87.
60. Yehuda S, Youdim MBH. Brain iron: a lesson for animal models. *Am J Clin Nutr*. 1989;50:618–620.
61. Yoshida T, Udo M, Chida M, Ichioka M, Makiguchi K. Dietary iron supplement during severe physical training in competitive female distance runners. *Sports Training Med Rehab*. 1990;1:279–285.
62. Zhu YI, Haas JD. Altered metabolic response of iron-depleted nonanemic women during a 15-km time trial. *J Appl. Physiol*. 1998;84:1768–1775.
63. Zoller H. Vogel W. Iron supplementation in athletes—first do no harm. *Nutrition*. 2004;20:615–619.

13

WHO (OR WHAT) IS SETTING THE PACE?

Scenario #1 Standing at the starting line of a 10-km road race awaiting the gun, runner A is considering just how he'll set his pace: "For me, I know it's usually best to maintain the same pace throughout the race. The course today is flat, not really any hills, so I think this strategy will work. I'll monitor my sensations of fatigue, particularly my breathing rate, and then I can adjust the pace. If there's too much stress—I won't make it to the end in any reasonable shape at this speed—then I'll back off on the pace. If I'm feeling too comfortable after the first mile, I'll choose to pick up my speed. I've done enough racing that I know what level of fatigue I should be feeling to optimize my 10K time, so I can make a decision about pace, based on how much distance there is yet to go."

Scenario #2 Standing next to runner A, sharing his pre-race jitters, runner B is unaware that his subconscious brain is also considering pacing strategy: "Throughout the race," it (the subconscious brain) says to itself, "I'm going to pay close attention to markers of fatigue, like breathlessness, leg muscle stress, and body heat. From experience, I know that my guy here can run this distance without excessive stress or generally disgracing himself if he runs at a pace of 7:30 per mile. I will set his stride length and frequency to achieve this velocity in an *anticipatory* manner from the start of the race. Through millions of years of evolution, I've learned to recognize the markers of fatigue that would put my man at risk, and when these occur I will *create* uncomfortable feelings in his conscious as well as reduce central neurologic drive to his leg muscles that will slow him down."

Two diametrically opposed models of how pace is regulated in an endurance race, a dichotomy harkening back to the classic philosophical dilemma—are one's actions a matter of conscious free will? Or are they dictated by deterministic forces outside our conscious decision-making? In scenario #1 the decision regarding the pace to be taken during the race rests squarely on the shoulders of the runner. Runner A makes a cognitive decision regarding a proper velocity, or pattern of velocities, based on sensory input reflecting the stress of the race. The sensations of fatigue he feels alert him to regulate consciously his pace as a means of optimizing overall performance. But, instead, are actions pre-determined by the subconscious mind, molded by experience, genetic endowment, and sociocultural influences, outside one's own cognitive decision-making? In scenario #2, sensations of stress felt by runner B are *created* by the subconscious brain with the goal of not only prescribing the optimal pace based on past experience of the runner but, in addition, protecting him against potentially catastrophic outcomes which exceed limits of homeostatic safety.

This chapter will explore the bases of each of these models of pacing during endurance competitions, reviewing the evidence supporting each, as well as the influence of extrinsic factors (such as ambient temperature, competitors, and sex). Theoretical constructs will be contrasted with empiric observations of how athletes actually pace in the real world of sports competition.

It is important to recognize that there exist two separate issues here: First, the speed that the race should be run, which can be modified as the race progresses, and, second, the specific pattern of changes in speed that will occur in the race as strategized by the athlete beforehand (49). While these may demand separate decision-making, both share in common the goal of delivering the athlete to the finish line in the shortest time within the constraints of the physiological mechanisms responsible for exercise fatigue.

Fatigue and Its Physiological Markers

The limiting factor in any endurance athletic performance is the progression of muscular fatigue, normally defined in this context as physiological events that effect a failure to sustain an expected or desired force or power output (21). All tactics employed by athletes—equipment, training regimens, nutritional manipulation, mental preparation, and pacing strategies—are specifically designed to delay or reduce fatigue during competition and thereby enhance performance. A full discussion of the complex nature and still-unresolved etiology of fatigue during sports play is well beyond the scope of this chapter. Still, since perception of physiological manifestations of fatigue are key in dictating pacing strategies—either by cognitive decision-making or subconscious biological control—it is important to at least provide a capsule summary here (see refs. 2 and 6 for in-depth reviews).

While a single unified construct of the genesis of fatigue with endurance exercise remains elusive, a number of mechanisms have repeatedly been demonstrated in certain experimental models to contribute (36,43):

- Energy supply/demand imbalance. Energy provided by both aerobic and anaerobic metabolic pathways is contingent on adequate supply of intracellular oxidative substrate (glycogen stores) and circulatory support (adequacy of blood flow for oxygen delivery), as well as the metabolic capacity (i.e., mitochondrial density) of contracting muscle. A failure of any of the mechanistic components results in an inadequate supply of adenosine triphosphate (ATP), the energy source for muscular contraction.

- Metabolite accumulation. At high exercise intensities, aerobic pathways are supplanted by anaerobic metabolism, which generates byproducts of [H^+] and other ions which can interfere with cross-bridge coupling of actin-myosin filaments, with a resulting reduction in power production.
- Heat accumulation. Heat generated by the relatively low efficiency of muscular contraction must be dispelled by the body's thermoregulatory mechanisms (evaporation of sweat, convection at the skin surface via increased cutaneous blood flow). Prolonged high intensity exercise can produce a heat load which overwhelms these responses, causing core temperature to rise. Increased body temperature adversely affects the operation of all body systems, including cardiac and skeletal muscle contraction and cerebral function.
- Depressed central drive. The control of voluntary muscular activity begins in the brain, with descending signals down the spinal cord and on to the skeletal muscle, adjusting recruitment and frequency of firing of motor units. A decrease in such central function can occur from neuronal dysfunction or the influence of certain central nervous system neurotransmitters (i.e., serotonin).
- Peripheral neuromuscular fatigue. Interference with normal neuromuscular excitation-contraction coupling can occur at several locations in the periphery. These include particularly failure of transmission at the neuromuscular junction and alterations in release and reuptake of ionized calcium by the sarcoplasmic reticulum.

Any one or a combination of these processes define the limits of endurance exercise performance, and the extent of their impact on such performance is dictated by the intensity and duration of the exercise. As pacing strategies are aimed at establishing an appropriate work rate for the distance of the event, appreciating the level of such fatigue becomes important. Unfortunately, it is impossible for the runner to have any direct knowledge of the status of these processes and thus must rely on indirect markers of fatigue levels via sensory input as the race progresses. In reviewing the mechanisms outlined above one can make a list of such "signalers" of fatigue: exaggerated breathlessness, leg muscle weakness (inability to pick up the pace), increased body heat (sweating), light-headedness, and a difficult-to-describe but commonly appreciated generalized miserable sense of body discomfort.

Pacing and the Work Rate-Endurance Time Connection

It is intuitively obvious even to the novice runner that the longer the race, the slower one must go. Indeed, one can generate a peak power output for only about 5–6 seconds (as during a 100-m dash) before a fatiguing muscle slows one down. As the race distance is extended, one must run at a progressively lower percent of maximal power to escape encountered disabling fatigue before the completion of the race. When such relationships are expressed as true *endurance*, the distance (D) a certain speed can be maintained before limited by fatigue is inversely related to the running velocity (V) (which is the pace) (4,40). The two are not linked linearly, however (that is, a doubling of one is not associated with a halving of the other). Instead, the mathematical equation is a non-linear, power function: $D \sim aV^b$ where a and b are constants, and graphically the association of the two describes a hyperbolic curve. This form of association has been observed in various forms of exercise, including swimming, cycling (where power replaces velocity as the independent variable), and even weight lifting. In the latter case, work is expressed as weight lifted (as a percentage of one-repetition maximum, and number of repetitions replaces distance) (40).

Not surprisingly, the same relationships are observed when pace (or velocity) over a particular distance (V_d) is related to the distance itself (d) (this mimicking the condition observed in real-world running competitions). As far back as 1906, Kennelly described this "law of fatigue" in humans (using world records at the time) and horses as $V_d \sim ad^b$, where a is a constant and b has a value between 0.125 and 0.111 (29). Plotted graphically, the relationship again defines a hyperbolic curve, as indicated when one plots running distance against running pace (velocity). This mathematical relationship between velocity to run a distance and the distance itself seems to be universal in the world of exercise science, having been observed in cycling, skating, running, rowing, hurdling, swimming, and even isokinetic activities. M.S. Townsend has presented a graph showing an identical hyperbolic relationship when isometric holding time of knee-extensor muscles in adult athletes is plotted against the load being resisted (58).

There would seem to be here a clue to some fundamental nature of fatigue and its limiting control of exercise performance. These hyperbolic curves are, in effect, an indicator of the fatigue threshold created by the factors which define the limits of exercise capacity. The key to understanding the genesis of exercise-limiting fatigue might well reside in understanding what factor(s) is responsible for the shape of the curve. In this respect, too, it is intriguing to note that the curve crosses energy domains (i.e., anaerobic-aerobic), suggesting some continuum of a determinant which is common to fatigue in all forms of exercise, from weight lifting to ultramarathon running (50). Billat et al. commented that "all agree that the ultimate goal is to give a biochemical explanation for all aspects of the speed/time curve" (4). A number of explanatory models have been proposed (see ref. 4 for discussion), without any clear resolution.

Pacing Essentials

So, the longer the race, the lower the pace should be set relative to maximal speed. Let us assume, for the sake of this discussion, that the combined influences of all the above contributors to fatigue can be expressed collectively as "energy."

Standing at the starting line, one has, let's say, 100 units of energy available for the race. To achieve a maximal performance—the greatest speed for the distance—one would like to utilize this store of energy at such a rate during the race such that it is totally depleted just as one crosses the finish line (49). It would be a mistake to arrive with a surplus, or, on the other hand, to exhaust the stores of energy a mile before the finish. To achieve this goal, one must utilize the energy at just the right rate—a Goldilocks affair of not too rapidly, nor too slowly. The degree of work—the velocity—must be adjusted to the length of the race.

This all sounds elementary and evident. But it's not easily accomplished, and selecting a proper pacing strategy is what often separates the good from the not-so-good competitors. Effective pacing is a skill, one that requires training through experience. Endurance events are not exactly marked by dramatic moments of action-driven decision-making. No play-calling, pick and rolls, end-around sweeps, drop shots, and so forth that provide the "color" of other sports. No, it's just one foot in front of the other, another stroke and feather, a turn of the crank, not much different than the last one. The ability to select pace is one variable that provides distance athletes with the opportunity to maximize performance.

In scenario #1 that decision-making lies with the athlete. He or she must estimate from past experience a particular pace that's appropriate for the distance and then monitor those indicators of fatigue—breathlessness, leg weakness, discomfort, and so on—that provide a measure of how much is left in the tank. These are telling him or her what is the rate of energy consumption. The athlete must interpret these sensory feelings in light of the distance of the race. Is it signaling at the 3-mile mark that the level of fatigue, or the rate of energy consumption, is excessive for that distance? Then slow down. Or, if these signals indicate low levels of fatigue, that the stores of energy are high, speed up. In this cognitive model of pacing, it is the responsibility—or better yet, the opportunity—of the athlete, out on the course, all by him- or herself, to monitor sensory input and wisely adjust pace in accord with the distance of the race.

In scenario #2 this decision-making is taken over by a subconscious controller in the brain that sets pace in the same way—relating sensory markers of fatigue with race distance. Optimal performance is an expected outcome, but this central governor has a larger priority—constraining the runner from excessive levels of physical effort that would prove harmful. It does this by limiting motor activities through a) depressing central neurological drive to exercising muscle, and b) creating unpleasant sensations that effect a decrease or discontinuance of exercise effort. In the sections that follow, these different models of pacing will be discussed in more detail.

The Cognitive Pacing Model

The traditional interpretation of race pacing holds that the athlete *self-selects* pace (i.e., race velocity, an expression of work rate) by means of an integration between peripheral sensory feedback and the distance of the race (that is, the expected remaining workload) (3). The effect of combined sensory information on sensations of fatigue has been defined during research investigations by the *rating of perceived exertion (RPE)*, in which a subject reports subjective feelings of exercise stress on a scale of 6–20. The RPE, then, is an effort to change subjective feelings into an objective numerical marker of perception of fatigue.

Not surprisingly, RPE rises directly in respect to work intensity. Moreover, supporting the cognitive pacing model, RPE increases in an approximately linear fashion in respect to the proportion of the exercise event which has been completed (15,44). De Koning et al. contended that "together these data suggest that the athlete is continuously comparing how they feel at any moment in a competition with how they expected to feel at that moment. If their RPE is larger than expected for that point in the event, then power output (i.e., running speed) will decrease, even if it means giving up on the competition. If RPE is less than expected, then power output will increase. The process of controlling muscular power output via RPE apparently occurs continuously throughout an exercise bout and almost certainly takes into account the amount of distance remaining to be covered as well as the momentary value of RPE" (12). Supporting this conclusion, these authors demonstrated that what they termed a "hazard score," calculated as the product of RPE and percentage of distance remaining, explained variations in pacing elected by runners and cyclists (12).

An extensive number of investigations have been conducted to determine just what physiological marker accounts for the rise in RPE. That is, the question is, what cues to level of fatigue does the athlete use—consciously or unconsciously—to decide on an appropriate pace? These studies have found that, in fact, *all* such markers—labored breathing, heart rate, muscle stress, body temperature, blood lactate level—are directly associated with RPE during exercise. The problem is that RPE and all these factors are expected to rise with increasing exercise intensity, thereby confounding any interpretation of causality for any one marker. Consequently, "the literature on perceived exertion shows that there is not a single physiological variable which consistently explains perception of effort. . . . It may be concluded that effort perception involves the integration of multiple signals from a variety of perceptual clues" (23).

The importance of the ability of the athlete to voluntarily control pace is indicated by studies in which subjects are asked to perform at a given workload (53). When such an assigned work rate is different than a self-selected one, performance declines (34). Slorski and Abbiss concluded that "forcing athletes to adopt a given pacing profile might remove self-choice, giving them less control over the situation and influence performance and motivation. . . . Enforced or externally placed strategies force athletes to abandon their pacing pattern and minimize opportunities for self-managing fatigue" (53).

The Brain and Fatigue

The common-sense soundness of the cognitive model notwithstanding, a number of observations have raised awareness that brain activity can play a critical primary role in both the development of performance-limiting fatigue with exercise and pacing strategies. These findings would indicate that pacing decisions might bypass the cognitive mind and suggest alternative approaches to "selection" regarding appropriate pace during endurance sports events.

- Amann et al. blocked sensory pathways from leg muscles without affecting motor nerve activity in subjects who then performed a 5-km time trial (1). Lacking sensory input on muscle fatigue, the cyclists maintained a higher central motor drive and consequently altered pace during the simulated race compared to a control condition.
- Administration of pharmacological agents can alter both pace and performance (49). Dopaminergic agents increase performance and pedaling rate, while administration of serotonin and noradrenaline reduce power production, with a fall in performance and pace.
- When exercise is performed in hot ambient conditions, a reduction of pedaling rate (compared with that in a normothermic environment) is often observed during the early stages of exercise, long before any critical rise in body core temperature (60). This speaks to an anticipatory function of pace regulation.

The Central Governor Hypothesis

Effective pacing, that which establishes a velocity which provides just the right amount of effort—not too much, nor too little—during endurance competitions, involves the integration of sensory information regarding level of fatigue with the duration of the work to be completed (i.e., the distance of the race). In the traditional cognitive model this is accomplished by a thinking, calculating athlete. By the *central governor hypothesis* determination of appropriate pace is instead the responsibility of a subconscious controller within the brain. By this concept "pacing strategy is organized in an anticipatory way designed not only to optimize performance but also to prevent unreasonably large homeostatic disturbances during the exercise bout" (12).

This idea is not a new one. In his historical review, Tim Noakes cites the Italian physiologist A. Mosso, who wrote in 1915 that "fatigue is a sensation . . . nervous fatigue is the prepondering phenomenon, and muscular fatigue also is at bottom an exhaustion of the nervous system" (41,46). Nine years later A.V. Hill and his colleagues suggested that during high intensity exercise a governor "causes slowing of the circulation as soon as a serious degree of [oxygen] desaturation occurs, since it would obviously be very dangerous for [the heart] to be able to exhaust itself very completely" (27). In 1996, Ulmer proposed the concept of "teleo-anticipation," whereby a central "programmer," by a feedback control system, is responsible for optimal adjustment of metabolic rate during the heavy exercise of athletic competition in respect to a finishing point (61).

Most recently, Noakes and his co-workers at the University of Cape Town in South Africa have extended this concept to contend that the brain serves as an involuntary central governor during competitive exercise in a tripartite manner—anticipatory, monitoring, and, ultimately, protective—all with the goal of optimizing individual performance and safety (46,55,60).

Anticipation

According to this hypothesis, at the starting line of a 10K race the central governor, acting subconsciously, has already anticipated an appropriate beginning pace, based on the distance of the race and prior racing experience, as well as factors such as environmental conditions, terrain, presence of particular competitors, and health status. [Indeed, a mathematically knowledgeable central controller would be aware, based on past races, of the non-linear equation for pace over a given distance (V_D) versus the distance itself (D) described above ($V_D \sim aD^b$) which is specific for that particular individual. The controller would then simply have to plug in the distance in order to know what pace to start the race.]

As evidence for this, it is noted that values for factors such as RPE, rate of glycogen utilization, and body temperature rise during a race (or with progressive exercise) in a linear fashion and are superimposable when expressed as percentage of the time duration of the event rather than in absolute terms (15,19). For example, Faulkner et al. compared RPE values in nine men and women during a 7-mile road race and then again in a half marathon (15). As expected, the rate of rise of RPE was greater in the shorter race, but there were no differences when RPE was expressed as percent time of the race, implying "the brain uses a scalar timing mechanism" (15). For this to happen, the central controller must be aware of the distance-energy requirement relationship *at the start of the race* (60).

By this concept, the central governor acquires such pacing intelligence through compiling past race experiences. The validity of such a learning process might be tested by examining the pacing of run-naïve subjects over non-instructed repeat distance runs. That is, will a central controller enhance pacing strategies by "learning" with repeated experience? It's an investigation that might appropriately be performed in children, and Lambrick et al. have done just that (33).

These authors examined the pacing behavior of 13 inexperienced children ages 9–11 years who, without instructional intervention or feedback, performed a series of three self-paced individual 800-m time trials (33). Intriguingly, the pace pattern did not differ among the three trials. The basic pattern consisted of a fast start in the first 200 m, then an approximate 20% slowing to a steady pace in the middle portion of trial, followed by slight acceleration at the finish. This study, then, revealed no evidence of any unconscious learning process in pace in race-naïve subjects. However, as the authors noted, the pace pattern adopted by these children mimicked that commonly selected by trained adult runners.

They considered the findings "quite remarkable" in that "the children in this study having never experienced running continuous 800-m distance before the initial trial, they were able to i) demonstrate an appropriate pacing strategy for the given relative distance and ii) regulate their pace to employ an end spurt to optimize performance, without prior training or familiarization to the exercise task" (33). Might, they speculated, these results reflect an inherent genetic, evolutionary-based strategy of energy conservation during physical exercise, as proposed by Noakes (45)?

Micklewright et al. observed the same pacing pattern in their study of 106 children in four age groups (5–6, 8–9, 11–12, and 14 years) (39) who performed self-paced runs of 450 m, 600 m, 750 m, and 900 m, respectively. The authors indicated that "pacing strategy in schoolchildren differs with age and cognitive development" (the title of their manuscript), but the pacing patterns were in fact similar among groups, with a rapid start (25% above average pace) and then a declining speed in the midportion of the run to about 10% below average pace. The difference between groups was evident at the end, when the oldest demonstrated a finishing spurt which was not evident in the younger children. Overall, then, the pace strategy selected by these inexperienced children, without instruction or feedback, was almost identical to that found by Lambrick et al. on repeated trials. A later study from the same research group of 12-year-old schoolchildren who performed a 750-m timed run indicated the same pattern with an average pace of 15 km/hr in the initial portion, falling to a steady 12 km/hr speed in the middle, and then a slight spurt to 13 km/hr at the finish (5).

Interpretation of these pacing data in race-naïve children is clouded. Still, one cannot fail to suspect that some key insight is hidden in the observation of a) the identical pacing patterns revealed in three separate independent studies and b) the similarity of that pattern to the strategy commonly employed by elite adult endurance athletes.

Monitoring

During the race, the central governor monitors pace in relation to physiological cues to assess the appropriateness of its previously selected pace in respect to the distance yet to be covered. It then adjusts: if the initial pace was too fast, indicating that exhaustion will occur before the end of the race, pace is reduced. And conversely, if in its anticipatory calculation the pace is too slow, one that would permit too much reserve at the finish, speed is increased. All of this re-calculation and pace adjustment is performed repeatedly during the race, below the level of the runner's consciousness. It has been pointed out that this controlling function of adjusting pace to race distance demands a keenly sensitive intrinsic biological clock (55). Such a timekeeper must, in fact, be responsible for the scalar time frame of physiological functions and RPE noted above.

Safeguard

A central feature of the central governor hypothesis is that RPE takes on a different meaning than that in the traditional self-selection pacing model (60). In that cognitive model, RPE is considered as the athlete's feelings reflecting the level of the physiological markers of fatigue, and these sensations are used by the athlete to set pace in accordance with the race distance. In the central governor hypothesis, RPE is also a subjective marker of how one feels, but this sense of level of fatigue is a construct of the subconscious central governor, not a physical event (46). Rather it is an "emotion," created by the brain to set the limits of exercise, thereby *protecting* the athlete from risk. By this concept, then, maximal exercise effort is defined by RPE produced by the brain rather than by physiological limits of function. At the end of exhaustive exercise, muscle ATP content, glycogen stores, myocardial function, etc., are not, in fact, observed to be depleted (16,25). According to Noakes, "there is no evidence that homeostatic control fails at exhaustion in any form of exercise. . . . By contrast, the single variable that is always maximal at exhaustion during exercise is the rating of perceived exertion" (45).

Besides utilizing sensations of extreme fatigue to limit exercise, there is evidence that a central governor may also act to reduce active muscle recruited during high intensity extended exercise. St Clair Gibson et al. found that power output and muscle electromyographic activity fell during time trials of highly trained cyclists (56). They postulated that "the progressive reduction in neuromuscular activity may be the cause of fatigue in this trial as an anticipatory mechanism occurring at a subconscious level" (56).

The role of the central governor as a protector against catastrophic outcomes of excessive physical activity exercise was introduced back in Chapter 5. The idea here is that exercise exceeding certain bounds carries distinct risk—heat stroke, bone fractures, muscle tetany, cardiac dysrhythmias, myocardial ischemia, rhabdomyolysis. Acting in accord with Darwinian dictates, the central governor is proposed to serve as a benevolent dictator, limiting exercise and avoiding risk by overwhelming the athlete with unbearable feelings of fatigue. That is, it would speak contrary to accepted evolutionary biological tenets that body locomotion be designed without protection against the dangers of excessive motor activity.

Part of the evidence for the protective power of a central governor in this role is that such adverse events are extraordinarily rare among the many millions of competing endurance athletes. At the finish line they are, for the most part, all nauseated, lighted-headed, dyspneic, staggering, confused, or maybe even near syncopal, but virtually none will experience a catastrophic outcome. Still, is it possible for a purported central governor to be overridden by human will? In extremely rare situations of extreme determination and motivation (i.e., the collapsed ultramarathoner crawling to cross the finish line), or in constrained, inescapable situations (the drill instructor or coach demanding inappropriate work outputs in adverse environmental conditions), the answer would seem to be "yes." In some of these, an underlying pathology might be suspected, such as abnormal thermogenesis of muscle; in others, the influence of drugs, such as the tragic death of the cyclist Tom Simpson during the 1967 Tour de France from a combination of hyperthermia and amphetamines, could be responsible.

As was pointed out in Chapter 5, there has been no lack of objections to the central governor hypothesis, some of it rather outspoken. To wit: Inzlicht and Marcora: "The central governor resembles the fabled homunculus and is another theoretical soup stone—it appears to do theoretical work, but upon closer inspection is actually does very little" (28). Shephard: "There seems to be mounting evidence against several key correlates of this hypothesis. . . . Until there is convincing experimental evidence of an underlying physiological mechanism, most sports scientists will continue to express skepticism concerning the existence of a 'Central Governor'" (52). Edwards and Polman: "[We] suggest that brain regulation of exercise performance occurs by considering that the brain regulates performance via relative states of awareness rather than in conscious or subconscious states. In this context, awareness relates to performance without the need for an elusive and perhaps implausible intelligent central regulator within the subconscious" (14).

To sum up, then, it comes down to the essential question: Agreed by all, the human body can only physically exercise to a certain limit of endurance and/or intensity. But in performing a bout of endurance exercise to exhaustion, what is it that defines that maximal effort—be it in the laboratory on a progressive cycle test, or in the competitive world of a 10K race? In the traditional model, ascribed to by proponents of the cognitive model of pacing, this limit represents the functional limits of all those elements that contribute to exercise work (cellular metabolic capacity, cardiac output, oxygen uptake, etc.). And those repulsive, insufferable feelings of fatigue experienced by the athlete at the point of exhaustion are manifestations of those physiological processes pushed to their utmost.

To the advocates of the central governor hypothesis, on the other hand, a maximal effort is defined by the brain, acting in a subconscious manner to limit exercise levels that would place the athlete at risk for harmful outcomes. In this case, those unpleasant findings of fatigue are *created* by the brain controller to prevent further exercise. To those supporters of this argument, then, there is, physiologically speaking, no such thing as a "maximal effort"—there is always some reserve capacity. At the end of a marathon there are always glycogen stores, etc. But to encroach on such reserve would pose risk (Figure 13.1).

Pacing Pattern Strategies

A competitor in an endurance athletic event has the option of choosing among several patterns of pace during the race. Most simply, a stable submaximal pace

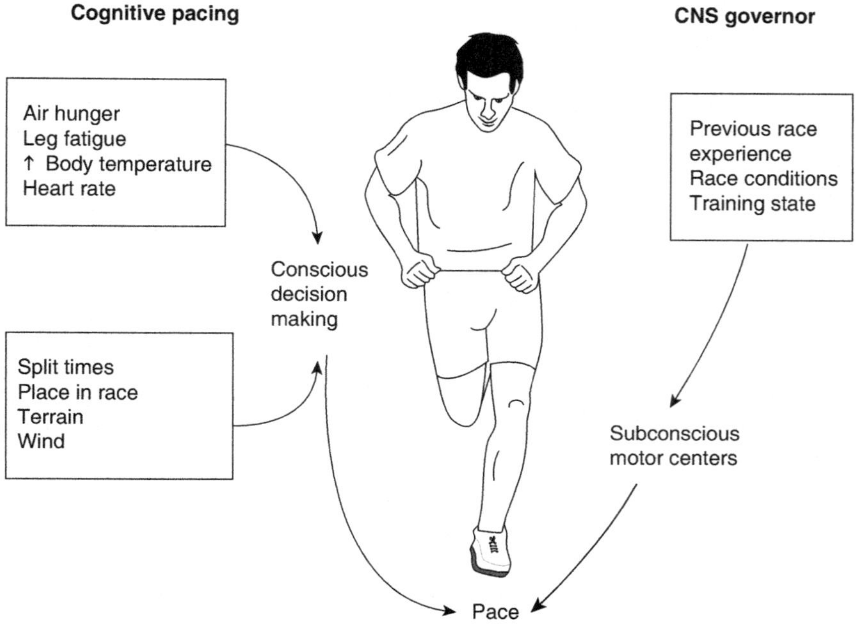

FIGURE 13.1 Two contrasting views on what determines "selection" of pace during distance running: the traditional cognitive approach whereby the runner dictates pace based on physiological signals of fatigue, and a proposed central governor which subconsciously controls pace based on optimizing performance and providing for runner safety.

Reprinted by permission from T.W. Rowland, *The Athlete's Clock: How Biology and Time Affect Sport Performance* (Champaign, IL: Human Kinetics, 2011), 10.

might be maintained throughout (even pacing). Or, a fast start, slowing to a steady slower pace during the central portion of the race, then a spurt toward the finish (positive pacing). Alternatively, a slow comfortable start, saving for a rapid finish (negative pacing).

A number of theoretical constructs have been advanced as to which strategy might be most effective, mostly based on sequences of temporally parceling out energy expenditure. Specifically, these have suggested advantages of certain patterns of pacing in respect to supply and utilization of anaerobic versus aerobic energy sources (3,18). It is difficult to discern any particular consistent take-away messages among these. What might be expected to be more relevant to the question are studies which have compared performance in endurance athletes relative to specific pacing strategies. Unfortunately, such reports have not revealed any consistent conclusions either, which has been attributed to the influence of many variables which might potentially affect distribution of energy expenditure during a race (weather, terrain, distance, individual fitness level, competitors, etc.).

Nonetheless, the general wisdom out in the sports world reflects the summary conclusions of reviews of these data by Foster et al. (18) and Abbiss and Laursen (3): For endurance events of relatively short duration, a positive pacing pattern with initial pace or power output after the start above average pace, while resulting in an early rate of carbohydrate depletion and lactate accumulation, can provide overall race benefits by shortening acceleration time (important particularly, for example, in rowing competitions). For races of longer duration, the customary advice is to not stray far from a constant pace throughout. That's because "as even minor fluctuations in speed can result in greater energy cost, it is possible that overall performance times during prolonged events may be optimized when acceleration and deceleration is minimized" (3).

At the same time, an early positive pacing strategy which is commonly elected by distance athletes may have no deleterious effect on performance. Gosztyla et al. reported that among 11 female distance runners, no differences were demonstrated in 5-km trial performance when employing even split times or early paces that were 3% and 6% above average pace (22). There are, in fact, reports indicating that a positive pacing start may offer certain overall metabolic advantages over the duration of the race (i.e., greater fraction of VO_2max) (51). Still, "it is possible that a relatively fast starting strategy during competition may be the result of unrealistic ambitious perceptions regarding personal athletic ability" (3).

Those who prefer a more comfortable start with negative pacing (with the joy of passing up competitors later in the race) can find comfort in the report by Mattern et al. (37). These investigators found that in 20-km cycling time trials, a low starting power output (15% less than self-selected power) resulted in lower lactate levels and improved trial performance compared to self-paced trials.

One of the problems with these kinds of studies is determining what constitutes a truly meaningful difference in performance between pacing strategies. For example, Hettinga et al. examined the effect of altering pacing strategy during 1,500-m time trials—even pacing in contrast to positive and negative pacing (115% and 95% of mean power output during the first 750 m, respectively [26]). Anaerobic and aerobic work each were not significantly different in the three trials. However, when combined, the total metabolic work was 2% greater in the even pacing trial compared to the other two, which the authors considered might "be relevant to sports performance" (26).

A "best" pacing strategy from these experimental data remains elusive. As St Clair Gibson et al. have concluded, "there appears to be no clear optimal pacing strategy identified by previous research, and it may be that each individual has a uniquely optimal pacing strategy" (55).

Empiric Observations

So, enough theory. Let's examine the observations of how endurance athletes actually elect to pace themselves during race competition. It should be noted that the great majority of these reports involve elite, highly trained athletes whose race strategies undoubtedly reflect volumes of experience and training. That is, these competitors are at the far end of the learning curve. Just how these approaches to race pacing strategies might be transposed to those of recreational athletes remains to be explored.

The most common preferred pace among endurance athletes appears to be that of a rapid start, slow to steady pace in the middle, and acceleration with a fast spurt as the finish line approaches. This pattern has been described in world record-holders for 1,500-, 5,000-, and 10,000-m events (47,59), competitors in open water 10-km world swimming championships (48), elite cross-country skiers (17,35), elite track cyclists (6), middle-distance speed skaters (42), and elite 400-m freestyle swimmers (38). (Theoretical considerations would dictate, however, that the latter would be best utilizing an even pacing strategy, since the resistance created by the water increases exponentially with swim velocity [57].)

Descriptions of these patterns in relation to race time often indicate that the portion of the pacing pattern that distinguishes the talented from not-so-talented athlete is the ability to perform that final spurt to the finish. This observation might suggest that if one is not among the top competitors in a race, an even pace would be best to enable a stronger finish. Still, which of these strategies would provide the best overall race time for those in the back of the pack is unclear.

Attempts to gain an early lead with a fast start strategy is common among rowers (13,20). This jump start serves to accelerate the boat but also provides tactical advantages, since the rowers can see the other boats and avoid their wake. An exception to this trend toward positive pacing are champion racewalkers, who often adopt a negative pacing strategy (24).

For Those Wondering About Racehorses

Do racehorses pace? This may seem like an odd moment to interject this question. But racehorses do not cognitively plan how to set pace during separate parts of a race. They do not spend the evening before plotting if they should go off at a brisk pace, then slow. Or keep it steady and hope this can be maintained for a fast finish. Or trail at the back of the pack, only to surge forward rounding the final turn. Perhaps there is something to be learned regarding pacing in mammals other than human beings. One could argue that, yes, racehorses are not cognitive beasts, but they have been bred to race and moreover are subjected to extrinsic factors, such as competing horses, and, most particularly, the controlling influence of a jockey.

These considerations notwithstanding, the report of Spence et al. of pacing strategies in 44,803 racehorses in 3,357 races using a radio tracking system are interesting and perhaps instructive (54). These involved races ranging in distance from 1,000 to 4,225 m in length with race times from 50 seconds to 5 minutes in duration. They found that a "breakpoint" occurred in the latter portions of the race when the speeds of the competing horses began to diverge. That is, races were won or lost in the last 500 m or so. Over 90% of the horses slowed after the breakpoint following a period in the middle portion of the race during which speed was increasing or stable. This deceleration amounted to, on the average, about 15% below peak pace. In effect, then, "the horse that slows down the least, wins" (54). (This is reminiscent of the same phenomenon in humans in short-distance sprints.) The authors considered that among Thoroughbred racehorses, "higher speeds ... may arise due to the nature of the pack racing itself, or may be a reflection of individual capabilities, that is, corresponding to horses that perform well in roles suited to their 'front running' or 'chaser' personality traits" (54).

Extrinsic Influences on Pacing

Questions of how and why distance athletes pace during competition are confounded by what to all competitors is obvious—*ça dépend* (it depends). That is, pacing decisions are influenced by a number of significant variables.

Heat

Clearly an increase in body core temperature during exercise performed in the heat diminishes performance. Still, the mechanism(s) for this decline remains controversial. Dehydration, diminished central drive, circulatory inadequacy, mental fatigue, and a direct depression of skeletal muscle function are among the candidates.

Pacing is also altered during progressive exercise in hot environmental conditions, which typically exhibits a progressive fall off of power output (8). This is evident from the early portions of a bout of exercise and then becomes more pronounced in the middle and later stages. It has been suggested that pacing is adjusted to avoid accelerated rises in core temperature, but other factors, such as rise in skin temperature, RPE, and thermal sensations could be involved (8).

However, allusion has already been made earlier in this chapter to the finding that power output and muscle electromyographic activity are diminished early during exercise in the heat at a point when core temperature, heart rate, and RPE are similar to that in cool conditions (60). This implies an anticipatory element to pacing in the heat.

Sex

The pacing strategies of females tend to be different from that of males. This has been reported in marathon running (10), 5-km high school cross-country running (11), 10-km road races (9), and triathlon events (30). In all these reports the sex difference is consistent—men are more likely to slow down during the middle stages of the race. For example, Deaner et al. examined percentage change in the second half of 14 marathon races compared to the pace in the first half (10). The average change in pace was −15.6% and −11.7% for males and females, respectively, a magnitude of difference that was observed in all 14 races.

The explanation for pacing differences during distance running in men and women is obscure. Metabolic differences between the sexes, such as rate of glycogen utilization, as well as anthropometric factors (such as limb length) have been proposed (30). However, as the same sex difference in pacing has been documented in a 5-km race, in which glycogen depletion is irrelevant, Deaner and Lowen suggested that "sex differences in pacing partly reflect a sex difference in some aspect of decision making, such as overconfidence, risk perception, or willingness to tolerate discomfort" (11).

Competitors

Corbett et al. examined the effects on pacing and performance in the laboratory of cycle power production in a 2,000-m time trial in the presence of a virtual competitor (simulated on a projected screen) (6). As expected, performance was improved while "competing" compared to a solo time trial. The basic pacing pattern were similar in the two conditions, with an initial peak in the first 500 m followed by a steady decline during the rest of the trial. No end spurt was observed in either case. During the "head-to-head" competition, however, the initial rise in power was greater. Similar findings were reported by Konings et al., who found that the presence of a virtual opponent triggered a faster, more aggressive strategy in the first half of a 4-km cycling time trial (32). Confirming this trend, a later study by Konings and Hettinga revealed that in short-track speed skating competitions, the number of competitors in a race was directly related to the velocity of initial pace (31).

Concluding Thoughts

It might be expected that very few competitive distance runners are willing to accept the idea that race pace is outside their individual control. Their common experience is to the contrary—it is obvious that consideration of run velocity is adjusted to race distance based on prior experience as well as sensory input signaling moment-to-moment level of fatigue. That an involuntary controller in the central nervous system is in reality dictating pace is an anathema, contrary to their concept of sports competition as a marker of individual free will and their personal identity as an athlete.

But, once again, as we've asked in other chapters in this book, are we being fooled? That the human brain is capable of independent action outside the realm of our conscious self, performing functions that common sense would indicate is an outcome of cognitive decision-making, is, in fact, a recurring theme in these chapters. The problem here is that very instrument we utilize to decide this point, the conscious thinking brain, is the same one that we are suggesting might be being deceived. That is, how would it be able to tell?

The likelihood that subconscious brain function controls much of our decision-making is consistent with contemporary views that the brain acts as a controller of mental function instead of serving as simply a passive, reflective organ acting in response to sensory input. This idea is supported by brain imaging studies which demonstrate that actions and decisions we once took for granted were cognitively derived are, in fact, manifestations of subconscious functions of which we are unaware. In this light, current concepts regarding control of race pacing by athletes may open up new windows of insight on the importance of cerebral function in controlling human function and behavior.

As for the pattern of pacing, the wisdom of dividing up pace by one means in a race over another is still unsettled. Perhaps the best conclusion has been provided by Carl Foster and his colleagues, that defining a "best" pacing strategy for any given race, considering distance, terrain, weather, fellow competitors, and training status, might be best considered a learning process for the individual athlete (18).

References

1. Amann M. Central and peripheral fatigue: interaction during cycling exercise in humans. *Med Sci Sports Exerc.* 2011;43:2039–2045.
2. Abbiss CR, Laursen PB. Models to explain fatigue during prolonged endurance cycling. *Sports Med.* 2005;35:865–898.
3. Abbiss CR, Laursen PB. Describing and understanding pacing strategies during athletic competition. *Sports Med.* 2008;38:239–252.
4. Billat LV, Koralsztein JP, Morton RH. Time in human endurance models: from empirical models to physiological models. *Sports Med.* 1999;27:359–379.
5. Chinnasamy C, St Clair Gibson A, Micklewright D. Effect of spatial and temporal cues on athletic pacing in schoolchildren. *Med Sci Sports Exerc.* 2013;45:395–402.
6. Corbett J. An analysis of the pacing strategies adopted by elite athletes during track cycling. *Int J Sports Physiol Perf.* 2009;4:195–205.
7. Corbett J, Barwood MJ, Ouzounoglou A, Thelwell R, Dicks M. Influence of competition on performance and pacing during cycling exercise. *Med Sci Sports Exerc.* 2012;44:509–515.
8. Davies MJ, Clark B, Welvaert M, et al. Effect of environmental and feedback interventions on pacing profiles in cycling: a meta-analysis. *Front Physiol.* 2016;7:e591.
9. Deaner RO, Addona V, Carter RE, Joyner MJ, Hunter SK. Fast men slow more than fast women in a 10 kilometer road race. *PeerJ.* 2016;4:e2235.
10. Deaner RO, Carter RE, Joyner MJ, Hunter SK. Men are more likely than women to slow in the marathon. *Med Sci Sports Exerc.* 2015;47:607–616.
11. Deaner RO, Lowen A. Males and females pace differently in high school cross-country races. *J Strength Cond Res.* 2016;30:2991–2997.
12. De Koning JJ, Foster C, Bakkum A, et al. Regulation of pacing strategy during athletic competition. *PLoS ONE.* 2011;6:e15863.
13. Edwards AM, Guy JH, Hettinga FJ. Oxford and Cambridge boat race: performance, pacing and tactics between 1890 and 2014. *Sports Med.* 2016;46:1553–1562.
14. Edwards AM, Polman RCJ. Pacing and awareness: brain regulation of physical activity. *Sports Med.* 2013;43:1057–1064.

15. Faulkner J, Parfitt G, Eston R. The rating of perceived exertion during competitive running scales with time. *Psychophysiol.* 2008;45:977–985.
16. Fitts RH. Cellular mechanisms of muscle fatigue. *Physiol Rev.* 1994;74:49–94.
17. Formenti D, Rossi A, Calogiuri G, Thomassen TO, Scurati R, Weydahl A. Exercise intensity and pacing strategy of cross-country skiers during a 10 km skating simulated race. *Res Sports Med.* 2015;23:126–139.
18. Foster C, Schrager M, Snyder AC, Thompson NN. Pacing strategy and athletic performance. *Sports Med.* 1994;17:77–85.
19. Gant N, Williams C, King J, Hodge BJ. Thermoregulatory responses to exercise: relative versus absolute intensity. *J Sports Sci.* 2004;22:1083–1090.
20. Garland SW. An analysis of the pacing strategy adopted by elite competitors in 2000 m rowing. *Br J Sports Med.* 2005;39:39–42.
21. Gibson H, Edwardes RHT. Muscular exercise and fatigue. *Sports Med.* 1985;2:120–132.
22. Gosztyla AE, Edwards DG, Quinn TJ, Kenefick RW. The impact of different pacing strategies on five-kilometer running time trial performance. *J Strength Cond Res.* 2006;20:882–886.
23. Hampson DB, St Clair Gibson A, Lambert MI, Noakes TD. The influence of sensory cues on the perception of exertion during exercise and central regulation of exercise performance. *Sports Med.* 2001;31:935–952.
24. Hanley B. An analysis of pacing profiles of world-class racewalkers. *Int J Sports Physiol Perf.* 2013;8:435–441.
25. Helge JW, Richter EA, Kiens B. Interaction of training and diet on metabolism and endurance during exercise in man. *J Physiol.* 1996;492:293–306.
26. Hettinga FJ, De Koning JJ, Meijer E, Teunissen L, Foster C. The effect of pacing strategy on energy expenditure during a 1500-m cycling time trial. *Med Sci Sports Exerc.* 2007;39:2212–2218.
27. Hill AV, Long CHN, Lupton H. Muscular exercise, lactic acid, and the supply of oxygen. *Proc Roy Soc Brit.* 1924;97:438–475.
28. Inzlicht M, Marcora SM. The central governor model of exercise regulation teaches us precious little about the nature of mental fatigue and self-control failure. *Front Psychol.* 2016;7:e656.
29. Kennelly AE. An approximate law of fatigue in the speeds of racing animals. *Proc Am Acad Arts Sci.* 1906;42:275–331.
30. Knechtle B, Nikolaidis PT. Sex differences in pacing during 'Ultraman Hawaii'. *Peer J.* 2016;4:e2509.
31. Konings MJ, Hettinga FJ. The impact of different competitive environments on pacing and performance. *Int J Sports Physiol Perf.* 2017;12:1–21.
32. Konings MJ, Schoenmakers PP, Walker AJ, Hettinga FJ. The behavior of an opponent alters pacing decisions in 4-km cycling time trials. *Physiol Behav.* 2016;158:1–5.
33. Lambrick D, Rowlands A, Rowland T, Eston R. Pacing strategies of inexperienced children during repeated 800 m individual time-trials and simulated competition. *Pediatr Exerc Sci.* 2013;25:198–211.
34. Lander PJ, Butterly RJ, Edwards. Self-paced exercise is less physically challenging than enforced constant pace exercise of the same intensity: influence of complex central metabolic control. *Br J Sports Med.* 2009;43:789–795.
35. Losnegard T, Kieldsen K, Skattebo O. An analysis of the pacing strategies adopted by elite cross-country skiers. *J Strength Cond Res.* 2016;30:3256–3260.
36. MacLaren DM, Gibson H, Parry-Billings M, Edwards RHT. A review of metabolic and physiological factors in fatigue. *Exerc Sport Sci Rev.* 1989;17:29–66.

37. Mattern CO, Kenefick RW, Kertzer R, et al. Impact of starting strategy on cycling performance. *Int J Sports Med.* 2001;22:350–355.
38. Mauger AR, Neuloh J, Castle PC. Analysis of pacing strategy selection in elite 400-m freestyle swimming. *Med Sci Sports Exerc.* 2012;44:22–25.
39. Micklewright D, Angus C, Suddaby J, St Clair Gibson A, Sandercock G, Chinnasamy C. Pacing strategy in schoolchildren differs with age and cognitive development. *Med Sci Sports Exerc.* 2012;44:362–369.
40. Morton RH, Hodgson DJ. The relationship between power output and endurance: a brief review. *Eur J Appl Physiol.* 1996;73:491–502.
41. Mosso A. *Fatigue.* London: Allen & Unwin Ltd.; 1915.
42. Muehlbauer T, Schindler C, Panzer S. Pacing and performance in competitive middle-distance speed skating. *Res Q Exerc Sport.* 2010;81:1–6.
43. Noakes TD. Physiological models to understand exercise fatigue and the adaptations that predict or enhance athletic performance. *Scand J Med Sci Sports.* 2000;10:123–145.
44. Noakes TD. Linear relationship between the perception of effort and the duration of constant load exercise that remains. *J Appl Physiol.* 2004;96:1571–1572.
45. Noakes TD. Is it time to retire the A.V. Hill model? A rebuttal to the article by Professor Roy Shepard. *Sports Med.* 2011;41:263–277.
46. Noakes TD. Fatigue is a brain-derived emotion that regulates the exercise behavior to ensure the protection of whole body homeostasis. *Front Physiol.* 2012;3:e82.
47. Noakes TD, Lambert MI, Hauman R. Which lap is the slowest? An analysis of 32 world mile record performances. *Br J Sports Med.* 2009;43:760–764.
48. Rodriguez L, Veiga S. Effect of the pacing strategies on the open water 10km world swimming championships performances. *Int J Sports Med.* 2017;12:1–19.
49. Roelands B, de Koning J, Foster C, Hettinga F, Meeusen R. Neurophysiological determinants of theoretical concepts and mechanisms involved in pacing. *Sports Med.* 2013;43:301–311.
50. Rowland T. Thoughts on a hyperbolic curve. *Pediatr Exerc Science.* 2007;19:1–5.
51. Sandals LE, Wood DM, Draper SB, et al. Influence of pacing strategy on oxygen uptake during treadmill middle-distance running. *Int J Sports Med.* 2006;27:37–42.
52. Shephard RJ. Is it time to retire the 'central governor'? *Sports Med.* 2009;39:709–721.
53. Skorski S, Abbiss CR. The manipulation of pace within endurance sport. *Front Physiol.* 2017;8:e102.
54. Spence AJ, Thurman AS, Maher MJ, Wilson AM. Speed, pacing strategy and aerodynamic drafting in Thoroughbred horse racing. *Biol Lett.* 2012;8:678–681.
55. St Clair Gibson A, Lambert EV, Rauch LHG, et al. The role of information processing between the brain and peripheral physiological systems in pacing and perception of effort. *Sports Med.* 2006;36:705–722.
56. St Clair Gibson A, Schabort EJ, Noakes TD. Reduced neuromuscular activity and force generation during prolonged cycling. *Am J Physiol.* 2001;281:R187–R196.
57. Thompson KG, MacLaren DP, Lees A, Atkinson G. The effect of even, positive and negative pacing on metabolic, kinematic and temporal variables during breaststroke swimming. *Eur J Appl Physiol.* 2003;88:438–443.
58. Townsend MS. *Mathematics in Sports.* Chichester: Ellis Horwood Ltd.; 1984.
59. Tucker R, Lambert MI, Noakes TD. An analysis of pacing strategies during men's world-record performances in track athletes. *Int J Sports Physiol Perf.* 2006;1:233–245.

60. Tucker R, Rauch L, Harley YX, Noakes TD. Impaired exercise performance in the heat is associated with anticipatory reduction in skeletal muscle recruitment. *Pflugers Arch.* 2004;448:422–430.
61. Ulmer HV. Concept of an extracellular regulation of muscular metabolic rate during heavy exercise in human by psychophysiological feedback. *Experientia.* 1996;52:416–420.

14

COURTS-MÉTRAGES (SHORT SUBJECTS)

What Causes Exercise-Associated Muscle Cramps?

Anyone who watches sports has witnessed the familiar scenario. The season has just started, and the climatic conditions happen to be hot, often unexpectedly so. In the midst of the competition, a player suddenly clutches his calf in the agonizing pain of a muscle spasm and collapses. The action is halted, a trainer races out to stretch the player's leg, and more often than not the sufferer limps off under support to the locker room for salutary therapies of electrolyte drinks and intravenous fluids. "I hope," says the television announcer, "that it's only a cramp."

What's going on here? What would cause all those muscle fibers to contract vigorously in one painful spasm, to deprive the home team from the services of its star point guard at a critical juncture of the game? The surprising answer is that nobody really knows. There exist two camps of opinion. One, the traditional viewpoint, is that a combination of heat, dehydration, and electrolyte imbalance are responsible. The other, one that its supporters consider a more enlightened perspective, holds that exercise-induced cramps are a manifestation of muscle fatigue, a disturbance of neurological activation and relaxation.

Frequency

The frequency of top athletes suffering from exercise-induced cramping during competition is remarkably high. A majority of triathletes report having experienced cramps (28). For example, Schwellnus et al. studied participants in the Two Oceans Ultramarathon, a 56-km race in South Africa (54). Of the 72 runners, 19 (26%) experienced muscular cramping during the race. All reported that their leg cramps had developed in the second half of the race, and two-thirds of these runners described cramping immediately after crossing the finish line. Most were located in the calf muscles (hamstrings), but over a third originated in the thigh (quadriceps). The runners reported that they could best relieve their cramps by decreasing the race pace (76%) or passive stretching (52%).

Pathogenesis

The mechanism underlying an exercise-induced muscle cramp is, to put it simply, a sudden burst of motor neuron activation of skeletal muscle contraction. But just *why* this occurs is uncertain. Some evidence supports a central basis; that is, that such a crescendo of neurologic stimulation originates in the spinal cord and central nervous system (37). Other data indicate a peripheral hyper-excitation, whereby abnormal discharges occur in the terminal branches of the motor axons.

It should be recognized that deciphering neuromuscular mechanisms underlying cramps is not an easy task, given their sporadic nature. In the laboratory, electrical stimulation has been most commonly utilized to induce cramps (37), but how findings in such studies might or might not accurately reflect exercise-induced cramping on the athletic field remains problematic.

As noted above, two theories have been disputed surrounding the etiology of muscle cramping during sports play. One holds that vigorous exercise in hot environments without adequate hydration depletes body fluid content and leads to electrolyte disturbances, the combined effect of which triggers muscle cramping. The other holds that the key issue is, instead, fatigue of neuromuscular processes. It is not inconceivable that the truth might lie in causative contributions from both processes.

Dehydration and Electrolyte Imbalance

The idea that exercise-induced muscle cramps reflect disturbances of body hydration and electrolyte balance probably originated in the observation of frequent cramping of dehydrated miners and sailors working in hot environmental conditions (9). As dehydration and alterations in serum electrolytes are observed following endurance sports events such as marathons (21), this concept was transferred to athletes and became generally accepted dogma, based largely on anecdotal evidence.

Two studies supported the idea that excessive sodium loss via sweating in athletes might predispose to muscle cramping (23,58). Stofan et al. studied sweating sodium losses in Division I American collegiate football players during a training camp (58). Compared to players with no history of muscle cramps, those who had experienced past cramps demonstrated over twice the sodium losses in sweat. Horswill et al. compared serum sodium changes in response to a 2-hour training session in hot conditions in six football players who had a history of cramps with extensive sweating to eight subjects without previous cramping (23l). Average sweat sodium concentration was 53 ± 29 mmol/L in the cramping-history group and 38 ± 18 mmol/L in the controls, a difference that did not reach statistical significance. During the training session the serum sodium concentration fell from 137.8 ± 2.3 to 135.7 ± 3.1 mmol/L in the cramping-history players and remained stable in the controls (138.9 ± 1.8–139.0 ± 2.0). The authors interpreted these results as indicating that the athletes with a past history of cramps and greater sodium sweat losses "tended to experience a decline in [serum sodium concentration] . . . [and that] these changes may place cramp-prone players at greater risks for developing acute sodium deficits during training."

In a 2007 article, Randy Eichner summarized the attitude of many trainers, coaches, and sports physicians in response to such findings:

> Three lines of evidence suggest heat cramping is caused by "salty sweating," specifically the triad of salt loss, fluid loss and muscle fatigue. The first line of evidence is historical. Dating back 100 years, heat cramping in industrial workers was alleviated by saline, and in a self-experiment, salt depletion provoked muscle cramping. The second line of evidence is from field studies of athletes. In tennis and football alike, heat crampers tend to be salty sweaters. . . . The third line of evidence is practical experience with therapy and prevention. Intravenous saline can reverse heat cramping, and more salt in the diet and in sports drinks can help prevent heat cramping. For heat cramping, the solution is saline.
>
> *(10)*

Michael Bergeron echoed these conclusions in considering factors underlying muscle cramps in tennis players: "Evidence suggests that, when a tennis player cramps in warm to hot weather, extensive and repeated sweating during the current and previous matches and a consequent sodium deficit are usually the primary contributing factors. . . . Appropriate and sufficient salt and fluid intake will enhance rehydration and fluid distribution throughout a player's body, so that heat cramps can be completely averted, even during long matches in the most challenging environments" (3).

In an intervention study, Jung et al. sought to determine if hydration and electrolyte supplementation would influence rate of cramping (27). College-aged men (n = 13) with a past history of exercise-associated cramping performed exercise to promote fatigue in calf muscles in a hot environment with and without consumption of a carbohydrate-electrolyte beverage. The frequency of triggered cramps was similar in the two conditions, but cramp onset was delayed when the drink was consumed (mean 37 minutes to 15 minutes).

On the other hand, Schwellnus outlined arguments against the electrolyte depletion/dehydration hypothesis for the genesis of exercise-associated muscle cramps (52):

- No study has ever demonstrated that serum electrolyte concentrations, level of hydration, or sweat electrolyte concentrations are abnormal in athletes at the time of their cramping.

- Although muscle cramping occurs more often in the heat, cramps are known to occur in athletes in cool ambient temperatures and during swimming competitions in extremely cold water.
- There exists no "suitable physiological explanation" by which electrolyte depletion could cause localized, episodic muscle spasms.

In the study by Schwellnus et al. noted earlier, no significant differences were observed in markers of hydration status (change in body weight or plasma volume) between runners who cramped and those who did not during a 56-km road race (54). The only differences in serum electrolytes were a significantly lower average post-race sodium concentration in the cramp group (140 mmol/L) compared to the control group (142 mmol/L) and the post-race serum magnesium was significantly higher in the cramp group compared to the controls (0.73 mmol/L versus 0.67 mmol/L, respectively). The authors considered these differences to be "too small to be of clinical significance."

Based on his review, then, Schwellnus concluded that "the 'electrolyte depletion' and 'dehydration' hypotheses do not offer plausible pathophysiological mechanisms with supporting evidence that could adequately explain the clinical presentation and management of EAMC [exercise-associated muscle cramps]" (52).

Muscular Fatigue

In a later study, Schwellnus et al. sought to examine factors associated with exercise-associated muscle cramps in 43 runners who reported cramping during an Ironman triathlon (53). Of the 43 athletes who experienced muscle cramping during the event (out of 210 participants), no significant differences were observed compared to non-cramping athletes in pre-race-post-race concentrations of serum electrolytes or changes in body weight (as evidence against differences in hydration status). The occurrence of cramping, however, was greater in those with faster race times, and a history of previous race-triggered muscle cramps was also predictive of cramping during this triathlon competition.

These findings, then, support the concept that greater intensity of muscular work serves as a triggering factor in the development of exercise-associated muscle cramps, without evidence for influence of electrolyte levels or body hydration status. This is the essence of the "altered neuromuscular control" hypothesis for muscle cramping in athletes, which holds that repetitive muscle contractions (intense sports play) → muscle fatigue → abnormalities of muscle relaxation that effect bursts of sustained contractions → the star point guard is assisted off the court in agonizing pain. This construct is supported by laboratory findings in which cramping could be induced by both voluntary muscle contractions as well as electrical stimulation (52).

This mechanistic theory of cramping holds that a combination of increased excitation of muscle afferents in combination with a decrease in inhibitory action of the Golgi tendon organ—both a consequence of muscle fatigue—results in sustained muscle motor activation. This concept is supported by the common observation that the best treatment for an acute cramp is stretching of the muscle, an act which would augment the inhibitory action of the Golgi apparatus on the sustained motor innervation of the muscle. Schwellnus concluded that "Whilst it is clear that further evidence to support the 'altered neuromuscular control' hypothesis is also required, research data are accumulating that support this as the principal pathophysiological mechanism for the aetiology of EAMC [exercise-associated muscle cramps]" (52).

In their review of this topic, Nelson and Churilla were in accord (39). "Based on the findings of several large prospective and experimental investigations, the available evidence indicates that EAMC is multifactorial and stems from an imbalance between excitatory drive from muscle spindles and inhibitory drive from Golgi tendon organs to the alpha motor neurons rather than dehydration or electrolyte deficits. This imbalance is believed to stem from neuromuscular overload and fatigue."

Prevention and Treatment

Given the uncertainties surrounding the etiology of exercise-associated muscle cramps, it is difficult to formulate specific recommendations for their prevention. It might be proposed that two groups of athletes—those with a prior history of cramping and those who sweat particularly profusely—are at greater risk for cramps. As such, these individuals might best be advised to pay particular attention to a proper diet, hydration status, and fitness training. Such a recommendation, of course, is hardly helpful to most committed athletes who already normally comply with such habits.

Although solid evidence for their efficacy is lacking, a number of pharmacological agents have found use in patients with cramping associated with chronic disease and in those with idiopathic cramping (i.e., not induced by exercise). These include calcium channel blockers, baclofen, carbamazepine, and phenytoin (30). The drug which has demonstrated the greatest success in treating idiopathic muscle cramps is quinine sulfate (8). Because of its potential side effects, however, this agent has been banned for use in muscle cramps in the United States.

The only "pharmacological" treatment which has been employed for exercise-induced muscle cramping has been, strange as it may seem, pickle juice. No consideration of prevention and treatment of muscle cramps in athletes would be complete without at least a brief discussion of this novel intervention which has received considerable popular attention. By anecdotal reports pickle juice ingested in small amounts (30–60 ml) can arrest a muscle cramp in about half a minute's time. Reportedly, athletic trainers not uncommonly utilize this salty-brine-like drink to treat cramps on the expectation that this serves to normalize electrolyte imbalance (35). (Pickle juice typically has a sodium concentration of 530–970 mmol/L and pH 3.2–3.6 [34,36].)

There exists some research evidence to support this drink's efficacy in the treatment of muscle cramps, but not for that reason (36). Miller et al. studied the effect of pickle juice ingestion on electrically stimulated cramps in 10 dehydrated young men (mean age 24 years), all who had experienced an exercise-associated muscle cramp in the previous six months (36). After consuming 1.0 ml/kg body weight of pickle juice the duration of the induced cramp was shortened by 37% when compared to consumption of water (84.6 ± 18.5 versus 133.7 ± 15.9 seconds, respectively). The authors contended that variables such as psychological factors (i.e., taste), changes in blood electrolyte concentrations, placebo effect, and loss of body fluids could not explain this difference. A key observation in this study was the rapidity of the effect of drinking the pickle juice, which would be far too brief to permit gastrointestinal absorption and subsequent systemic effect. The authors postulated that, instead, the effect of pickle juice ingestion could be explained by a neurally mediated reflex in the oropharyngeal region which could inhibit firing of motor neurons.

Muscle Cramps in the Rest of Us

Given all this information, one might reflect on the origin of those agonizing night-time cramps that almost all of us nonathletes have experienced during sleep. (These have been termed "benign cramps," but they're hardly so for recurrent sufferers or those runners who are about to compete in a marathon race the next morning.) Do these nocturnal cramps share the same pathogenesis as exercise-induced cramps? One might be immediately skeptical, given that, at least usually, one is not dreaming at the time of competing against Rafa Nadal in a fifth set in 95° sunshine at Indian Wells. That is, in restful slumber one is normally neither dehydrated nor fatigued, and it might be assumed that one's serum electrolyte concentrations are probably spot on. Regrettably, the answer is, once again, nobody knows (5,63).

Why do Tennis Players Scream/Grunt when Striking the Ball?

There was once a time when the game of tennis was a very quiet sport. On placid Sunday afternoons on the lush lawns of English country estates, players in long skirts and baggy pants traded gentle shots across a high-slung net. Serving underhand was *de rigeur*, and proper etiquette was disturbed if one sprinted to reach a well-placed ball. As one British Lieutenant Colonel Robert Olson described it:

> The scene should be laid on a well-kept garden lawn. There should be a bright warm sun overhead, and just sufficient breeze whispering through the trees . . . to prevent the day from being sultry. Near at hand, under the cool shadow of a tree, there should be strawberries and cream, an iced

> claret mug, and a few spectators who do not want to play but are lovers of the game, intelligent and appreciative. If all these conditions are present, an afternoon spent at lawn tennis is a highly Christian and beneficent pastime. *(59)*

No longer. Nowadays, amidst the booming power game of professional tennis, spectators and players alike are assaulted by the shrieks and grunts of top level players emitted as they strike the ball. And they're loud. Levels as high as 100 decibels have been reached by some competitors, equivalent to the noise created by a riveting machine at a distance of 30 feet. As Farhead and Punt have put it, "grunting has become a familiar although generally unwelcome element of tennis" (12).

While simply annoying to some, certain players have voiced the opinion that such outcries unfairly serve to distract the opponent. What's more, they say, when the sound of the ball striking the racket is so masked, the opponent loses an auditory clue as to how the ball has been struck, which can permit anticipation of spin and direction. Others have interpreted all this on-court noise as nothing more than a means of self-encouragement, a sort of "Come on!!" or fist pump. Certainly, one expects that the games people play—as they reflect the realities of daily living—should be just and fair. Ethical issues, as well as input on financial earnings, might well be considered in this cacophony (51).

There could be, too, an underlying explanation that the player who shrieks is actually, in doing so, improving performance, perhaps by generating greater force of the stroke. That is, there may be a physiological advantage which accounts for all these shrieks/screams/squeals. The scientific community has begun to address this very issue. In this section, the limited research data will be reviewed which examine the question: why do they do this?

A Distraction?

To start with, Takeuchi supplied three experienced tennis players with ear plugs to determine if lack of auditory input would have an impact on their playing skills (60). With ear plugs in place, the players lost more games than without blocked sound, and their ability to receive serve suffered. However, there was no effect of "playing deaf" on service delivery. The author concluded that "these observations suggest that multisensory information is used in an adaptive manner when playing tennis." That is, such findings would be interpreted as supporting the idea that grunting, by removing certain auditory information available to the opponent (the sound of how the ball was struck), provides a competitive advantage. (Or, by an alternative explanation, here was evidence that wearing ear plugs itself detracts from tennis play and should be avoided in such competitions.)

There does exist, in fact, evidence in the psychophysiological literature that auditory cues can facilitate visual search performance, at least in the laboratory setting (42). Ngo and Spence found that auditory cues improved subjects' ability to follow color changes in a moving target compared to a no-cue baseline (42). In this study the presentation of auditory cues close to the visual search target resulted in significantly improved performance over those delivered via headphones.

Farhead and Punt examined the ability to make judgments of speed of tennis serves when accompanied by a grunt or not (12). Serves were presented on a computer screen, and accuracy and response time of appraisal as to speed were measured in 38 subjects. Grunting caused disruption of serve-speed perception for both above and below average serves. In the below average serves, response time was also diminished in the grunt condition. These findings, concluded the authors, indicate that "grunting provides a complex perceptual challenge."

In the study of Sinnett and Kingstone, subjects (who were not tennis players) watched a video recording of professional players striking a ball toward the left or right side of the court and were asked to decide as rapidly as possible the direction of the shot (55). A simulated grunt (a burst of white noise) at the time of racquet contact with the ball was included in one-half of the videos. When this sound accompanied the stroke, time to estimations of ball direction were longer (by 21–33 milliseconds) and more often erroneous (by 3–4%) than without the noise. Although these were not major decrements, the authors suggested the negative effect of noise on visual perception could amount to important differences in effectiveness of actual tennis play.

In a later study, Sinnett and colleagues confirmed that grunting may serve as a means of distracting an opponent (56). In this investigation, subjects' abilities to recognize the direction of a martial artist kicking on a video were impaired when a simulated grunt was included.

An Ergogenic Aid?

In a study of 32 collegiate tennis players, O'Connell and his colleagues demonstrated that the velocity and force of tennis serves and forehand strokes were significantly enhanced when players grunted (45). Stroke speed and applied forces were measured with a radar gun and dynamometer, respectively. Electromyographic measurements indicated as well that peak muscle activity in the external oblique and pectoralis major muscles was superior in grunting versus non-grunting for both serves and forehand strokes.

When one lifts a heavy object, the abdominal muscles tighten, the upper airway is closed up by the vocal cords, and this is all accompanied by a tense grunt. That's what is termed a "Valsalva maneuver," a forceful exhalation against a closed glottis. During such a maneuver the pressure within both the abdomen and the thoracic cavity are heightened, and blood return to the heart is transiently slowed. (A Valsalva maneuver that occurs during weight lifting has been known to cause intracranial bleeding due to exaggerated increases in blood pressure in the head.)

In effect, a tennis who player lets out with a sudden shriek when straining to strike the ball is performing a brief but forceful Valsalva maneuver. This may bear importance, since, for unexplainable reasons, increased muscle force has been observed experimentally in those executing this maneuver. Some have felt this can be explained by the effect of such pressure changes in the abdomen and chest on the stability and rigidity of the trunk when striking a tennis ball (13). However, this effect could not be confirmed by Hagins et al. who found that the Valsalva maneuver was not related to increased extension force of the trunk (20).

More likely this Valsalva-muscle force relationship is driven by some yet to be understood link between breathing pattern and motor drive within the central nervous system. A number of investigations have supported this idea, revealing a variety of changes, their magnitudes, and muscle-specific effects on muscle strength in humans during expiratory and inspiratory resistive breathing (2,14).

Ikeda and her colleagues at the University of Montana demonstrated this effect in ten subjects who performed maximal contractions of large muscle groups in four different conditions—normal breathing, non-resistive forced inhalation and exhalation (i.e., without airway obstruction), and Valsalva maneuver (without exhalation) (24). Effects varied somewhat according to muscle group and breathing pattern, but forced exhalation and the Valsalva maneuver both augmented peak force production during knee extension, elbow extension, and shoulder adduction compared to the other breathing conditions.

A subsequent investigation by O'Connell et al. provided some tennis-specific insights on this issue (44). The influence of forced expiration and inspiration, Valsalva maneuver, and—importantly—the act of grunting itself was examined on air volume, maximal force production, and muscle recruitment as collegiate tennis players simulated a forehand stroke. The effect on muscle activity varied among the different breathing conditions. In the deltoid muscle greater activity was observed in forced expiration and grunting than in the Valsalva maneuver. Grunting created a more accentuated activity of the internal oblique muscles compared to forced inspiration or Valsalva. Grunting caused greater muscle forces than forced inspiration or Valsalva maneuver. The authors suggested that "either grunting or a more quiescent forced expiration can be used to enhance force production [while hitting a tennis ball]."

To Sum Up

The volume of the scientific literature examining grunting in tennis players is scant, and some studies are obviously hampered by methodological weaknesses (small number of subjects, failure to examine the question in the real world of tennis play, etc.). Still, one cannot escape the observation that, taken collectively, these studies support a conclusion that grunting can, in fact, a) distract an opponent and b) proffers benefits of increased stroke velocity and force.

Purposeful distraction of an opponent violates the rules of professional tennis. A referee can penalize violators by awarding points to the more tight-lipped opponent. However, enforcing such a prohibition is practically difficult. Probably a majority of tennis player emit some noise when they strike the ball. How loud is too loud for the rules? Would referees need to monitor a decibel meter at courtside? Too, some of the world's greatest tennis players are among those most notorious for grunting. There has not—at least as of this writing—been a great rush to expel them from the game.

Is There a Limit to World Records for Athletic Performance?

The question would seem to be perhaps rhetorical, even a bit provocative. Of course, the answer is "yes." No one will ever sprint 100 m in 2 seconds, or pole vault a bar set at 100 feet, or throw a shot put 200 yards. There must therefore be, de facto, limits on athletic performance. (It is not often that one would expect the pop artist Andy Warhol to contribute to such a discussion, but, in fact, in his *Philosophy*, he did just that. While watching Olympic meets on the television, he mused that "if somebody runs at 2.2, does that mean that people will next be able to do it at 2.1 and 2.0 and 1.9 and so on until they can do it in 0.0? So, at what point will they not break a record? Will they have to change the time or change the record?" (62).

From one viewpoint this concern can easily be dispensed with if one is content in assuming a sufficiently accurate clock and the addition of some decimal points. That is, suppose 9.00 seconds is an absolute limit to performance on a 100-m sprint. The human physiological machinery, restricted by chemical-physical laws, cannot ever function faster. Now, in year one, a sprinter sets the world record by running it in 9.1 seconds. Next year, the record is broken when he does it in 9.05. Next year 9.005, then 9.0042, the 9.00035, and so, to infinity, a new world's record is achieved. So, by this argument, "no," there is no limit to world's records in a timed athletic event. It is possible to continuously break such records, forever even, without reaching a particular limiting performance time. The only limiting factor in this case is the discriminatory power of a means for timing performance.

Beneath these simplistic mathematical considerations, however, lie some deeper meanings surrounding the achievement of world record performance. The superb athletes who accomplish such astounding and singular performances are, of course, "outliers." They have set their physical capacity bar far above that of the billions of other human beings on this planet. What is it that sets them apart? What can we learn by teasing out the factors that have established such incredible physical prowess? Why should we even want to know this? How do differences between the sexes influence such a superior athletic performance? How does one account for the improvements in peak performance with time? Do societal values and even political influences play on reaching the pinnacles of athletic success?

A great number of analyses have been performed to address these queries as well as quantify progressive changes in top performance over time in a variety of sports, including track and field (32,38,64), swimming (41), speed skating (43), cycling (11), and so forth. In these publications various mathematical models to express trends in performance have been employed, largely with the goals of comparing male and female athletes and predicting record-breaking patterns in the future. A number of these reports have provided conflicting results, which Mognoni et al. attributed to the observation that "probably such a difficulty is the direct consequence of a complex interaction among the various factors that are at the basis of the continuous growth of the records. . . . We agree with Lloyd when he wrote 'one beauty of this field (i.e., the study of records) is that the athletic authorities of the world provide one with scientific impeccable data, usually accurate to a fraction of one percent, and the guinea pigs select, house and feed themselves,' but these data are often as difficult to understand as those coming from the guinea pigs of our laboratory" (33,38).

Trends in Running Performance

While analyses of trends in record-breaking run performances have varied in regard to event, epoch, gender, and mathematical models, all have demonstrated one finding in common: Championship athletic performance has steadily improved over time. Table 14.1, for example, is extracted from data in the 2015 *World Almanac and Book of Facts* depicting finishing times for the gold medal winning men in the 100-m dash, 1,500-m run, and marathon in the summer Olympic Games dating back to the turn of the 20th century (25). Improvements over that time have ranged from 12.5% to 19.7%, all rather striking magnitudes of increase in respect to finishing times. For the 1,500-m run, the top finisher in 2012 crossed the line almost half a minute faster than the medal recipient in 1900. And the winner of the marathon in 2012 dropped the winning time by 50 minutes over the Olympic champion in 1900.

Others have described similar patterns of improvement in running events (7,32,38,40,64). For example, Nevill and Whyte converted world record finish times into running velocities and found that between the years 1920 and 2000 that men's mile, 5,000-m, 10,000-m, and marathon speeds increased by 14.2%,

TABLE 14.1 Selected Gold Medal Winning Times in the Summer Olympic Games, 1900–2012 (Men)

Year	*100-m Dash*	*1,500-m Run*	*Marathon*
1900	0:11.0	4:00.2	2:59:45
1920	0:10.8	4:01.8	2:32:36
1948	0:10.3	3:49.8	2:34:52
1960	0:10.2	3:35.6	2:15:16
2000	0:09.87	3:32.1	2:10:11
2012	0:09.63	3:34.1	2:08:01
Cumulative improvement	12.5%	16.5%	19.7%

15.8%, 16.7%, and 21.2%, respectively (40). Weiss et al. calculated a combined average improvement of 25% in men's finish times between 1896 and 2014 in all Olympic running events (100-, 200-, 400-, 1,500-, 5,000-, and 10,000-m, as well as the marathon) (64).

What accounts for these temporal trends in improved championship run performance? One might be assured that the intrinsic structure and functional processes in the human body which contribute to athletic success have not altered in the past century; that is, the physical-chemical laws which underlie motor performance and athletic success in the year 1900 are no different than those in 2000. The agents responsible for improvement must be sought, then, in factors which influence the magnitude of physiological change (e.g., responses to training methods), improvements in equipment, and technical aspects of sports competition (e.g., the switch from manual to electric timing significantly lowered finish times in events such as the 100-m and 200-m runs). Table 14.2 catalogs some of these factors.

Broader sociocultural issues may be at play as well. Lippi et al. have written that "economic advances and broader coverage of sports by the media have contributed to enhance the base number of athletes, including those at higher levels. This has increased the chance that 'extreme outliers' will occur in a normal distribution of athletes and may partly account for an improvement in records" (32).

One determinant not typically included in such a list, that of *experience*, might play an important role in temporal advances in athletic performance. Weiss et al. contended that "improvements in sprint and distance running may follow experience curve patterns and could be understood as the outcome of experience accumulated by athletes, coaches and the manufacturers of equipment, nutrition and drugs" (64). Measuring "experience" as the total accumulated distances of races run by all athletes in a given event, however, was considered unfeasible. These

TABLE 14.2 Potential Factors Underlying Improvements in Championship Athletic Performance Over Time

Improved training methods (periodization, fitness-specificity, increased volume)
Secular changes in body stature and composition (48)
Global widening of sports participation (larger pool)
Changes in sports equipment (fiberglass poles, klapskates, synthetic tracks)
Improvements in sports nutrition (carbohydrate loading)
Ergogenic aids (legal or illegal)
Earlier sport specialization (50)
Changes in timing methods
Pacing strategies (15)
Improved coaching (and support team)
Changes in rules
Financial incentives
"Selective breeding" (athletes marrying athletes)

authors thus chose to estimate experience by a surrogate measure, the number of Olympic athletes participating in each of these events. Using this approach, they estimated that each doubling of cumulative experience could account for an average of 3% and 6% of improvements in run performance over time in women's and men's events, respectively.

Sex Differences in World Records in Running Events

Comparisons of Olympic gold medal times for running events from the 100-m run to the marathon over the past century have typically revealed lower finishing times in males compared to females by approximately 10% (25). Such sex differences in endurance running capacity have been traditionally attributed to the influence of physiological factors (limitation of oxygen carrying capacity in women due to lower blood hemoglobin concentration) and differences in body composition (greater percent body fat in females). However, two articles—one in 1992, the other in 2004—suggested that the *rate* of improvement in run performances over time was greater among women (61,66). The authors of these publications provocatively suggested, based on future projections of these trends, that future performance of female runners might well surpass that of their male brethren.

In the 1992 article, Whipp and Ward plotted run velocity for the Olympic gold medal winners by sex since 1920 in run events from the 200-m up to the marathon (66). By their analysis, trends for both male and females were linear, and the slope of year versus winning velocity was almost double for the women compared to the men. In fact, such regression lines intersected in the future, predicting that females would out-do males in the marathon by the year 1998, and for other run events by the mid-21st Century. "The suggestion that women could, so soon, be running these races as fast as men seems improbable," stated the authors. "However, it is the *rates* of improvement that are so striking—the gap is progressively closing."

In the later article, Tatem et al. supported this conclusion. Their plot of winning Olympic 100-m sprint times by year in men and women revealed a linear decrease in both males and females (61). Again, the slope of improved times was greater in the females, and projected forward into the future the finish times by sex intersected at the year 2156. The authors contended that "It is the winner of the event in the 2156 Olympics whose name will be etched in sporting history forever, because this may be the first occasion on which the race is won in a faster time [in the women's] than the men's event."

A number of authors have subsequently disputed these analyses and their conclusions, which "taken to their logical extremes make absurd predictions: negative race times, speeds in excess of Mach 1" (7). Nevill and Whyte agreed that the linear regression modeling of the above two papers was inappropriate since the derived plots eventually would predict finish times in negative values (i.e., before the firing of the gun) and also implied the lack of any limit of human performance (40). They found that winning running speeds during the 20th century were best modeled instead as a flattened S-shaped curve in which the finish times eventually would reach a plateau. That is, by this analysis, "there are indeed limits to human performance" at predicable asymptotic speeds and times. The erroneous conclusions based on the previous linear analysis of times achieved by male and female champions could be explained, then, by the fact that women, with more recent participation in Olympic running competitions, are still on the steep acceleration phase of the S-shaped curve compared to men.

Sparling et al. examined sex differences in race velocity for the world best and the 100th best times in the 1,500-m run and marathon between the years 1980 and 1996 (57). No changes in the gap in race pace was observed by sex over this period, in which performance in men was 11% greater than women.

Others have supported this interpretation of the running data. Based on an exponential time series analysis, Weiss et al. indicated that females will continue to demonstrate running race times 10–15% slower than males (64). According to their logistical analysis, Denny et al. suggested that both men and women are approaching a maximal speed in race competitions (1–5% "remaining" in men and 0.4–2.4% in women) (7). They predicted that this ultimate maximum limit is 9.3–13.4% slower in females than males.

The final—or, at least, most recent—account of this male-female comparison might have been best summarized by Constance Holden in an article in *Science*: "Absent unforeseen genetic or hormonal interventions, men, it seems, will maintain an advantage. That's due largely to their steady supply of a performance drug that will never be banned: endogenous testosterone, which boosts muscle power and oxygen capacity" (22).

Limits of Performance

To return to the essential issue at hand, does there exist a maximal limit of speed at which the human machinery can run? One would expect so. Ionic transfer across cell membranes can only happen so fast. The metabolic cascades within the skeletal muscle cells can only turn over an energy supply at a certain peak constraining rate. Actin-myosin filaments can only slide so rapidly. Nerve conduction velocity is not unlimited. And so forth.

Efforts have been made to identify the limits of such physiological-biochemical determinants of athletic excellence as a means of calculating the ultimate limit to a given sports performance (i.e., 26,33,46). That is, the peak ability to generate oxygen delivery (VO_2max) or the highest percent utilization of VO_2max over a race should be expected to define a ceiling of endurance performance. And the maximum strength that a human muscle can develop should predict an absolute limit of weight-lifting capacity. However, the lack of a firm understanding of all the factors that contribute to athletic success in any particular event, as well as inter-individual variability and the difficulty in accurately measuring these processes, serve as distinct barriers to any such approach. This observation notwithstanding, Péronnet and Thibault were able to generate equations which were closely predictive of world running records based on considerations of aerobic and anaerobic metabolic capacities (46).

Too, there are those who espouse a belief that such physiological markers *never* explain a true peak performance. That every "maximal" performance is, in fact, submaximal. That Usain Bolt could have always run faster. This line of thought is based on the idea, as described earlier in Chapter 13, that a protective central governor within the brain limits motor activity before such efforts would prove detrimental (hyperthermia, muscle damage, cardiac arrhythmias, etc.). By this concept, then, those who set world records in sports events are those with the extraordinary capacity to make the most of these limitations. But, limitations they remain. The human body is actually capable of doing more.

To sum up, certainly, there will always exist individuals—those "outliers"—who possess an extraordinary capacity to perform such functions well beyond that of the rest of mortal men (and women). Still, in the final analysis there must, it would be supposed, be an ultimate limit. Examining the patterns of improvement in world record performances has been an optimal means of "assessing the potentiality of the human body, which also reflects how society has evolved over time" (32), and, in doing so, such performance curves "represent an optimal proxy for the study of human limits in sports performance" (47).

Mathematical Models

A number of analyses of world record performances in running events have produced mathematical models which describe such advances over the past century. Some have reported that such improvements are best described as a linear progression of improvements over time in the past (1,31,32), but the majority of these also demonstrate a slowing in performance gains in recent years with a trend for finish times to plateau or approach a limit in an asymptotic manner. A similar plateau is observed in models of logistical analysis (7,40) and exponential time series (64) as well. In general, then, such analyses by different mathematical approaches have consistently predicted the existence of an ultimate absolute ceiling of performance.

Some of these analyses have suggested, in fact, that such limits of performance have already been attained in certain events (32,64). The curves produced by Kruse et al. indicated that between 1980 and 2013, men's top performances in the 10,000-m and 5,000-m races demonstrated a linear improvement until 2005 but have plateaued since (31). Nevill and Whyte contended (while expressing caution in the interpretation of such curves) that a limit to performance has currently been met by women in the 1,500-m event (40). These authors felt that in males the limits to performance had not yet been achieved, but the margin for improvement before reaching such a ceiling was small, ranging from 0.7% in the 10,000-m run to 3.3% in the 5,000-m event. Denny described similar findings (7). In summary, "these analyses suggest a declining performance improvement over time and a persistent gap between women's and men's performances" (64).

In a particularly interesting approach, Mark Denny compared the trends of peak human running performance over time with that of competitive greyhounds and Thoroughbred racehorses, animals which have been bred for speed and endurance performance (7). Similar to the human data, performance gains of both competitive animals improved linearly during the first portion of the 20th Century. The winning speed in the Kentucky Derby was 13% greater in the 1975 race than that in 1908. The top velocity in the greyhound English Grand National race rose by almost 15% in approximately the same period.

However, during the last 40–60 years the winning race velocities of Thoroughbred racehorses and greyhounds, despite selective breeding for speed, have not substantially increased. Thus, the biologically based locomotor limit of these animals seems to have been reached. As noted above, human beings are not far behind, with patterns of performance increments with time beginning to plateau in a number of events and with only a few percentage differences between present and predicted maximal finishing times. Denny concluded that "extreme-value analysis of race speeds during each plateau [in animals] suggests that there is an absolute upper limit to speeds in each of these races" and that the same is true for human athletes (7).

Berthelot et al. added as evidence a recent plateau in jumping distance in the Calaveras frog jump contest, held since 1920 (4). They concluded that "sports performance appears to have reached a state of stagnation in recent years, suggesting that the physical capacities of humans and other athletic species, such as greyhounds and thoroughbreds, cannot progress indefinitely."

Deeper Meanings

Denny wrote that "my results are as unsatisfying as those of previous statistical analyses: they tell us that speed has limits, but not what accounts for these limits. . . . It is striking that the predicted scope for increased speed in humans is similar across distances ranging from 100 to 42,195 m [the marathon]. This distance-independent scope for increase suggests that some sort of higher order constraint may act on the suite of physiological and mechanical factors to limit speed" (7). Others as well have proposed that the mathematical expressions of world-record athletic performances might hold key insights into general principles that define human motor performance (16,65). This line of thinking leads us into the fascinating world of fractals, complex systems, and chaos theory, a direction which is well beyond the scope of this discussion. Still, considering its potential importance, a brief summary is in order. (For those seeking a more extensive review of this topic, references 16 and 65 will be particularly helpful.)

As Denny recognized (7), such ideas have surrounded the negative relationship between the distance of a running event and the time (or speed) taken for its completion. That is, the greater the race distance, the slower the pace one runs it. (This was addressed in the preceding chapter in respect to pacing strategies. These mathematical concepts bear repeating here in considering the meaning of mathematical relationships between world record performances and race distance.) The relationship between this speed and the race distance is not linear but follows a hyperbolic curve which represents a *power law* in the form

$$\mathbf{V} = \mathbf{aD}^{b}$$

where velocity run (V) is related to race distance (D) by the scaling exponent b, which like a is a constant. That the velocity-distance relationship follows this power law equation is confirmed by the linear nature of its logarithmic derivation $\log V = \log a + b(\log D)$. (Here a is the Y-intercept, and the scaling exponent b is the slope of the regression line.)

That velocity is related to race distance by a power law indicates that this relationship possesses the nature of a *fractal*, meaning that it is independent of scale. In other words, when examined from any size perspective the relationship holds true. This means that if the race distance is changed by a factor z, the velocity or time changes by a factor of z^b.

Why is this an important observation? What does finding a power law illustrating a scale-free fractal nature of a relationship tell us? As Geoffrey West has stated, when assessing physiological processes one is confronted with a myriad of influencing variables, network interactions, hierarchical levels, and emergent phenomena that are simply too overwhelming to decipher (65). But the identification that such a system corresponds to a power law and acts as a fractal strongly suggests that there is some underlying general principle that governs the functions of a system.

(The reader is cautioned here not to be confused. Previously in this section, the relationships between top performances in a given athletic event were plotted against year of performance. The analysis, then, was peak performance in a given event over time. We are now addressing a different aspect, the relationship of top velocity in championship performance and the distance of the event.)

Katz and Katz found that power laws appropriately described best performance by men in events from the 100- to 10,000-m run between the years 1925 and 1995 (29). During that period the scaling exponent b decreased slightly with time (1.141 in 1925 and 1.123 in 1995). Garcia-Manso et al. found the power law scaling exponent of 0.0745 in the velocity-distance equation of world records in events ranging from 1,500 m to the marathon up to the year 2003 (17).

Interestingly, when Carbone and Savaglio performed a similar analysis, a biphasic pattern emerged (6). In the males, the initial scaling law with an exponent b of 0.165 was observed for distances of 200–1,000 m, and a second law was evident for distances 1,500 m to the marathon with a scaling exponent of 0.072. Respective values for the women were 0.175 and 0.071. The authors suggested that these two separate scaling laws, different for short and long races, might reflect the relative contributions of anaerobic versus aerobic metabolic pathways at these distances.

That there exists a mathematical relationship which links the limits of peak performance at distances from 100 m to the marathon suggests a commonality of mechanisms which serve as limiting factors in running events. Indeed, that hyperbolic curve is *defined* by performance-limiting fatigue. If one could be provided the physiological determinants of the curve, the secret of what controls the limits of human motor performance might well be revealed. In this regard, the observation is intriguing that this "fatigue continuity" curve crosses domains traditionally considered to be influenced by different physiological determinants (e.g., muscle strength and explosiveness defining sprint performance, oxygen supply and substrate availability limiting factors for distance running such as the marathon).

As noted above, Carbone and Savaglio proposed that their analysis revealing two separate power laws for world record run performance could be explained by the switch from reliance on anaerobic to aerobic metabolism at longer race distances (6). However, as noted by Garcia-Manso et al. (17), this breakpoint does not correspond with the physiological data indicating relative metabolic contributions at this speed: "According to [previously published data] the anaerobic metabolism is responsible for 35–40% of the energy required to run 1,000 m at world record pace, while the remaining 60% or more is provided by the aerobic metabolism."

Investigations into the physiological "meaning" of power law relationships in top athletic performances may serve to provide a "window" into understanding the determinants of athletic prowess. On the other hand, such research may reveal an increasingly complicated web of networks, system inter-relationships, emergent behaviors, and hierarchical structures typical of complex systems in human beings which may create even greater challenges to such insights. Time will tell.

The Future

The argument in the foregoing discussion that the physiological limits which dictate human performance have been—or are soon about to be—reached ignores the likelihood that new technological advances, training techniques, rule changes, and pharmacological innovations will continue to advance physical performance beyond such biological constraints (4). With each such "advance" the bar of peak performance times will be lifted, with new asymptotic relations to record-setting performances. From this standpoint, then, it is difficult to leave this discussion assuming that, yes, there exists a limit to world record performances.

Such modifications are likely to provoke ethical considerations. As Lippi and colleagues have concluded, "future limits to athletic performance will be determined less and less by the innate physiology of the athlete and more and more by scientific and technological advances and by the still evolving judgment on where to draw the line between what is 'natural' and what is artificially enhanced" (32).

Particularly ominous in this regard "are the approaching dark clouds of genetic selection and manipulation that will tax our ideas of the meaning of sports talent and performance as they touch all other aspects of human existence" (49). Elisavet Gazidou and her colleagues at the University of Athens have addressed this issue in an insightful article entitled "Genetically transformed world records: A reality or in the sphere of fantasy?" (18). They concluded that "given the modern lucrative nature of competitive sports and the appeal of an undetectable and effective method of athletic performance enhancement, it seems likely that gene doping will enter the athletic arena. . . . However, its misappropriation in athletics appears to be as hazardous and unethical as any type of traditional doping. Gene doping is not yet a reality in the world of sports, but it is not beyond the realm of imagination."

References

1. Atkinson M, Hay SI, Stephens P, Hunter C, Bignell G. Momentous sprint at the 2156 Olympics? *Nature*. 2004;431:525–526.
2. Balzamo E, Vuillon-Cacciuttolo G, Burnet H, Jammes Y. Influence of respiratory afferents upon the proprioceptive reflex of skeletal muscles in healthy humans. *Neurosci Lett*. 1997;236:127–130.
3. Bergeron MF. Heat cramps: fluid and electrolyte challenges during tennis in the heat. *J Sci Med Sport*. 2003;6:19–27.
4. Berthelot G, Sedeaud A, Marck A, et al. Has athletic performance reached its peak? *Sports Med*. 2015;45:1263–1271.
5. Brown TM. Sleep-Related leg cramps: a review and suggestions for future research. *Sleep Med Clin*. 2015;10:85–92.
6. Carbone V, Savaglio S. Scaling laws and forecasting in athletic world records. *J Sport Sci*. 2001;19:477–484.
7. Denny MW. Limits to running speed in dogs, horses and humans. *J Exp Biol*. 2008;211:3836–3849.
8. Diener HC, Dethlefsen U, Dethlefsen-Gruber S, Verbeek P. Efficacy of quinine in treating muscle cramps: a double-blind, placebo-controlled, parallel-group multicentre trial. *Int J Clin Pract*. 2002;56:243–246.
9. Edsall DL. New disorder from heat: a disorder due to exposure to intense heat. *JAMA*. 1908;11:1969–1971.
10. Eichner ER. The role of sodium in "heat cramping." *Sports Med*. 2007;37:368–370.
11. El Helou N, Berthelot G, Thibault V, et al. Tour de France, Giro, Vuelta, and classic European races show a unique progression of road cycling speed in the last 20 years. *J Sport Sci*. 2010;28:789–796.
12. Farhead N, Punt TD. Silencing Sharapova's grunt improves the perception of her serve speed. *Percept Mot Skills*. 2015;120:722–730.

13. Findley BW, Keating T, Toscano L. Is the Valsalva maneuver a proper breathing technique? *Strength Cond J.* 2003;25:47–52.
14. Fontanari P, Vuillon-Cacciuttolo G, Balzamo E, et al. Resistive loaded breathing changes the motor drive to arm and leg muscles in man. *Neurosci Lett.* 1996;210:130–134.
15. Foster C, de Koning JJ, Thiel C. Evolutionary pattern of improved 1-mile running performance. *Int J Sports Physiol Perf.* 2014;9:715–719.
16. Garcia-Manso JM, Martin-Gonzalez JM, Davila N, Arriaza E. Middle and long distance athletics races viewed from the perspective of complexity. *J Theor Biol.* 2005;233:191–198.
17. Garcia-Manso JM, Martin-Gonzalez JM, Vaamonde D, Da Silva-Grigoletto ME. The limitations of scaling laws in the reduction of performance in endurance events. *J Theor Biol.* 2012;300:324–329.
18. Gatzidou E, Gatzidou G, Theocharis S. Genetically transformed world records: a reality or in the sphere of fantasy? *Med Sci Monit.* 2009;15:RA41–47.
19. Gisinger T. Scale invariance in biology: coincidence or footprint of a universal mechanism? *Biol Rev Camb Philos Soc.* 2001;76:161–209.
20. Hagins M, Pietrek M, Sheikhzadeh A, Nordin M. The effects of breath control on maximum force and IAP during a maximum lifting task. *Clin Biomech.* 2006;21:775–780.
21. Hiller WD, O'Toole M, Laird RH, et al. Electrolyte and glucose changes in endurance and ultra-endurance exercise: results and medical implications. *Med Sci Sports Exerc.* 1986;18 Suppl:S62–S63.
22. Holden C. An everlasting gender gap? *Science.* 2004;305:639–640.
23. Horswill CA, Stofan JR, Lacambra M, et al. Sodium balance during U.S. football training in the heat: cramp-prone vs. reference players. *Int J Sports Med.* 2009;30:789–794.
24. Ikeda ER, Borg A, Brown D, et al. The Valsalva maneuver revisited: the influence of voluntary breathing on isometric muscle strength. *J Strength Cond Res.* 2009;23:127–132.
25. Janssen S. *The World Almanac and Book of Facts, 2015.* New York: Infobase Learning; 2015. pp. 872–877.
26. Joyner MJ. Modeling optimal marathon performance on the basis of physiological factors. *J Appl Physiol.* 1991;70:683–687.
27. Jung AP, Bishop PA, Al-Nawwas A, Dale RB. Influence of hydration and electrolyte supplementation on incidence and time to onset of exercise-associated muscle cramps. *J Athl Train.* 2005;40:71–75.
28. Kantarowski P, Hiller W, Garrett W. Cramping studies in 2600 endurance athletes. *Med Sci Sports Exerc.* 1990;22 Suppl 2:S104.
29. Katz JS, Katz L. Power laws and athletic performance. *J Sports Sci.* 1999;17:467–476.
30. Katzberg HD. Neurogenic muscle cramps. *J Neurol.* 2015;262:1814–1821.
31. Kruse TN, Carter RE, Rosedahl JK, Joyner MJ. Speed trends in male distance running. *PLoS ONE.* 2014;9:e112978.
32. Lippi G, Banfi G, Favaloro J, Rittweger J, Maffuli N. Updates on improvement of human athletic performance: focus on world records in athletics. *Br Med Bull.* 2008;87:7–15.
33. Lloyd BB. Energetics of running: an analysis of the records. *Adv Sci.* 1966;22:515–530.
34. McKenney MA, Miller KC, Deal JE, Garden-Robinson JA, Rhee YS. Plasma and electrolyte changes in exercising humans after ingestion of multiple boluses of pickle juice. *J Athl Train.* 2015;50:141–146.
35. Miller K, Knight K, Williams R. Athletic trainers' perceptions of pickle juice's effects on exercise associated muscle cramps. *Athl Ther Today.* 2008;13:31–34.

36. Miller KC, Mack GW, Knight KL, et al. Reflex inhibition of electrically induced muscle cramps in hypohydrated humans. *Med Sci Sports Exerc.* 2010;42:953–961.
37. Minetto MA, Holobar A. Botter A, Farina D. Origin and development of muscle cramps. *Exerc Sport Sci Rev.* 2013;41:3–10.
38. Mognoni P, Lafortuna C, Russo G, Minetti A. An analysis of world records in three types of locomotion. *Eur J Appl Physiol.* 1982;49:287–299.
39. Nelson NL, Churilla JR. A narrative review of exercise-associated muscle cramps: factors that contribute to neuromuscular fatigue and management implications. *Muscle Nerve.* 2016;54:177–185.
40. Nevill AM, Whyte G. Are there limits to running world records? *Med Sci Sports Exerc.* 2005;37:1785–1788.
41. Nevill AM, Whyte GP, Holder RL, Peyrebrune M. Are there limits to swimming world records? *Int J Sports Med.* 2007;28:1012–1017.
42. Ngo MK, Spence C. Auditory, tactile, and multisensory cues facilitate search for dynamic visual stimuli. *Aten Percept Psychophys.* 2010;72:1654–1665.
43. Noordhof DA, van Tok E, Joosten FS, et al. Historical improvement in speed skating economy. *Int J Sports Physiol Perform.* 2017;12:175–181.
44. O'Connell DG, Brewer JF, Man TH, Weldon JS, Hinman MR. The effects of forced exhalation and inhalation, grunting, and Valsalva maneuver on forehand force in collegiate tennis players. *J Strength Cond Res.* 2016;30:430–437.
45. O'Connell DG, Hinman MR, Hearne KF, Michael ZS, Nixon SL. The effects of "grunting" on serve and forehand velocities in collegiate tennis players. *J Strength Cond Res.* 2014;28:3469–3475.
46. Péronnet F, Thibault G. Mathematical analysis of running performance and world running records. *J Appl Physiol.* 1989;67:453–465.
47. Radicchi F. Universality, limits and predictability of gold-medal performances at the Olympic Games. *PLoS ONE.* 2012;7:e40335.
48. Rowland T. The ascendancy of the modern athlete: a virtual roundtable. *Pediatr Exerc Science.* 2002;14:111–117.
49. Rowland T. *The Athlete's Clock.* Champaign, IL: Human Kinetics; 2011. pp. 90–91.
50. Rowland T. *Tennisology.* Champaign, IL: Human Kinetics; 2014. pp. 73–84.
51. Rowland T. *A Philosophy of Tennis.* The Hague: Kemper Conseil Publishing; 2018. pp. 39–54.
52. Schwellnus MP. Cause of exercise associated muscle cramps (EAMC)—altered neuromuscular control, dehydration or electrolyte depletion? *Br J Sports Med.* 2009;43:401–408.
53. Schwellnus MP, Drew N, Collins M. Increased running speed and previous cramps rather than dehydration or serum sodium changes predict exercise-associated muscle cramping: a prospective cohort study in 210 Ironman triathletes. *Br J Sports Med.* 2011;45:650–656.
54. Schwellnus MP, Nicol J, Laubscher R, Noakes TD. Serum electrolyte concentrations and hydration status are not associated with exercise associated muscle cramping (EAMC) in distance runners. *Br J Sports Med.* 2004;38:488–492.
55. Sinnett S, Kingstone A. A preliminary investigation regarding the effect of tennis grunting: does white noise during a tennis shot have a negative impact on shot perception? *PLoS ONE.* 2010;5:e13148.
56. Sinnett S, Maglinti CJ, Kingstone A. Grunting's competitive advantage: considerations of force and distraction. *PLoS ONE.* 2018;13:e0192939.

57. Sparling PB, O'Donnell EM, Snow TK. The gender difference in distance running performance has plateaued: an analysis of world rankings from 1980 to 1996. *Med Sci Sports Exerc.* 1998;30:1725–1729.
58. Stofan JR, Zachwieja JJ, Horswill CA, et al. Sweat and sodium losses in NCAA football players: a precursor to heat cramps? *Int J Sport Nutr Exerc Metab.* 2005;15:641–652.
59. Sumner A. *Court on Canvas: Tennis in Art.* London: Philip Wilson; 2011.
60. Takeuchi T. Auditory information in playing tennis. *Percept Mot Skills.* 1993;76:1323–1328.
61. Tatem AJ, Guerra CA, Atkinson PM, Hay SI. Momentous sprint at the 2156 Olympics? *Nature.* 2004;431:525.
62. Warhol A. *The Philosophy of Andy Warhol. From A to B and Back Again.* Orlando, FL: Harcourt; 1975.
63. Weiner IH, Weiner HL. Nocturnal leg muscle cramps. *JAMA.* 1980;244:2332–2333.
64. Weiss M, Newman A, Whitmore C, Weiss S. One hundred and fifty years of sprint and distance running—Past trends and future prospects. *Eur J Sport Sci.* 2016;16:393–401.
65. West G. *Scale.* New York: Penguin Press; 2017.
66. Whipp BJ, Ward SA. Will women soon outrun men? *Nature.* 1992;25:355.

CLOSING COMMENTS

In these pages the reader has been presented an eclectic mixture of topics comprising a collection of "controversies"—or, perhaps better yet, "mysteries"—in exercise science. The subjects have been diverse, including conundrums in basic science, such as the nature of biological variability and physiological time, as well as challenging clinical questions, as the physician dealing with the uncertainty surrounding the collapse of a young athlete. As predicted in the Preface, however, they all share in common the expectation that in resolving such issues, new insights into the essential nature of living beings—just how the human machine "works"—might be revealed. This seems evident.

As each of these topics have filed by, however, a number of deeper, more substantive issues of a distinct philosophical nature have arisen. One would not customarily expect, of course, any conversational proximity between physiological controversies and philosophical dilemmas. Still, the link throughout the chapters of this book between these two odd bedfellows—the "objective" and the "subjective"—is quite inescapable.

To start with, there is the issue of *uncertainty*. No one needs to be convinced that in the flow of daily life, little seems entirely predictable, and that the unexpected often derails the best-laid plans. Uncertainty is the norm. But over 250 years ago, the physical laws laid out by Sir Isaac Newton—and confirmed by his later followers—implied an incontestable, deterministic universe. Living beings are somehow uniquely different from inanimate objects, but they, too, must adhere to the same predictable physical-chemical laws that govern physical matter. It might be assumed that when at that magic moment the key to understanding the unique nature of life is revealed, it, too, will involve a certainty previously attributed to non-living materials.

Of course, the historical development of physics and mathematics has revealed this to be true only in a particular macroscopic corner of the real world. We now have theories of relativity, and quantum mechanics, and Gödel's Incompleteness Theorem, and Heisenberg's Uncertainty Principle, and the recognition of dependence on initial conditions on deterministic outcomes (chaos), all indicating that a) "certainty" exists only in very particular contexts, and that b) "uncertainty" is a central characteristic of the physical world, particularly at the subatomic level. Once again, can such perspectives of physical reality—an expansion of assumed certainty into a more realistic picture of uncertainty—be transferred to biological function, including exercise? As described in these chapters, a recognition of the extraordinarily complicated nature of complex systems and the ubiquity of organized variability inherent in living beings would say "almost certainly yes."

Akin to dealing with uncertainty is the recognition that the closer one examines the scientific evidence surrounding the controversies in this book, the more complicated the matter becomes, and the more distant—instead of closer—appears to be any ultimate resolution to the issue. One can grow disillusioned here. Does ultimate scientific truth truly exist? Can it be appreciated? Are scientific methods up to the task of providing a final answer to *any* biological controversy? Or are we (meaning the brain provided us by Darwinian processes to address such issues) constrained in our abilities to ultimately understand a true nature of the "real world"? (Somewhat comforting, at least, is the recognition that philosophers have been wrestling with such issues for a greater many years, without consensus.) The take-away message here must be that one should best be wary of accepting simplistic explanations.

By our direct everyday experience, the Earth is flat, and the Sun unquestionably revolves (like the stars) around the Earth. Lesson: "Common sense" is not always a guide to truth. So, we are convinced that we can consciously decide how fast to run a road race, or to engage in physical activity. That would make common sense, too. So, we ask ourselves, does common sense, based on experience and cognitive thought, provide us with a realistic picture of what is actually going on in the world around us? The problem, as outlined in several locations in these pages, is that the instrument one is using to judge (i.e., the conscious brain) is exactly the same one whose role in such decision-making is being assessed. There is, in fact, increasing evidence on a number of fronts that the subconscious acts beneath the level of consciousness, and what we feel intuitively is under our conscious control is not always the case.

So, again, in examining physiological issues in exercise science, we are confronted with another classical philosophical dilemma: Does one have free will to make conscious decisions? Or are we driven by deterministic processes that subconsciously make decisions, surreptitiously, for us. In the opening chapter we examined a different take on the same issue—are we limited in our ability to improve athletic performance with training by a deterministic, fixed ceiling of genetic endowment? Or do we have free will to train harder and better without such a biologically established limit, one out of our control?

The point here is that one finds oneself in this book's survey of controversial areas in exercise science not infrequently confronted by deeper philosophical issues invading the more comfortable and customary physiological ones. It's an important bottom line to *Controversies in Exercise Science*. As the British philosopher of biology Tim Lewens has written:

> Scientists cannot make plausible pronouncements about the repercussion of evolutionary theorizing for human morality, they cannot assess the fate of free will in the face of work in neuroscience, unless they have well-formulated views about what morality, or freedom of the will, involve. In other words, whether they like it or not, scientists end up running into exactly the same conceptual issues that have puzzled philosophers for centuries.
>
> *(1)*

And to emphasize this sentiment, a quote from Albert Einstein, written in a letter to a graduate student:

> A knowledge of the historic and philosophical background gives that kind of independence from prejudices of his generation from which most scientists are suffering. This independence created by philosophical insight is—in my opinion—the mark of distinction between a mere artisan or specialist and a real seeker after truth.
>
> *(1)*

Reference

1. Lewens T. *The Meaning of Science: An Introduction to the Philosophy of Science*. New York: Basic Books; 2016.

INDEX

Page numbers in *italic* indicate figures; those in **bold** indicate tables.